Postmenopausal Endocrinology

Editors

NANETTE SANTORO
LUBNA PAL

ENDOCRINOLOGY AND METABOLISM CLINICS OF NORTH AMERICA

www.endo.theclinics.com

Consulting Editor
DEREK LeROITH

September 2015 • Volume 44 • Number 3

ELSEVIER

1600 John F. Kennedy Boulevard • Suite 1800 • Philadelphia, Pennsylvania, 19103-2899

http://www.theclinics.com

ENDOCRINOLOGY AND METABOLISM CLINICS OF NORTH AMERICA Volume 44, Number 3
September 2015 ISSN 0889-8529, ISBN 13: 978-0-323-39561-8

Editor: Jessica McCool
Developmental Editor: Meredith Clinton

Endocrinology and Metabolism Clinics of North America (ISSN 0889-8529) is published quarterly by Elsevier Inc., 360 Park Avenue South, New York, NY 10010-1710. Months of issue are March, June, September, and December. Periodicals postage paid at New York, NY and additional mailing offices. Subscription prices are USD 330.00 per year for US individuals, USD 581.00 per year for US institutions, USD 165.00 per year for US students and residents, USD 415.00 per year for Canadian individuals, USD 718.00 per year for Canadian institutions, USD 480.00 per year for international individuals, USD 718.00 per year for international institutions, and USD 245.00 per year for international and Canadian and foreign students/residents. To receive student/resident rate, orders must be accompanied by name of affiliated institution, date of term, and the signature of program/residency coordinator on institution letterhead. Orders will be billed at individual rate until proof of status is received. Foreign air speed delivery is included in all *Clinics* subscription prices. All prices are subject to change without notice. **POSTMASTER:** Send address changes to *Endocrinology and Metabolism Clinics of North America*, Elsevier Health Sciences Division, Subscription Customer Service, 3251 Riverport Lane, Maryland Heights, MO 63043. **Customer Service: Telephone: 1-800-654-2452** (U.S. and Canada); **1-314-447-8871** (outside U.S. and Canada). **Fax: 1-314-447-8029. E-mail: journalscustomerservice-usa@elsevier.com (for print support); journalsonlinesupport-usa@elsevier.com (for online support).**

Reprints. For copies of 100 or more, of articles in this publication, please contact the Commercial Rights Department, Elsevier Inc., 360 Park Avenue South, New York, NY 10010-1710; phone: +1-212-633-3874; fax: +1-212-633-3820; E-mail: reprints@elsevier.com.

Endocrinology and Metabolism Clinics of North America is covered in *MEDLINE/PubMed (Index Medicus), EMBASE/Excerpta Medica, Current Contents/Clinical Medicine, Current Contents/Life Sciences, Science Citation Index, ISI/BIOMED, BIOSIS,* and *Chemical Abstracts.*

Contributors

CONSULTING EDITOR

DEREK LEROITH, MD, PhD
Director of Research, Division of Endocrinology, Diabetes and Bone Diseases, Icahn School of Medicine at Mt Sinai, New York, New York

EDITORS

NANETTE SANTORO, MD
Professor and E Stewart Taylor Chair of Obstetrics and Gynecology, University of Colorado School of Medicine, Aurora, Colorado

LUBNA PAL, MBBS, MRCOG, MS, FACOG
Associate Professor, Division of Reproductive Endocrinology and Infertility, Department of Obstetrics, Gynecology and Reproductive Sciences, Yale University School of Medicine, New Haven, Connecticut

AUTHORS

JEFFREY R. BENDER, MD
Robert I. Levy Professor of Preventive Cardiology; Professor of Medicine and Immunobiology; Director, Section of Cardiovascular Medicine, Cardiovascular Research Center, Raymond and Beverly Sackler Cardiovascular Laboratory, Yale University School of Medicine, New Haven, Connecticut

JUDI CHERVENAK, MD
Associate Professor of Obstetrics and Gynecology and Women's Health, Department of Obstetrics and Gynecology, Montefiore Medical Center, Albert Einstein College of Medicine, Bronx, New York

MARK H. EINSTEIN, MD
Professor, Division of Gynecologic Oncology, Department of Obstetrics and Gynecology and Women's Health, Montefiore Medical Center; Albert Einstein Cancer Center, Albert Einstein College of Medicine, Bronx, New York

C. NEILL EPPERSON, MD
Professor of Psychiatry, Perelman School of Medicine, University of Pennsylvania, Philadelphia, Pennsylvania

VALERIE A. FLORES, MD
Women and Infants Hospital, Warren Alpert Medical School of Brown University, Providence, Rhode Island

KATHLEEN M. GAVIN, PhD
Postdoctoral Fellow, Division of Geriatric Medicine, Department of Medicine, University of Colorado Anschutz Medical Campus, Aurora, Colorado

JANET E. HALL, MD
Reproductive Endocrine Unit, Massachusetts General Hospital, Harvard Medical School, Boston, Massachusetts; National Institute of Environmental Health Sciences, Research Triangle Park, North Carolina

KARL INSOGNA, MD
Professor of Medicine; Director, Yale Bone Center, Department of Internal Medicine, Yale University School of Medicine, New Haven, Connecticut

WENDY M. KOHRT, PhD
Professor of Medicine, Division of Geriatric Medicine, Department of Medicine, University of Colorado Anschutz Medical Campus, Aurora, Colorado

NANCI F. LEVINE, MD
Division of Gynecologic Oncology, Department of Obstetrics and Gynecology and Women's Health, Montefiore Medical Center, Bronx, New York

BEATRICE C. LUPSA, MD
Assistant Professor of Medicine, Department of Internal Medicine, Yale Bone Center, Yale University School of Medicine, New Haven, Connecticut

SARAH B. MATHEWS, MD
Assistant Professor of Clinical Psychiatry, Perelman School of Medicine, University of Pennsylvania, Philadelphia, Pennsylvania

GENEVIEVE NEAL-PERRY, MD, PhD
Division Director, Reproductive Endocrinology and Infertility, Department of Obstetrics and Gynecology, University of Washington, Seattle, Washington

NICOLE S. NEVADUNSKY, MD
Associate Professor, Division of Gynecologic Oncology, Department of Obstetrics and Gynecology and Women's Health, Montefiore Medical Center; Albert Einstein Cancer Center, Albert Einstein College of Medicine, Bronx, New York

CHILESHE NKONDE-PRICE, MD
Director, Penn Heart and Vascular Center for Women's Cardiovascular Health; Assistant Professor of Medicine, Perelman School of Medicine, University of Pennsylvania, Philadelphia, Pennsylvania

LUBNA PAL, MBBS, MRCOG, MS, FACOG
Associate Professor, Division of Reproductive Endocrinology and Infertility, Department of Obstetrics, Gynecology and Reproductive Sciences, Yale University School of Medicine, New Haven, Connecticut

MARIA RODRIGUEZ, MD
Department of Obstetrics and Gynecology, Cedars-Sinai Medical Center, Los Angeles, California

NANETTE SANTORO, MD
Professor and E Stewart Taylor Chair of Obstetrics and Gynecology, University of Colorado School of Medicine, Aurora, Colorado

DONNA SHOUPE, MD, MBA
Professor of Obstetrics and Gynecology, Keck School of Medicine of University of Southern California, Los Angeles, California

CYNTHIA A. STUENKEL, MD
Clinical Professor of Medicine, Deparment of Medicine, University of California, San Diego, School of Medicine, La Jolla, California

HUGH S. TAYLOR, MD
Professor and Chair, Department of Obstetrics, Gynecology and Reproductive Sciences, Yale University School of Medicine, New Haven, Connecticut

MAIDA TAYLOR, MD, MPH, FACOG
Clinical Professor, Department of Obstetrics, Gynecology and Reproductive Sciences, University of California San Francisco, San Francisco, California

KIMBERLEY THORNTON, MD
Reproductive Endocrinology and Infertility Fellow, Department of Obstetrics and Gynecology, Montefiore Medical Center, Albert Einstein College of Medicine, Bronx, New York

SAIOA TORREALDAY, MD, FACOG
Staff Physician, Reproductive Endocrinology and Infertility, Department of Obstetrics and Gynecology, Womack Army Medical Center, Fort Bragg, North Carolina

RACHAEL E. VAN PELT, PhD
Associate Professor of Medicine, Division of Geriatric Medicine, Department of Medicine, University of Colorado Anschutz Medical Campus, Aurora, Colorado

Contents

In women, age-related changes in ovarian function begin in the mid-30s with decreased fertility and compensatory hormonal changes in the hypothalamus-pituitary-gonadal axis that maintain follicle development and estrogen secretion in the face of a waning pool of ovarian follicles. The menopause transition is characterized by marked variability in follicle development, ovulation, bleeding patterns, and symptoms of hyper- and hypoestrogenism. The menopause, which is clinically defined by the final menstrual period, is followed by the consistent absence of ovarian secretion of estradiol.

The menopause transition is associated with various symptoms, which can interact to produce morbidity. Vasomotor symptoms are the most commonly reported, but vaginal dryness/dyspareunia, sleep difficulties and adverse mood changes have all been shown to worsen as women approach menopause. For postmenopausal women changes in cognition are more likely to be related to aging and not to hormones. This article reviews the symptoms of hot flashes (vasomotor symptoms), vaginal dryness/dyspareunia, adverse mood, poor sleep/insomnia, and cognitive complaints, describing their epidemiology, diagnosis, and treatment. This article thus reviews the epidemiology, pathophysiology, diagnosis, and treatment of these common menopausal symptoms.

Osteoporosis is characterized by low bone mass and microarchitectural deterioration of bone tissue leading to decreased bone strength and an increased risk of low-energy fractures. Central dual-energy X-ray absorptiometry measurements are the gold standard for determining bone mineral density. Bone loss is an inevitable consequence of the decrease in estrogen levels during and following menopause, but additional risk factors for bone loss can also contribute to osteoporosis in older women. A well-balanced diet, exercise, and smoking cessation are key to maintaining bone health as women age. Pharmacologic agents should be recommended in patients at high risk for fracture.

In addition to the common symptoms that occur after natural menopause, special considerations apply to women who have had their ovaries removed, particularly when oophorectomy occurs before age 45 years. Women with premenopausal oophorectomy have more severe and prolonged menopausal symptoms. Their risks of adverse mood, heart disease, excessive bone resorption, sexual dysfunction, and cognitive disorders are increased compared with the general population. Retention of the ovaries carries a survival benefit for women at low risk of ovarian malignancy. Women facing oophorectomy should understand the balance of risks and benefits in order to make an informed decision.

A heterogeneous disorder, premature menopause is not an uncommon entity, affecting approximately 1% of women younger than 40 years. Multisystem implications are recognized as sequelae to the premature deprivation of ovarian steroids, posing unique health-related challenges in this population. An integrated management approach that addresses both the physical and psychological health concerns and the overall well-being of this relatively chronologically young population is paramount.

Cardiovascular disease is the leading cause of death in postmenopausal US women. The contribution of postmenopausal hormone replacement therapy to cardiovascular risk is one of the most controversial women's health topics. Strikingly discordant results, between observational and randomized clinical trials, have been reported. Remaining questions regarding time of hormone therapy initiation are discussed, as are ongoing trials focused on these questions. Cardiovascular concerns, cautions, and current recommendations for use are delineated.

Menopausal hormone therapy (MHT) is the most effective treatment for vasomotor and vaginal symptoms. Today, symptomatic women younger than 60 years of age or less than 10 years since onset of menopause yield the greatest benefit of MHT with the lowest risks when compared with older women remote from menopause. Careful assessment before initiating therapy includes severity of bothersome symptoms, treatment preferences, medical history, presence of contraindications to MHT, and personal risk of cardiovascular disease and breast cancer. Considerations of type of MHT, dosing, and route of administration, and recommendations regarding duration of therapy are discussed.

Estrogen and progestogen treatment results in greater risk of breast cancer than placebo. Treatment with estrogen alone does not increase the risk of breast cancer, may be used by women who have had a hysterectomy, and may even result in a decreased risk of breast cancer. Continued research seeks to improve the understanding of the interplay between estrogen and progestogens that predispose to adverse effects on breast tissue. Caution over this hypothesized benefit is warranted until it is substantiated by data on the incidence of breast cancer in tissue selective estrogen complex users.

Cancer is a disease of aging, and therefore is more prevalent after menopause. Menopausal symptoms resulting from cancer treatments are an important survivorship issue in cancer care. This article reviews the preventive strategies, utilization of health resources, and management of menopausal symptoms after cancer treatment. Preventive screening as informed by genetic and lifestyle risk, and lifestyle modification, may mitigate the risk of cancer and cancer mortality. Despite potential benefits to quality of life, hormone replacement is rarely prescribed to survivors of gynecologic malignancies. Special considerations are needed for the treatment and supportive care of menopausal symptoms in cancer survivors.

Given the persistent confusion about the risks and benefits of hormone therapy since 2002 and the first publication from the Women's Health Initiative's primary findings, women and health care providers are increasingly motivated to find effective, nonhormonal approaches to treat menopause-related symptoms. Complementary and alternative medicine has grown increasingly popular in the last decade. A wide array of botanic medicines is offered as an alternative approach to hormone therapy for menopause, but data documenting efficacy and safety are limited. None of the available botanicals is as effective as hormone therapy in the management of vasomotor symptoms.

Sexuality is an important component in the lives of menopausal women. Despite the importance of sexual function in menopausal women, sexual dysfunction increases with age. Age-related decline in sexual function

ENDOCRINOLOGY AND METABOLISM CLINICS OF NORTH AMERICA

FORTHCOMING ISSUE

December 2015
**Reproductive Consequences of
Pediatric Disease**
Peter Lee and
Christopher P. Houk, *Editors*

RECENT ISSUES

June 2015
Adrenal Cortical Neoplasia
Alice C. Levine, *Editor*

March 2015
Pituitary Disorders
Anat Ben-Shlomo and Maria Fleseriu,
Editors

December 2014
Lipids
Donald A. Smith, *Editor*

RELATED INTEREST

Obstetrics and Gynecology Clinics, Volume 42, Issue 1 (March 2015)
Reproductive Endocrinology
Michelle L. Matthews, *Editor*
Available at: http://www.obgyn.theclinics.com/

Foreword

Postmenopausal Endocrinology

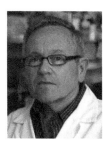

Derek LeRoith, MD, PhD
Consulting Editor

Drs Santoro and Pal have compiled a number of articles involving the important topic of the menopause. The articles cover the pathophysiology, diagnosis, and therapeutic options available to women as well as future directions and newer agents currently being tested to overcome many of the complications introduced by the menopause.

In the introductory article, Dr Hall describes the endocrine changes associated with the menopause. Menopause is associated with amenorrhea and a decrease in circulating sex hormone levels such as estradiol. There is a marked decrease in ovarian follicles that lead to changes in estradiol levels and a compensatory rise in luteinizing hormone (LH) and follicle stimulating hormone (FSH), the latter secondary to a reduction in inhibin B levels as well.

The menopause is associated with a variety of symptoms that vary in intensity between women. One of the more immediate and troublesome is the vasomotor "hot flash" that is directly related to the loss of estradiol secretion. As discussed in the article by Drs Santoro, Epperson, and Mathews, hot flashes were initially thought to be of limited duration, although there is strong evidence that hot flashes may last up to ten years or more for some women. Fortunately, there are hormonal and non-hormonal therapies for hot flashes.

Drs Lupsa and Insogna discuss the important problem of postmenopausal osteoporosis that is very common in women and begins even prior to and increases after the menopause. They describe in detail normal bone mineralization and the changes that occur primarily secondary to the fall in estradiol levels; however, other causes need to be identified that may exacerbate the changes occurring during the menopause. As osteoporosis develops, there are clear changes on DEXA scanning, and there is a marked increase in fragility fractures, which may be devastating and even fatal. Some degree of protection can be afforded by supplementing the diet with vitamin D and calcium; however, therapeutic intervention is often required.

Drs Rodriguez and Shoupe describe how surgical menopause differs from naturally occurring menopause. The removal of the ovaries leads to a sudden onset of

Endocrinol Metab Clin N Am 44 (2015) xiii–xv
http://dx.doi.org/10.1016/j.ecl.2015.07.002
0889-8529/15/$ – see front matter © 2015 Published by Elsevier Inc.

endo.theclinics.com

menopausal symptoms as opposed to the gradual onset seen with natural menopause, and the symptoms are often more severe. When oophorectomy is performed premenopausally, there are consequences related to the secondary effects of menopause such as osteoporosis, cardiovascular disease, and cognitive decline. Studies have suggested that there is an increased survival benefit with retention of the ovaries as long as possible; however, many women prefer removal of the ovaries to avoid ovarian cancer.

Premature menopause should be considered in women under the age of 40 years who present with secondary amenorrhea for more than three cycles. As described by Drs Torrealday and Pal, reduced circulating estradiol and elevated FSH and LH are confirmatory as well as low inhibin B and AMH levels. The causes of the condition include multiple causes that require investigation. Probably the most practical investigation is for autoimmune disorders, including autoantibodies for thyroid, type 1 diabetes, and adrenal, thus implicating autoimmune oophoritis as the cause for the premature menopause. Therapy requires hormone replacement to prevent the complications of hypoestrogenism.

One of the most controversial aspects of the menopause that still remains is the question of cardiovascular disease and its prevention. As discussed by Drs Nkonde-Price and Bender, one the one hand, the reduction in the protective effects of ovarian steroids after the menopause is the etiologic reason for the worsening of cardiovascular disease, while on the other hand, whether estrogen replacement therapy protects the cardiovascular system at all postmenopausally is still controversial. It may be reasonable to consider menopausal hormone therapy (MHT) early after onset of the menopause and use the lowest dose and limit to 5 years in women who are symptomatic. In older women, hormone replacement therapy use is probably not the wisest choice, since its harms seem to outweigh its benefits after a certain, ill-defined age.

In a further exposition on the consideration of MHT for menopausal symptoms, Dr Stuenkel discusses the question of choices, including early treatment of vasomotor symptoms of women under the age of 60 years. In addition, there are new options such as the selective estrogen receptor modulators, bazedoxifene (in combination with conjugated equine estrogens), and ospemifene.

A major concern with MHT regimens that include progestins is an increased risk for breast cancer. Drs Flores and H.S. Taylor describe the results of the Women's Health Initiative (WHI) that support this concern. It is important to realize that this complication is particularly related to combined estrogen and progesterone use, whereas estrogen alone does not seem to have the same relationship to breast cancer risk. As discussed, women with an intact uterus should not use estrogen alone because of the complication of endometrial hyperplasia and possible endometrial cancer. For women with a uterus, the recently approved SERM, bazedoxifene, combined with conjugated estrogens provides a progestin-free regimen, and other such regimens may become available to avoid this potential harm of combined MHT.

Drs Einstein, Levine, and Nevadunsky discuss the increased incidence of cancers other than breast cancer in postmenopausal women. This increase may, of course, be an age-related phenomeno. Gynecologic cancers, such as endometrial, ovarian, and vaginal, should be constantly screened for by the practicing physician. On the other hand, many cancers are treated by chemotherapeutic agents that may affect both ovarian and reproductive function, and raises the issue of counseling for these patients, since it may also affect sexual function.

Dr M. Taylor discusses the alternative treatments that are commonly used by women who prefer to avoid MHT, following the WHI published results, and their publicity. The article goes into detail on the various agents that have been tested and found to be no more effective than placebo: a rather disappointing finding, since these products are so widely used worldwide.

Menopause and sexual issues are important problems presenting to health care providers. The lack of estradiol is well known to result in vaginal changes such as atrophy. However, less well discussed is the loss of libido commonly experienced by postmenopausal women. As discussed by Drs Thornton, Chervenak, and Neal-Perry, therapy for vaginal atrophy is available using multiple options that utilize very low-dose estrogen. Therapy for lack of libido should include counseling, and more recently, physicians have been considering testosterone therapy. In addition, there are nonhormonal therapies that are being tested; most are centrally acting drugs.

Drs Van Pelt, Gavin, and Kohrt discuss the commonly seen increase in weight and particularly abdominal fat in postmenopausal women. While this is definitely a self-image and esthetic problem, it also increases the risk for diabetes and cardiovascular complications. In preclinical studies, there is a definite association of increased body fat and estrogen deficiency. Estrogen replacement, by activating the estrogen receptor, can prevent or reverse this effect. In human studies, the effect of loss or replacement with estrogen on body composition is yet to be well-defined.

I am indebted to the issue editors and the authors for contributing to this important and practical issue that I believe the practicing health care provider will find interesting, with relevant updates that will be useful in their practice.

Derek LeRoith, MD, PhD
Director of Research
Division of Endocrinology, Diabetes and Bone Diseases
Icahn School of Medicine at Mt Sinai
1 Gustave Levy Place (1055)
Atran B4-35
New York, NY 10029, USA

E-mail address:
derek.leroith@mssm.edu

Preface

Menopause and Perimenopause

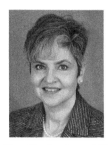 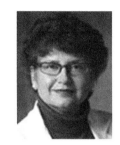

Nanette Santoro, MD   Lubna Pal, MBBS, MRCOG, MS, FACOG
Editors

In just a decade, the field of menopause has seemingly traversed a millennial journey! A number of longitudinal studies have helped define the natural history of the menopausal transition, and racial and ethnic nuances in the spectrum and the severity of symptomatology are now recognized. Through a series of well-conducted clinical trials, the ambiguities of decades past regarding the promise and the place of hormone therapy in menopause management are all but expunged, and the risks and the benefits of various hormonal and nonhormonal therapies to treat the symptoms and attendant health problems of menopausal and postmenopausal women are better understood than ever before.

In this issue of *Endocrinology and Metabolism Clinics of North America*, we have attempted to merge the natural history data that describe this normal life passage (the transition into menopause) with clinical trial data that inform treatment of largely finite, yet bothersome symptoms, and finally, to provide the clinician with information to help partner with patients in optimizing their quality of life and overall health, as menopause intersects with and influences a variety of diseases of aging. We have marshaled experts in their fields to bring the most up-to-date findings to bear on this fascinating field of endocrinology, and we are profoundly thankful for their contributions, as we are sure you will agree.

Nanette Santoro, MD
University of Colorado School of Medicine
12631 East 17th Avenue
AO1, Room 4010
Aurora, CO 80045, USA

Endocrinol Metab Clin N Am 44 (2015) xvii–xviii
http://dx.doi.org/10.1016/j.ecl.2015.07.003
0889-8529/15/$ – see front matter © 2015 Published by Elsevier Inc.

Lubna Pal, MBBS, MRCOG, MS, FACOG
Yale University School of Medicine
Department of Obstetrics, Gynecology
and Reproductive Sciences
333 Cedar Street
New Haven, CT 06510, USA

E-mail addresses:
Nanette.Santoro@ucdenver.edu (N. Santoro)
lubna.pal@yale.edu (L. Pal)

Erratum

Please note that in the article "Adrenocortical Carcinoma," by Eric Baudin, MD, PhD, which appeared on pages 411-434 of the June 2015 issue (Volume 44, Issue 2), co-authors included the following from the Endocrine Tumor Board of Gustave Roussy (Department of Endocrine Oncology and Nuclear Medicine): Segolene Hescot, MD; Amandine Berdelou, MD; Isabelle Borget, PharmD; Caroline Caramella, MD; Frederic Dumont, MD; Desirée Deandreis, MD; Frederic Deschamps, MD; Eric Deutsch, MD, PhD; Abir Al Ghuzlan, MD; Marc Lombes, MD, PhD; Rossella Libe, MD; Angelo Paci, PharmD; Jean-Yves Scoazec, MD, PhD; Jacques Young, MD, PhD; Sophie Leboulleux, MD, PhD; and Martin Schlumberger, MD, PhD. These authors were originally listed in an Acknowledgements section.

Endocrinol Metab Clin N Am 44 (2015) xix
http://dx.doi.org/10.1016/j.ecl.2015.07.001
0889-8529/15/$ – see front matter Published by Elsevier Inc.

endo.theclinics.com

Endocrinology of the Menopause

Janet E. Hall, MD[a,b,*]

KEYWORDS

- Ovary • Hypothalamus • Pituitary • Menopause • Estradiol
- Follicle-stimulating hormone

KEY POINTS

- Menopause is defined by the final menstrual period (FMP), but this diagnosis can only be made retrospectively after a year of amenorrhea.
- Reproductive aging in women is largely due to the loss of ovarian function, which is marked by decreased levels of inhibin B and antimullerian hormone (AMH).
- In the early stages of reproductive aging, there is an increase in follicle-stimulating hormone (FSH) as inhibin B levels decline, which serves to maintain folliculogenesis and estradiol secretion.
- With further loss of ovarian function, these compensatory changes are not always sufficient and result in marked variability in cycle dynamics and in estradiol and FSH levels.
- Estradiol levels stabilize at very low levels after the FMP.

Menopause is a signal event in a woman's life that marks the end of reproductive competence. Although the age-related loss of vaginal bleeding in women has been described throughout history, the studies of Block,[1] published in 1952, documented the dramatic decrease in the number of follicles within the ovary as a function of age, demonstrating that the loss of both germ cells and the hormone-producing cells that support them is key to the loss of menstrual function in women. Menopause is defined retrospectively by the FMP and occurs at an average age of 51. The process of reproductive aging, however, is gradual, begins much earlier than the FMP, and can be conceptualized as encompassing (1) an initial period in which compensatory changes in the hypothalamus, pituitary, and ovary help to maintain both reproductive competence and gonadal hormone secretion; (2) a period characterized by marked variability in follicle development, ovarian secretion, and consequent symptomatology

The author has nothing to disclose.
[a] Reproductive Endocrine Unit, Massachusetts General Hospital, Harvard Medical School, 55 Fruit Street, Boston, MA 02460, USA; [b] National Institute of Environmental Health Sciences, 111 TW Alexander Drive, Research Triangle Park, NC 27709, USA
* Reproductive Endocrine Unit, Massachusetts General Hospital, Harvard Medical School, 55 Fruit Street, Boston, MA 02460, USA
E-mail addresses: hall.janet@mgh.harvard.edu; janet.hall@nih.gov

Endocrinol Metab Clin N Am 44 (2015) 485–496
http://dx.doi.org/10.1016/j.ecl.2015.05.010
endo.theclinics.com

leading up to the FMP; and (3) stable and low ovarian hormone secretion. In this article these 3 phases of reproductive aging are discussed on the background of a discussion of normal reproductive cycle function and the changes that occur at all levels of the reproductive axis with aging.

REPRODUCTIVE FUNCTION IN NORMAL WOMEN

Regular reproductive cycles are established within the first 1 to 3 years after the first menstrual period in normal women.[2] Although cycles between 25 and 35 days (from the first day of menses in 1 cycle to the first day of menses in the subsequent cycle) are considered normal,[3] cycle-to-cycle variability in an individual woman is considerably smaller ($\pm$2 days).

Normal menstrual cycle function requires tightly integrated interactions between the hypothalamus, pituitary, and ovary whereas the endometrium serves as a gonadal steroid end organ and clinical marker of reproductive cycles (**Fig. 1**). Estradiol secretion from developing follicles causes follicular phase proliferation of the endometrium. After ovulation, the combination of progesterone and estrodial produces the secretory changes that prepare the endometrium for implantation if conception occurs. In the absence of pregnancy, the function of the corpus luteum declines, hormonal support of the endometrium is lost, and menses results (for review see Hall[4]).

At the beginning of each cycle, increasing levels of FSH are necessary for recruitment of a new cohort of follicles while restraint of FSH is required to ensure that only a single

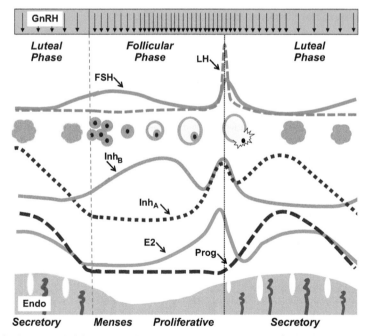

Fig. 1. The hormonal, follicular, and endometrial (Endo) dynamics of the normal menstrual cycle from the late luteal phase through menses and the beginning of a new cycle of follicle development, ovulation, and corpus luteum function and decline. Inh$_A$, inhibin A; Inh$_B$, inhibin B; E2, estradiol; Prog, progesterone. (*From* Hall JE. Neuroendocrine control of the menstrual cycle. In: Strauss JF, Barbieri RL, editors. Yen and Jaffe's reproductive endocrinology. 7th edition. Philadelphia: Elsevier Publishing; 2013. p. 148; with permission.)

follicle reaches the preovulatory stage to ensure optimum pregnancy outcomes for women. Estradiol secretion from developing follicles contributes to the negative feedback control of FSH, acting at both the hypothalamus and, to a lesser degree, the pituitary. Ovarian secretion of inhibin B and inhibin A provides an additional level of control through selective inhibition of FSH at the pituitary. In the late follicular phase, rising levels of estradiol result in generation of the preovulatory luteinizing hormone (LH) surge that is necessary for ovulation. The LH surge requires ongoing pulsatile gonadotropin-releasing hormone (GnRH) secretion but is otherwise fully dependent on the marked augmentation of gonadotropin responses to GnRH that occur at the level of the pituitary in response to the exponential rise in estradiol secretion from the dominant follicle.[4]

Progesterone secretion from the corpus luteum is maintained by LH secretion and inhibits GnRH pulse frequency.[5,6] In the early and midluteal phase, slow-frequency GnRH pulses are hypothesized to increase synthesis of FSH over that of LH, as has been shown in animal models,[7] although secretion of FSH is inhibited by estradiol and probably inhibin A. In the late luteal phase, the loss of this negative feedback from the waning corpus luteum[8] results in a preferential rise in FSH over LH. Increased hypothalamic GnRH secretion, made possible by the loss of progesterone and estradiol-negative feedback, is also necessary during the luteal-follicular transition to achieve levels of FSH that are adequate for the next wave of follicular recruitment.[9]

OVARIAN AGING IN WOMEN

In women, the finite pool of resting follicles in the ovary reaches its maximum in neonatal life. Thereafter, there is a steady decline due to atresia such that, at birth, only 1 million follicles remain, with a further reduction to 250,000 by the time of puberty (for review see Gougeon[10]). During and after puberty, follicles leave the pool of resting follicles by activation of further growth or by degeneration. Rising levels of FSH provide a critical stimulus for recruitment of resting follicles into the growing follicle pool whereas AMH, produced in granulosa cells from small growing follicles, restrains this effect of FSH within the ovary.[11] Throughout early reproductive life, the number of growing follicles is highly correlated with the size of the resting pool. Between the ages of 30 and 35, however, the percentage of growing follicles increases[12–14] and the trajectory of follicle loss is accelerated until the pool of resting follicles is reduced to between 100 and 1000, when there is cessation of reproductive cycles.[15] Age-related changes in oocyte quality parallel the decrease in follicle number, with reported decreases in fertilization and conception rates and higher rates of pregnancy loss. Chemotherapy, radiation, and smoking are all factors that accelerate follicle loss through damage to the oocyte and/or dividing granulosa cells.[16–19]

One of the most powerful predictors of age at menopause is family history, however, with twin studies estimating that a remarkable 44% to 85% of the variance in age at natural menopause is heritable.[20–22] At least 17 genes functioning in diverse pathways, including hormonal regulation, DNA repair, and immune function, have been associated with the age at natural menopause in genome-wide association studies (GWAS).[23–26] There is further evidence of gene-environment interactions,[27] raising the possibility that the wide range in age at menopause in normal women will be found to result from such interactions.

CHANGES IN THE HYPOTHALAMUS AND PITUITARY WITH REPRODUCTIVE AGING

Response to the Loss of Ovarian Feedback

During normal reproductive life, the ovarian hormones and peptides restrain gonadotropin secretion through mechanisms that are operative at both the hypothalamus and pituitary. At the hypothalamus, progesterone has a profound GnRH pulse frequency as measured by pulsatile LH levels. Estradiol does not seem to influence pulse frequency in women but does decrease the overall quantity of GnRH secretion and thus the amount of GnRH secreted with each pulse. At the level of the pituitary, estradiol decreases the gonadotrope response to GnRH, with an effect that is greater for FSH than LH; inhibin B plays an additional pituitary role in the selective inhibition of FSH over LH.

The earliest hormonal evidence of ovarian aging is the selective increase in FSH that results from decreasing levels of inhibin B, a marker of granulosa cell number. With a further decrease in ovarian function and the loss of ovulatory cycles, GnRH pulses occur more frequently.[28] In addition, declining levels of estradiol permit increases in both GnRH[29] and in the gonadotropin responses to GnRH.[30] Autopsy studies confirm an increase in GnRH expression in the medial basal hypothalamus after menopause[31] and suggest that this effect is mediated by an increase in the stimulatory neuropeptides, neurokinin B, and kisspeptin and a decrease in the inhibitory neuropeptide, dynorphin.[32] Finally, the half-life of LH and FSH disappearance is prolonged in postmenopausal women as a result of alterations in the isoform composition of these 2 glycoprotein hormones with the loss of estradiol.[33,34] Taken together, declining levels of ovarian steroids and peptides with ovarian aging result in a 15-fold increase in FSH and a 10-fold increase in LH in postmenopausal women in the early years after their FMP.[35]

Aging of the Hypothalamus and Pituitary: Possible Contribution to Menopause

In rodents, ovaries from old donors undergo folliculogenesis and ovulation when transplanted to young ovariectomized hosts,[36] providing evidence for a central contribution to reproductive failure with aging in rodents. Further studies have pointed to the importance of age-related alterations in estrogen-positive feedback on GnRH secretion as at least 1 contributing mechanism.[37] An important question is whether similar central mechanisms contribute to reproductive failure in women.

Studies in younger and older postmenopausal women suggest that there are effects of aging on the hypothalamus and pituitary that are independent of the loss of steroid feedback. After menopause there is a 30% to 40% decrease in LH and FSH between the ages of 50 and 75.[35,38] Underlying these gonadotropin changes are complex effects of aging on GnRH secretion, with a 22% decrease in GnRH pulse frequency[39] that is partially compensated by a 14% increase in the overall amount of GnRH secreted over that due to the loss of ovarian function alone.[29] There are also age-related effects at the pituitary, with a 30% decrease in both LH and FSH responses to GnRH in older compared with younger postmenopausal women.[30]

Estrogen-negative feedback at the hypothalamic level remains intact in older compared with younger postmenopausal women; low-dose estrogen administration is associated with a significant decline in circulating levels of LH, FSH, and free alpha-subunit and a parallel decrease in the overall amount of GnRH, with no effect on pulse frequency.[28] Addition of progesterone decreased pulse frequency in younger and older postmenopausal women with a concomitant decrease in overall amount of GnRH.[28,29] The effect of estrogen-negative feedback on the LH response to GnRH is not influenced by aging although the FSH response to GnRH is attenuated with aging.[30]

Several studies have suggested that sensitivity to estrogen-positive feedback may be lost with aging in women[40,41] as it is in rodents.[42] An LH surge and increased progesterone were not evident in a small percentage of women who collected daily urine samples for variable periods of time during the menopause transition, despite similar peak late follicular phase estradiol levels.[43] In further studies, a controlled and graded steroid infusion paradigm that recreated early and late follicular phase levels of estradiol in younger and older postmenopausal women demonstrated attenuation of the LH surge with age in the face of identical preovulatory patterns of estradiol.[44] There is now ample evidence for the overriding importance of increased pituitary responsiveness to GnRH in generation of the LH surge in women and, thus, attenuation of the steroid induced-surge with aging is consistent with the age-related decrease in pituitary responsiveness to GnRH.[45]

INTEGRATION OF HORMONAL CHANGES WITH REPRODUCTIVE AGING IN WOMEN

Our clinical and mechanistic understanding of the process of ovarian aging has progressed dramatically since the classic studies of Block[1] in the 1950s demonstrated follicle loss across the reproductive lifespan in women, and novel markers of ovarian aging have been developed have also changed. FSH levels are increased in older women even before their FMP[46] and for many years the selective rise in FSH on day 3 of the menstrual cycle was the only clinically available marker of fertility potential. Although the discovery of inhibin B elucidated its critical roles in ovarian-negative feedback on FSH and as a marker of ovarian aging,[47,48] measurement of inhibin B was unable to serve as a better marker of fertility potential than FSH itself.[49] Since that time, however, AMH has been established as an unexpected marker of the number of ovarian follicles, and AMH and antral follicle count have been used as prognostic markers in infertility programs (for review see Broekmans and colleagues[50]). Studies of these new ovarian factors not only has contributed to fertility prognosis but also has provided important insights into the integrated changes that occur with reproductive aging.

Maintenance of Follicle Development and Estrogen Secretion in Early Ovarian Aging

The existence of compensatory hormonal and intraovarian mechanisms that are operative in the early stages of ovarian aging is evidenced by continued follicle development and maintenance of estradiol levels well beyond the time at which other markers indicate declining ovarian function.[51–54] The age-related decrease in the number of follicles in the ovary is reflected in the number of antral follicles seen on ultrasound[55]; in declining levels of AMH,[12] which is expressed only in small growing follicles[11]; and in decreased levels of inhibin B, which is constitutively secreted from granulosa cells in FSH-dependent growing follicles.[56]

Inhibin B plays an extremely important role as a gonadal feedback modulator of FSH secretion in early ovarian aging, with declining levels of inhibin B associated with increasing levels of FSH.[48,57] Higher levels of FSH drive increased recruitment of follicles into the growing pool, the percentage of growing follicles increases,[13,14] and there is an increase in the rate of follicle loss.[15] It is likely that increased FSH is responsible both for the increased rate of spontaneous dizygotic twinning in older women[58] and for the increased follicular phase estradiol levels in early reproductive aging even when only 1 preovualtory follicle develops.[59] AMH restrains the stimulatory actions of FSH on recruitment of primordial follicles into the growing pool[11] and on the FSH-dependent stimulation of aromatase;[60] the age-related decline in AMH, therefore, facilitates the actions of FSH on follicle recruitment and aromatase. Up-regulation of aromatase in older cycling women is suggested by an increase in the ratio of serum levels of estrone to androstendione in the follicular phase in regularly cycling women older than 34 compared with their younger counterparts,[61] and supported by the finding of increased aromatase expression in granulosa cells aspirated from the dominant follicle in older compared with younger normal women.[62]

Taken together, these data support the hypothesis that lower levels of AMH in conjunction with elevated levels of FSH drive the accelerated depletion of the resting follicle pool after age 35 and that these hormonal and autocrine/paracrine changes are important for maintaining estradiol levels in the face of declining ovarian function and serve, serving to extend fertility and maintain reproductive cycles and estrogen levels early in reproductive aging.

Hormonal Variability of the Menopause Transition

With ongoing follicle loss, the compensatory mechanisms, described previously, are no longer adequate and cycles become irregular, signifying the onset of the menopause transition. Large-scale cohort studies describe the overall hormonal changes, characterized by the reciprocal relationship between decreasing inhibin B and increasing FSH levels early on and a later decline in estradiol that may not reach its nadir until 1 to 2 years after the FMP.[52,63,64]

These aggregate changes, however, do not reflect the marked variability in hormone levels that occur between women and within an individual woman (**Fig. 2**) from month to month over the 2 to 5 years of the menopause transition. Estrogen levels may fluctuate between undetectable and many times normal for variable periods of time, with these anovulatory hormonal patterns interspersed with ovulatory cycles.[65] Although the inconsistent estrogen response to FSH is not well understood, there is evidence of a mismatch between the progressively decreasing and scattered follicles in the ovary and their blood supply; Doppler studies indicate reduced ovarian blood supply in the aging ovary[66,67] and there are higher levels of vascular endothelial growth factor, a marker of tissue hypoxia, in older reproductive aged women.[68]

FSH levels are dramatically increased when estrogen levels are low due to the loss of steroid and inhibin feedback at the pituitary and also because of a marked decrease in gonadotropin clearance in the face of hypoestrogenism.[34] Age-related slowing of

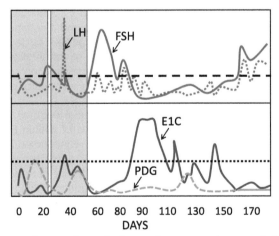

Fig. 2. Daily urine samples over 6 months in a perimenopausal woman indicate marked variability in the pattern of LH, FSH, estrone conjugates (E1C), and progesterone diglucuronide (PDG). The dashed line in the upper panel indicates the upper limit of normal for FSH in young women whereas the dotted line in the lower panel indicates the upper limit of normal E1C in young women. Shaded bars indicate cycles in which levels of PDG are consistent with ovulatory cycles. (*Data from* Santoro N, Brown JR, Adel T, et al. Characterization of reproductive hormonal dynamics in the perimenopause. J Clin Endocrinol Metab 1996;81(4):1495–501.)

GnRH pulse frequency also favors synthesis and secretion of FSH over LH.[7,39] Prior to the complete loss of ovarian follicles, consistently increased FSH levels drive follicle development and estrogen synthesis and secretion to levels that may be many times higher than ever seen in normal cycles.[65]

In the year before the FMP, 60% to 70% of cycles are either anovulatory or have prolonged follicular phases[69,70] consistent with hormonal data indicating that a significant number of increases in estradiol are not followed by an LH surge and an increase in progesterone. Generation of a preovulatory surge requires a highly specific pattern of increasing estrogen levels over an adequate duration,[71,72] both of which are likely to be altered in the face of asynchronous FSH and ovarian function.[43] Attenuation of the pituitary response to GnRH with aging[45] may further contribute to the abnormal cycle dynamics of the perimenopause. Irregular bleeding patterns, varying breast tenderness, hot flashes, sleep disturbance, and possible mood changes are a frequent accompaniment of the variability in hormonal patterns in the menopause transition.

Stability of Hormone Secretion after Menopause

In the first 1 to 2 years after the FMP, occasional follicle development is evident in individual women. Consistent with these observations, epidemiologic studies using sensitive estradiol assays[54] demonstrate a further decrease from the FMP to the estradiol nadir 2 years later. Thereafter, estradiol levels remain low and stable. FSH levels also remain stable between 2 and 8 years after the FMP[54] but decline over time such that FSH decreases by 30% by approximately age 75, as does LH.[73] Although women are no longer bothered by irregular bleeding and breast tenderness, hot flashes may persist for up to 7 years after the FMP,[74] and with prolonged hypoestrogenism, the genitourinary syndrome of menopause (GSM) may emerge as a new clinical symptom.

	REPRODUCTIVE		MENOPAUSE TRANSITION		POSTMENOPAUSE	
	Peak	Late	Early	Late	Early	Late
PRINCIPAL CRITERIA						
Menstrual cycle	Regular	Subtle changes	Variable length	Interval of amenorrhea ≥ 60 d		
SUPPORTIVE CRITERIA						
Endocrine						
FSH	low	variable	high variable	high >25 IU/L	high variable	stable
AMH	low	low	low	low	low	very low
Inhibin B		low	low	low	low	very low
Antral follicle count	low	low	low	low	very low	very low
Estradiol	normal	normal	normal	highly variable	stable	low stable

Final menstrual period

Fig. 3. Qualitative changes in estradiol superimposed in relation to the STRAW+10 system for reproductive aging[76] reflect the result of initial compensatory changes that preserve folliculogenesis and estrogen section and the progressive loss of compensation (*graded arrow*) with marked hormonal variability leading up to the FMP, followed by low and stable estrogen secretion.

Clinical Assessment of Reproductive Aging and Menopause

In 2001, the first Stages of Reproductive Aging Workshop (STRAW) used the findings from important cohort studies of women across the menopause transition, based primarily on changes in menstrual bleeding patterns and qualitative changes in FSH, and introduced standardized terminology referenced to the FMP.[75] This staging system provided a critical scaffold for further studies and was updated a decade later (STRAW+10) to incorporate the results of longitudinal studies across the menopause transition and studies of fertility in older women.[76] FSH cutoff levels are now possible because of international standardization of this measure. AFC and AMH have been limited to qualitative descriptors because these measures have not been standardized across centers and are used primarily in infertility populations and particularly in women over 35.[77]

Addition of changes in estradiol to this schema permits understanding the clinical symptoms of changes in menstrual cyclicity, vasomotor symptoms and GSM,[78] in the context of evolving hormonal changes with progressive loss of ovarian function (**Fig. 3**).

SUMMARY

Reproductive aging in women is primarily due the progressive, and ultimately accelerating, loss of ovarian follicles. The associated decline in inhibin B secretion from the ovaries results in the loss of negative feedback on FSH. Within the ovary, FSH-stimulated follicle growth and estrogen synthesis and secretion. With further follicle loss, these compensatory hormonal mechanisms are no longer adequate and follicle development becomes unpredictable before further loss of ovarian function results in the stable but very low estradiol levels that characterize the postmenopause.

REFERENCES

1. Block E. Quantitative morphological investigations of the follicular system in women; variations at different ages. Acta Anat (Basel) 1952;14(1–2):108–23.
2. Legro RS, Lin HM, Demers LM, et al. Rapid maturation of the reproductive axis during perimenarche independent of body composition. J Clin Endocrinol Metab 2000;85(3):1021–5.
3. Treloar AE, Boynton RE, Behn BG, et al. Variation of the human menstrual cycle through reproductive life. Int J Fertil 1967;12(1 Pt 2):77–126.
4. Hall JE. Neuroendocrine control of the menstrual cycle. In: Strauss JF, Barbieri RL, editors. Yen and Jaffe's reproductive endocrinology. 7th edition. Philadelphia: Elsevier Publishing; 2013. p. 141–56.
5. Filicori M, Butler JP, Crowley WF Jr. Neuroendocrine regulation of the corpus luteum in the human. Evidence for pulsatile progesterone secretion. J Clin Invest 1984;73(6):1638–47.
6. Soules MR, Steiner RA, Clifton DK, et al. Progesterone modulation of pulsatile luteinizing hormone secretion in normal women. J Clin Endocrinol Metab 1984; 58(2):378–83.
7. Dalkin AC, Haisenleder DJ, Ortolano GA, et al. The frequency of gonadotropin-releasing-hormone stimulation differentially regulates gonadotropin subunit messenger ribonucleic acid expression. Endocrinology 1989;125(2):917–24.
8. Hall JE, Schoenfeld DA, Martin KA, et al. Hypothalamic gonadotropin-releasing hormone secretion and follicle-stimulating hormone dynamics during the luteal-follicular transition. J Clin Endocrinol Metab 1992;74(3):600–7.

9. Welt CK, Martin KA, Taylor AE, et al. Frequency modulation of follicle-stimulating hormone (FSH) during the luteal-follicular transition: evidence for FSH control of inhibin B in normal women. J Clin Endocrinol Metab 1997;82(8):2645–52.

10. Gougeon A. Regulation of ovarian follicular development in primates: facts and hypotheses. Endocr Rev 1996;17(2):121–55.

11. Durlinger AL, Gruijters MJ, Kramer P, et al. Anti-Mullerian hormone attenuates the effects of FSH on follicle development in the mouse ovary. Endocrinology 2001; 142(11):4891–9.

12. Bentzen JG, Forman JL, Johannsen TH, et al. Ovarian antral follicle subclasses and anti-mullerian hormone during normal reproductive aging. J Clin Endocrinol Metab 2013;98(4):1602–11.

13. Gougeon A, Ecochard R, Thalabard JC. Age-related changes of the population of human ovarian follicles: increase in the disappearance rate of non-growing and early-growing follicles in aging women. Biol Reprod 1994;50(3):653–63.

14. Gougeon A. Ovarian follicular growth in humans: ovarian ageing and population of growing follicles Regulation of ovarian follicular development in primates: facts and hypotheses. Maturitas 1998;30(2):137–42.

15. Gosden RG, Faddy MJ. Ovarian aging, follicular depletion, and steroidogenesis. Exp Gerontol 1994;29(3–4):265–74.

16. Soleimani R, Heytens E, Darzynkiewicz Z, et al. Mechanisms of chemotherapy-induced human ovarian aging: double strand DNA breaks and microvascular compromise. Aging (Albany NY) 2011;3(8):782–93.

17. Mattison DR, Shiromizu K, Nightingale MS. The mechanisms of action of reproductive toxins Oocyte destruction by polycyclic aromatic hydrocarbons Effects of toxic substances on female reproduction. Am J Ind Med 1983;4(1–2): 65–79.

18. Cramer DW, Xu H. Predicting age at menopause. Maturitas 1996;23(3):319–26.

19. Gold EB, Bromberger J, Crawford S, et al. Factors associated with age at natural menopause in a multiethnic sample of midlife women. Am J Epidemiol 2001; 153(9):865–74.

20. de Bruin JP, Nikkels PG, Bruinse HW, et al. Morphometry of human ovaries in normal and growth-restricted fetuses. Early Hum Dev 2001;60(3):179–92.

21. Treloar SA, Do KA, Martin NG. Genetic influences on the age at menopause. Lancet 1998;352(9134):1084–5.

22. Snieder H, MacGregor AJ, Spector TD. Genes control the cessation of a woman's reproductive life: a twin study of hysterectomy and age at menopause. J Clin Endocrinol Metab 1998;83(6):1875–80.

23. He C, Kraft P, Chen C, et al. Genome-wide association studies identify loci associated with age at menarche and age at natural menopause. Nat Genet 2009; 41(6):724–8.

24. Schuh-Huerta SM, Johnson NA, Rosen MP, et al. Genetic markers of ovarian follicle number and menopause in women of multiple ethnicities. Hum Genet 2012; 131(11):1709–24.

25. Stolk L, Perry JR, Chasman DI, et al. Meta-analyses identify 13 loci associated with age at menopause and highlight DNA repair and immune pathways. Nat Genet 2012;44(3):260–8.

26. Titus SA, Southall N, Marugan J, et al. High-throughput multiplexed quantitation of protein aggregation and cytotoxicity in a huntington's disease model. Curr Chem Genomics 2012;6:79–86.

27. Butts SF, Sammel MD, Greer C, et al. Cigarettes, genetic background, and menopausal timing: the presence of single nucleotide polymorphisms in cytochrome

P450 genes is associated with increased risk of natural menopause in European-American smokers. Menopause 2014;21:694–701.

28. Gill S, Lavoie HB, Bo-Abbas Y, et al. Negative feedback effects of gonadal steroids are preserved with aging in postmenopausal women. J Clin Endocrinol Metab 2002;87(5):2297–302.

29. Gill S, Sharpless JL, Rado K, et al. Evidence that GnRH decreases with gonadal steroid feedback but increases with age in postmenopausal women. J Clin Endocrinol Metab 2002;87(5):2290–6.

30. Shaw ND, Histed SN, Srouji SS, et al. Estrogen negative feedback on gonadotropin secretion: evidence for a direct pituitary effect in women. J Clin Endocrinol Metab 2010;95(4):1955–61.

31. Rance NE, Uswandi SV. Gonadotropin-releasing hormone gene expression is increased in the medial basal hypothalamus of postmenopausal women. J Clin Endocrinol Metab 1996;81(10):3540–6.

32. Rance NE, Krajewski SJ, Smith MA, et al. Neurokinin B and the hypothalamic regulation of reproduction. Brain Res 2010;1364:116–28.

33. Sharpless JL, Supko JG, Martin KA, et al. Disappearance of endogenous luteinizing hormone is prolonged in postmenopausal women. J Clin Endocrinol Metab 1999;84(2):688–94.

34. Wide L, Eriksson K, Sluss PM, et al. Serum half-life of pituitary gonadotropins is decreased by sulfonation and increased by sialylation in women. J Clin Endocrinol Metab 2009;94(3):958–64.

35. Hall JE. Neuroendocrine physiology of the early and late menopause. Endocrinol Metab Clin North Am 2004;33(4):637–59.

36. Krohn PL. Review lectures on senescence. II. Heterochronic transplantation in the study of ageing. Proc R Soc Lond B Biol Sci 1962;157:128–47.

37. Wise PM, Smith MJ, Dubal DB, et al. Neuroendocrine influences and repercussions of the menopause. Endocr Rev 1999;20(3):243–8.

38. Santoro N, Banwell T, Tortoriello D, et al. Effects of aging and gonadal failure on the hypothalamic-pituitary axis in women. Am J Obstet Gynecol 1998;178(4):732–41.

39. Hall JE, Lavoie HB, Marsh EE, et al. Decrease in gonadotropin-releasing hormone (GnRH) pulse frequency with aging in postmenopausal women. J Clin Endocrinol Metab 2000;85(5):1794–800.

40. van Look PF, Lothian H, Hunter WM, et al. Hypothalamic-pituitary-ovarian function in perimenopausal women. Clin Endocrinol (Oxf) 1977;7(1):13–31.

41. Fujimoto VY, Klein NA, Battaglia DE, et al. The anterior pituitary response to a gonadotropin-releasing hormone challenge test in normal older reproductive-age women. Fertil Steril 1996;65(3):539–44.

42. Wise PM, Kashon ML, Krajnak KM, et al. Aging of the female reproductive system: a window into brain aging. Recent Prog Horm Res 1997;52:279–303.

43. Weiss G, Skurnick JH, Goldsmith LT, et al. Menopause and hypothalamic-pituitary sensitivity to estrogen. JAMA 2004;292(24):2991–6.

44. Shaw ND, Srouji SS, Histed SN, et al. Differential effects of aging on estrogen negative and positive feedback. Am J Physiol Endocrinol Metab 2011;301(2):E351–5.

45. Shaw ND, Srouji SS, Histed SN, et al. Aging attenuates the pituitary response to gonadotropin releasing hormone. J Clin Endocrinol Metab 2009;94:3259–64.

46. Sherman BM, West JH, Korenman SG. The menopausal transition: analysis of LH, FSH, estradiol, and progesterone concentrations during menstrual cycles of older women. J Clin Endocrinol Metab 1976;42(4):629–36.

47. Muttukrishna S, Sharma S, Barlow DH, et al. Serum inhibins, estradiol, progesterone and FSH in surgical menopause: a demonstration of ovarian pituitary feedback loop in women. Hum Reprod 2002;17(10):2535–9.
48. Welt CK, McNicholl DJ, Taylor AE, et al. Female reproductive aging is marked by decreased secretion of dimeric inhibin. J Clin Endocrinol Metab 1999;84(1):105–11.
49. Hall JE, Welt CK, Cramer DW. Inhibin A and inhibin B reflect ovarian function in assisted reproduction but are less useful at predicting outcome. Hum Reprod 1999;14(2):409–15.
50. Broekmans FJ, Soules MR, Fauser BC. Ovarian aging: mechanisms and clinical consequences. Endocr Rev 2009;30(5):465–93.
51. Burger HG. The endocrinology of the menopause. Maturitas 1996;23(2):129–36.
52. Sowers MR, Zheng H, McConnell D, et al. Estradiol rates of change in relation to the final menstrual period in a population-based cohort of women. J Clin Endocrinol Metab 2008;93(10):3847–52.
53. Sowers MR, Eyvazzadeh AD, McConnell D, et al. Anti-mullerian hormone and inhibin B in the definition of ovarian aging and the menopause transition. J Clin Endocrinol Metab 2008;93(9):3478–83.
54. Randolph JF Jr, Zheng H, Sowers MR, et al. Change in follicle-stimulating hormone and estradiol across the menopausal transition: effect of age at the final menstrual period. J Clin Endocrinol Metab 2011;96(3):746–54.
55. La Marca A, Spada E, Sighinolfi G, et al. Age-specific nomogram for the decline in antral follicle count throughout the reproductive period. Fertil Steril 2011;95(2):684–8.
56. Welt CK, Schneyer AL. Differential regulation of inhibin B and inhibin a by follicle-stimulating hormone and local growth factors in human granulosa cells from small antral follicles. J Clin Endocrinol Metab 2001;86(1):330–6.
57. Santoro N, Adel T, Skurnick JH. Decreased inhibin tone and increased activin A secretion characterize reproductive aging in women. Fertil Steril 1999;71(4):658–62.
58. Beemsterboer SN, Homburg R, Gorter NA, et al. The paradox of declining fertility but increasing twinning rates with advancing maternal age. Hum Reprod 2006;21(6):1531–2.
59. Hansen KR, Thyer AC, Sluss PM, et al. Reproductive ageing and ovarian function: is the early follicular phase FSH rise necessary to maintain adequate secretory function in older ovulatory women? Hum Reprod 2005;20(1):89–95.
60. di Clemente N, Goxe B, Remy JJ, et al. Inhibitory effect of AMH upon aromatase activity and LH receptors of granulosa cells of rat and porcine immature ovaries. Endocirne 1994;2:553–8.
61. Welt CK, Jimenez Y, Sluss PM, et al. Control of estradiol secretion in reproductive ageing. Hum Reprod 2006;21(8):2189–93.
62. Shaw ND, Srouji SS, Welt CK, et al. Compensatory increase in ovarian aromatase in older regularly cycling women. J Clin Endocrinol 2015. [Epub ahead of print].
63. Randolph JF Jr, Sowers M, Gold EB, et al. Reproductive hormones in the early menopausal transition: relationship to ethnicity, body size, and menopausal status. J Clin Endocrinol Metab 2003;88(4):1516–22.
64. Burger HG, Hale GE, Robertson DM, et al. A review of hormonal changes during the menopausal transition: focus on findings from the Melbourne Women's Midlife Health Project. Hum Reprod Update 2007;13(6):559–65.
65. Santoro N, Brown JR, Adel T, et al. Characterization of reproductive hormonal dynamics in the perimenopause. J Clin Endocrinol Metab 1996;81(4):1495–501.

66. Pan HA, Cheng YC, Li CH, et al. Ovarian stroma flow intensity decreases by age: a three-dimensional power doppler ultrasonographic study. Ultrasound Med Biol 2002;28(4):425–30.

67. Ng EH, Chan CC, Yeung WS, et al. Effect of age on ovarian stromal flow measured by three-dimensional ultrasound with power Doppler in Chinese women with proven fertility. Hum Reprod 2004;19(9):2132–7.

68. Klein NA, Battaglia DE, Woodruff TK, et al. Ovarian follicular concentrations of activin, follistatin, inhibin, insulin-like growth factor I (IGF-I), IGF-II, IGF-binding protein-2 (IGFBP-2), IGFBP-3, and vascular endothelial growth factor in spontaneous menstrual cycles of normal women of advanced reproductive age. J Clin Endocrinol Metab 2000;85(12):4520–5.

69. Van Voorhis BJ, Santoro N, Harlow S, et al. The relationship of bleeding patterns to daily reproductive hormones in women approaching menopause. Obstet Gynecol 2008;112(1):101–8.

70. O'Connor KA, Ferrell R, Brindle E, et al. Progesterone and ovulation across stages of the transition to menopause. Menopause 2009;16(6):1178–87.

71. Keye WR Jr, Jaffe RB. Strength-duration characteristics of estrogen effects on gonadotropin response to gonadotropin-releasing hormone in women. I. Effects of varying duration of estradiol administration. J Clin Endocrinol Metab 1975; 41(06):1003–8.

72. Young JR, Jaffe RB. Strength-duration characteristics of estrogen effects on gonadotropin response to gonadotropin-releasing hormone in women. II. Effects of varying concentrations of estradiol. J Clin Endocrinol Metab 1976;42(3): 432–42.

73. Hall JE. Neuroendocrine changes with reproductive aging in women. Semin Reprod Med 2007;25(5):344–51.

74. Avis NE, Crawford SL, Greendale G, et al. Duration of menopausal vasomotor symptoms over the menopause transition. JAMA Intern Med 2015;175(4):531–9.

75. Soules MR, Sherman S, Parrott E, et al. Executive summary: Stages of Reproductive Aging Workshop (STRAW). Fertil Steril 2001;76(5):874–8.

76. Harlow SD, Gass M, Hall JE, et al. Executive summary of the Stages of Reproductive Aging Workshop + 10: addressing the unfinished agenda of staging reproductive aging. Fertil Steril 2012;97(4):843–51.

77. Freeman EW, Sammel MD, Lin H, et al. Anti-mullerian hormone as a predictor of time to menopause in late reproductive age women. J Clin Endocrinol Metab 2012;97(5):1673–80.

78. Santora N, Epperson CN, Mathews SB. Menopausal Symptoms and Their Management. Endocrinol Metab Clin North Am 2015, in press.

Menopausal Symptoms and Their Management

Nanette Santoro, MD[a,*], C. Neill Epperson, MD[b], Sarah B. Mathews, MD[b]

KEYWORDS

- Menopause • Perimenopause • Vasomotor symptoms • Vaginal dryness
- Dyspareunia • Depression • Cognitive impairment • Insomnia

KEY POINTS

- The late menopause transition (when women begin to experience 60 or more days of amenorrhea) is the point in time when hot flashes, adverse mood, vaginal dryness, and sleep complaints accelerate in prevalence.
- The duration of hot flashes (vasomotor symptoms) maybe longer than previously thought, with newer studies indicating durations of as long as 10 or more years.
- There are nonestrogenic alternatives that are now approved by the US Food and Drug Administration (FDA) for the treatment of menopause-related vulvovaginal atrophy.
- Both depression and anxiety increase in prevalence as women traverse the menopause, and the most vulnerable women are those without any prior episodes.
- Cognitive changes related to estrogen withdrawal include deficits in verbal and working memory, with almost three-fourths of women having a subjective sense of memory loss.

INTRODUCTION

The menopause transition is experienced by 1.5 million women each year and often involves troublesome symptoms, including vasomotor symptoms, vaginal dryness, decreased libido, insomnia, fatigue, and joint pain.[1–3]

In one population-based assessment of 386 Australian women, 86% consulted a clinician at least once to discuss menopausal symptoms.[4] Several symptoms bear an obvious relationship to the changing hormonal milieu associated with menopause, and most women make direct linkages between menopause and the common symptoms of hot flashes, vaginal dryness, and disrupted sleep (with or without associated

N. Santoro has investigator-initiated grant support from Bayer and stock options in Menogenix. C.N. Epperson and S.B. Matthews have nothing to disclose.
[a] Department of Obstetrics & Gynecology, University of Colorado School of Medicine, 12631 East 17th Avenue, AO1, Room 4010, Aurora, CO 80045, USA; [b] Department of Psychiatry Perelman School of Medicine, University of Pennsylvania, 3535 Market Street, 3rd Floor, Philadelphia, PA 19104-3309, USA
* Corresponding author.
E-mail address: Nanette.Santoro@ucdenver.edu

Endocrinol Metab Clin N Am 44 (2015) 497–515
http://dx.doi.org/10.1016/j.ecl.2015.05.001
0889-8529/15/$ – see front matter © 2015 Elsevier Inc. All rights reserved.

endo.theclinics.com

night sweats). In addition, during menopause, women may develop depressive symptoms and cognitive difficulties, which are more subtly and inconsistently linked to hormones. Depression and cognitive impairment can be burdensome for women and also compound the burden of medical illness for the aging female population. As postmenopausal women are already at risk for osteoporosis and cardiovascular disease, it is important to address potentially changeable psychiatric issues that may make medical issues more difficult to treat. An understanding of the risk factors, clinical presentation, and management of these common menopausal symptoms allows for improved patient care and health outcomes for older female patients.

THE CORE 4 SYMPTOMS: VASOMOTOR, VAGINAL, INSOMNIA, AND MOOD
Epidemiology

Population-based, epidemiologic studies of menopausal women have recently been conducted and are yielding reliable and consistent information about the incidence, prevalence, and severity of several menopausal symptoms. However, the field is relatively new, and it is likely that there are subsets of women who are more or less vulnerable to particular symptoms or sets of symptoms. In 2005, a state-of-the-science conference on menopausal symptoms was convened, with a worldwide panel of expert evaluators who were tasked with determining which among the large set of midlife symptoms are most likely to be due to menopause. Symptoms were evaluated for their proximity to menopause, apart from the aging process, and the likelihood that estrogen is effective in relieving symptoms.[2] Based on this evidence review, 3 symptoms emerged as having good evidence for linkage to menopause: vasomotor symptoms, vaginal dryness/dyspareunia, and difficulty sleeping/insomnia. After this conference and based on 3 seminal studies,[3,5,6] adverse mood/depression was added to the list. Adequate longitudinal studies on cognitive function during the menopause were not yet available but have also become subsequently widely reported.[2,3,5,7,8]

It is clear that there are many other symptoms that are reported by menopausal women. These include joint and muscle aches, changes in body contour, and increased skin wrinkling.[1] Several studies have examined the associations between these symptoms and menopause. Given the methods of ascertainment, the subjective nature of the complaints, the likelihood that there is publication bias (wherein positive studies demonstrating linkage to menopause are more likely to be published than negative studies), and their variation over time, it has been difficult to establish a true relationship between these symptoms and menopause. Other symptoms, such as urinary incontinence (UI) and sexual function, have mixed data for efficacy of estrogen treatment and linkage to menopause, apart from the aging process. For these reasons, this article addresses the core 4 symptoms and includes cognitive issues because they are of great importance and concern to aging women.

Vasomotor symptoms

Vasomotor symptoms afflict most women during the menopausal transition, although their severity, frequency, and duration vary widely between women. Hot flashes are reported by up to 85% of menopausal women.[7] Hot flashes are present in as many as 55% of women even before the onset of the menstrual irregularity that defines entry into the menopausal transition[9] and their incidence and severity increases as women traverse the menopause, peaking in the late transition and tapering off within the next several years.[10–12] The average duration of hot flashes is about 5.2 years, based on an analysis of the Melbourne Women's Health Project, a longitudinal study that included 438 women.[11] However, symptoms of lesser intensity may be present for a longer period. Approximately 25% of women continue to have hot flashes up to 5 or more years after menopause. A meta-analysis of 35,445 women taken from 10 different studies confirmed a 4-year duration of hot flashes, with the most bothersome symptoms beginning about 1 year before the final menstrual period and declining thereafter.[10]

The exact cause of the hot flash has not been elucidated. The most accessible theory purports that there is a resetting and narrowing of the thermoregulatory system in association with fluctuations in or loss of estrogen production. In the past, hot flashes were thought to be related solely to a withdrawal of estrogen; however, there is no acute change in serum estradiol during a hot flash. Others have related hot flashes to variability in both estradiol and follicle-stimulating hormone (FSH) levels.[6] It is thought that decreased estrogen levels may reduce serotonin levels and thus upregulate the 5-hydroxytryptamine (serotonin) ($5\text{-}HT_{2A}$) receptor in the hypothalamus. As such, additional serotonin is then released, which can cause activation of the $5\text{-}HT_{2A}$ receptor itself. This activation changes the set point temperature and results in hot flashes.[13] Regardless of the exact cause of the hot flash, both hormone therapy and nonhormonal regimens can help to relieve vasomotor symptoms (**Table 1**).

Vulvovaginal atrophy

Urogenital tissues are exquisitely sensitive to estrogen, and the fluctuations in estrogen that occur during the menopausal transition, followed by sustained low levels after menopause, can render these tissues fragile and cause distressing symptoms. Multiple population- and community-based studies confirm that about 27% to 60% of women report moderate to severe symptoms of vaginal dryness or dyspareunia in association with menopause.[14,15] In addition to vaginal atrophy, narrowing and shortening of the vagina and uterine prolapse can also occur, leading to high rates of dyspareunia. Furthermore, the urinary tract contains estrogen receptors in the urethra and bladder, and as the loss of estrogen becomes evident, patients may experience UI. Unlike vasomotor symptoms, vulvovaginal atrophy does not improve over time without treatment.

Menopausal hormone therapy (MHT) is an effective treatment of vaginal atrophy and dryness. For this purpose, systemic or vaginal estrogen can be used, although locally applied estrogen is recommended and can be administered in very low doses (**Table 2**). These low doses are believed to be safe for the uterus, even without concomitant use of a progestin. Data are currently insufficient to define the minimum effective dose, but vaginal rings, creams, and tablets have all been tested and demonstrated to reduce vaginal symptoms.[16]

Although MHT is effective in reversing changes associated with vaginal atrophy,[17,18] it is not beneficial for UI. The Women's Health Initiative Hormone Trial found that women who received MHT and who were continent at baseline had an increase in the incidence of all types of UI at 1 year. The risk was highest for women in the conjugated equine estrogens (CEE)-alone arm. Among women experiencing UI at baseline, the frequency of symptoms worsened in both arms, and these women reported that UI limited their daily activities. This evidence clearly shows that the use of MHT increases the risk of UI among continent women and worsened the characteristics of UI among symptomatic women after 1 year of use.[19]

Women who have urogenital atrophy symptom require long-term treatments. Over-the-counter lubricants and moisturizers may have some effectiveness for milder symptoms; however, for those with severe symptoms, hormonal treatment is the mainstay. Vaginal estrogen can be given locally in very small doses (see **Table 2**). Until recently, there were no alternatives available. However, the FDA approved

Table 1
Hormonal and nonhormonal formulations for the treatment of hot flashes

Trade Name	Estrogen	Progestin	FDA Approved	Dose
Hormonal Therapies				
Premarin	CEE	—	Yes	0.3–1.25 mg po daily
Cenestin	Synthetic CE	—	Yes	0.3–1.25 mg po daily
Menest	Esterified estrogen	—	Yes	0.3–1.25 mg po daily
Estrace	17β-estradiol	—	Yes	1–2 mg po daily
Estinyl	Ethinyl estradiol	—	Yes	0.02–0.05 mg po 1–3 times daily
Evamist	17β-estradiol	—	Yes	1–3 sprays daily
Alora, Climara, Esclim, Menostar, Vivelle, Vivelle-Dot, Estraderm	17β-estradiol	—	Yes	1 patch weekly to twice weekly
EstroGel	17β-estradiol	—	Yes	1.25 g daily transdermal gel (equivalent to 0.75 mg estradiol)
Estrasorb	17β-estradiol	—	Yes	2 foil pouches daily of transdermal topical emulsion
Activella	Estradiol 1 mg	NETA 0.5 mg	Yes	1 tablet po daily
Femhrt	Ethinyl estradiol 5 μg	NETA 1 mg	Yes	1 tab po daily
Ortho-Prefest	17β-estradiol 1 mg	Norgestimate 0.09 mg	Yes	First 3 tablets contain estrogen, next 3 contain both hormones; alternate pills every 3 d
Premphase	CEE 0.625 mg	MPA 5 mg	Yes	First 14 tablets contain estrogen only and remaining 14 tablets contain both hormones. 1 tab po daily
Prempro	CEE 0.625 mg	MPA 2.5 or 5 mg	Yes	1 tab po daily
CombiPatch	17β-estradiol	NETA	Yes	1 patch transdermal twice weekly
Climara Pro	17β-estradiol	LNG	Yes	1 patch weekly

(continued on next page)

Table 1
(continued)

Trade Name	Estrogen	Progestin	FDA Approved	Dose
Estrace	17β-estradiol vaginal cream	—	Yes	2–4 g daily for 1 wk, then 1 g 3 times weekly
Femring	Estradiol vaginal ring	—	Yes	1 ring inserted vaginally every 3 mo
Duavee	CEE 0.45 mg/ bazedoxifine 20 mg	—	Yes	1 tablet daily
Nonhormonal Therapies				
Brisdelle	Paroxetine[a] 7.5 mg	—	Yes	7.5 mg daily
Effexor	Venlafaxine 36.5–300 mg	—	No	37.5–75 mg daily
Pristiq	Desvenlafaxine	—	No	50–100 mg daily
Lexapro	Escitalopram	—	No	10–20 mg daily
Celexa	Citalopram	—	No	10 mg daily
Prozac	Fluoxetine[a]	—	No	10–20 mg daily
Zoloft	Sertraline	—	No	50–100 mg daily
Neurontin	Gabapentin	—	No	300–900 mg up to tid
Lyrica	Pregabalin	—	No	50–10 mg tid

Abbreviations: CE, conjugated estrogen; CEE, conjugated equine estrogen; LNG, levonorgestrel; MPA, medroxyprogesterone acetate; NETA, norethindrone acetate.
[a] Inhibitor of CYP2D6; unsafe for use in conjunction with tamoxifen.

ospemifene, a systemically administered selective estrogen receptor modulator, for vulvovaginal atrophy in 2013. Dehydroepiandrosterone vaginal preparations are also being tested for effectiveness in treating menopausal urogenital atrophy.[20] These 2 compounds may be particularly helpful for women who have estrogen-sensitive cancers, such as breast cancer, in whom exogenous estrogen use is contraindicated. It is too early to evaluate the comparative effectiveness of these treatments.

Table 2
Treatments for vulvovaginal atrophy

Trade Name	Hormone	FDA Approved	Dose
Premarin vaginal 0.625 gm	Conjugated equine estrogens	Yes	0.5–2 gm qd × 2–3 wk, off 1 wk, repeat prn[a]
Estrace vaginal 0.01% cream	Estradiol	Yes	1 gm biweekly to triweekly
Estring 2 mg	Estradiol	Yes	One ring every 3 mo
Osphena	Ospemifene	Yes	60 mg po qd

[a] Lower dosing/less-frequent application may be appropriate per patient preference.

Sleep disturbances and insomnia

Sleep quality generally deteriorates with aging, and menopause seems to add an additional, acute layer of complexity to this gradual process. Women report more trouble sleeping as they enter into the menopausal transition, and sleep has been shown to be worse around the time of menses, both by self-report as well as by actigraphy.[21,22] Actigraphy studies indicate that as much as 25 minutes of sleep per night can be lost when a woman is premenstrual in her late reproductive years.[21]

Women report sleep difficulties approximately twice as much as do men.[23] Further compromise in sleep quality is associated with the hormonal changes associated with the menopausal transition and with aging, apart from hormones. Over time, reports of sleep difficulties increase in women such that by the postmenopause more than 50% of women report sleep disturbance.[2] Women seem to experience more detrimental effects on sleep in association with aging, when compared with men.[24]

Hormonal changes alone are not likely to provide the complete explanation for the relationship between sleep difficulty and menopause. Consistent with this concept is the fact that hormones are not always successful in treating sleep problems in midlife and beyond.[25] Chronic poor sleep hygiene habits and mood disorders contribute further to sleep problems.

The nature of the sleep disturbance can help guide the clinician to appropriate treatment. Women who report nighttime awakening in association with night sweats are candidates for hormone therapy. However, the clinical history is not often so simple. Women with mood disorders, particularly anxiety and depression, may experience difficulty falling asleep and/or early awakening. Women aged 40 years and older also frequently report difficulty staying asleep. Lower socio-economic status (SES), white race, and low marital happiness are social factors that have all been associated with worse sleep.[26] Disorders such as sleep apnea and restless leg syndrome need to be considered. The clinical consequences of a poor night's sleep include daytime fatigue and sleepiness, which can be subjectively measured and form the basis for a referral for a sleep study. **Table 3** displays a clinically useful scale that can help the clinician estimate the daytime impact of the sleep complaint.

Polysomnography has become a clinically useful tool for assessing sleep complaints.[26] When polysomnography is not available, clinicians can use sleep questionnaires to ascertain the principal issues surrounding the sleep complaint. Using

Table 3
The Epworth sleepiness scale

Situation	Chance of Dozing
Sitting and reading	
Watching television	
Sitting inactive in a public place (eg, a theater or meeting)	
As a passenger in a car for an hour without a break	
Lying down to rest in the afternoon when circumstances permit	
Sitting and talking to someone	
Sitting quietly after a lunch without alcohol	
In a car, while stopped for a few minutes in traffic	

Responses are recorded on a 4-point scale of 0 to 3 (0, no; 1, light; 2, moderate; 3, high chance of dozing). A total score of greater than 9 merits further evaluation.
Adapted from Johns MW. A new method for measuring daytime sleepiness: the Epworth sleepiness scale. Sleep 1991;14:541; with permission.

polysomnography, investigators in the Study of Women's Health Across the Nation (SWAN) study observed 20% of women with clinically significant apnea/hypopnea and 8% with periodic leg movements.[26]

Treatment of sleep complaints depends on the clinical findings. For insomnia, the reader is referred to the practical clinical review by Buysse.[27] Sleep apnea is often treated with continuous positive airway pressure devices. Restless leg syndrome can be treated with dopamine agonists, gabapentin, and opioids.[28] Hormone therapy can be considered for women with difficulty maintaining sleep because of vasomotor symptoms but seems to be effective mostly in postmenopausal women with surgically induced menopause.

Adverse mood

One-fifth of the US population will have an episode of depression in their lifetime, and women are twice as likely to be affected.[29] Although depression is more likely to occur in young adults, with peak onset in the fourth decade of life, there is evidence that the perimenopause represents another period of vulnerability for women. Several large prospective cohort studies have shown an increased risk of depressed mood during the menopause transition and an approximately 3-fold risk for the development of a major depressive episode during perimenopause compared with premeno-pause.[3,5,30,31] Although a previous episode of depression has been shown to confer an increased risk, women with no previous episode of depression are still 2 to 4 times more likely to experience a depressive episode during the menopause transition compared with the premenopause. Anxiety symptoms have been found to precede depression in some instances, and anxiety may also be viewed as increasing a woman's vulnerability to a midlife depressive episode.[32]

Other independent risk factors for the development of depressed mood during the menopause transition include poor sleep, stressful or negative life events, lack of employment, higher body mass index, smoking, younger age, and race (African Americans twice as likely to have depressive symptoms). In addition, there is evidence that hormonal changes occurring during menopause play a role, as evidenced by increased risk for depression in association with variability in estradiol levels, increasing FSH levels, surgical menopause, the presence of hot flashes, and a history of premenstrual syndrome. Contrary to prior belief, hot flashes are not necessary to the development of depression. Some have proposed the cascade theory, in which hot flashes lead to sleep disturbance and then to daytime fatigue, poor quality of life, and then depressive symptoms. Research instead shows that depressive symptoms more often precede hot flashes when they co-occur.[33]

There may also be significant environmental stressors present at the time that a woman reaches menopause. During midlife, a woman may be faced with changes in her marriage and family structure, with children no longer living in the home. She may experience changes in her career path, possibly returning to work or retiring. She may be taking on new responsibilities as a caregiver to her parents or in-laws, a well-known risk factor for depression. Although these factors do not likely cause depression on their own, they can certainly contribute and should be considered, particularly if supportive resources may be of help (**Box 1**).

As the menopause transition involves significant instability in estrogen levels, with intense irregular fluctuations, many researchers have focused on understanding the association between estrogen level and mood changes. As stated above, in longitudinal prospective studies, women who developed depression were more likely to have increased variability in estrogen levels, particularly in the early to midperimeno-pause.[30] The absolute level of estrogen is not associated with risk, however. Some

---

Box 1
Science revisited

Estrogen affects the mood-regulating pathways of the brain: Depression is thought, albeit in part, to be caused by dysregulation of the monoaminergic pathways in the central nervous system, and changing estrogen levels can lead to alterations of these serotonergic and noradrenergic systems. In animal models, estrogen administration can induce changes in serotonin neurotransmission in the amygdala, hippocampus, and hypothalamus, brain regions that are involved in affect regulation. In humans, studies of menopausal women undergoing estrogen treatment showed changes in mood as well as serotonin transmission relative to hormonal status.[34]

---

studies have used gonadotropin-releasing hormone (GnRH) agonists in order to induce menopausal changes in premenopausal women, so that measurement of hormones, evaluation for mood symptoms, and response to add-back hormone therapy can be more easily determined.[35] In a group of healthy premenstrual women, without a psychiatric history, administration of a GnRH agonist did not uniformly precipitate depressive symptoms. In another related study involving withdrawal of estradiol treatment in women with and without a history of perimenopausal depression, those with history of this type of depression were more likely to experience depressive symptoms as a result of withdrawal of estradiol therapy (**Box 2**).

A major depressive episode is defined by the *Diagnostic and Statistical Manual of Mental Disorders* (Fourth Edition) (*DSM-IV*) (1994) as 5 or more of the following symptoms, present most of the day nearly every day for a minimum of 2 consecutive weeks. At least 1 symptom is either depressed mood or loss of interest or pleasure.

The DSM-IV criteria for depressive disorders, as for other mental disorders, require that the depressive episode cause significant distress or dysfunction. A depressive episode can be classified as mild, moderate, or severe, with or without psychotic symptoms. Psychotic symptoms can include hallucinations (usually auditory perceptual disturbances) and delusions (false beliefs). A depressive disorder may be recurrent if a patient has had an episode in the past. A person whose depressive symptoms do not meet criteria for a major depressive episode may be classified as having minor depression or/and adjustment disorder with depressed mood if a significant recent stressor is present. Chronic symptoms of depression not meeting criteria for a major depressive episode may represent a dysthymic disorder.

A depressive episode can also occur in the setting of bipolar disorder, a mood disorder that also involves at least 1 previous manic episode. Before treatment of depression, a bipolar-type disorder should be ruled out because of different effective treatment regimens. As anxiety disorders are very common in women with depression, assessment for panic symptoms, generalized worry, as well as obsessive thoughts

---

Box 2
Evidence at a glance

Timing is everything: A 4-year cohort study by Freeman and colleagues,[30] involving a balanced randomly identified sample of African American and white women aged 35 to 47 years showed an increased risk for depressive symptoms in early menopause (with variable cycle length more than 7 days) compared with late menopause (at least 2 skipped cycles and >60 days of amenorrhea) and no elevated risk in the postmenopause. Other researches have suggested that the late menopause transition represents a time of increased risk for depression[5,30,31]; overall, perimenopause seems to pose more risk than premenopause or postmenopause.

and compulsive behaviors should be included. In addition, evaluation for substance abuse and dependence, which can significantly affect mood, should be included. Medical workup for illnesses that can present with depressive symptoms, such as hypothyroidism and anemia, is also appropriate.

A complete interview for depressive symptoms in every perimenopausal patient is not necessary or time efficient. Screening tools can be used to determine who will need further evaluation. Referral of patients to a mental health specialist depends on the primary care provider's level of expertise in assessment and treatment of depression, the availability of mental health resources, and patient/family preference. Even if a provider initiates treatment, there may be reason for referral at a later point (**Table 4**).

First-line treatment of a major depressive episode may involve psychotherapy, antidepressants, or a combination thereof. Treatment is often tailored to patient preference and severity of depression. Certainly, a more severe episode would require combined psychotherapy and pharmacotherapy. A mild to moderate episode may respond to either psychotherapy or an antidepressant alone, and if a patient is interested in a trial of medication, it may benefit significantly if this is started soon after the diagnosis is made. Primary care practitioners frequently make the initial diagnosis of depression and are in a position to begin this treatment in a timely manner when possible.

Selective serotonin reuptake inhibitors (SSRIs) are the first-line medications used in the treatment of depression. These SSRIs include fluoxetine (Prozac), citalopram (Celexa), escitalopram (Lexapro), sertraline (Zoloft), and paroxetine (Paxil). Each of these medications is equally likely to be effective and share similar side effect profiles. Patients often describe gastrointestinal upset, jitteriness, or headache, but these symptoms usually abate in the first few weeks of therapy. Once initiated, it may take 6 to 8 weeks for a patient to respond; however, often, patients notice a difference within the first month of treatment. Dosage can be titrated to achieve improved effectiveness, with increases approximately every month as tolerated. Of particular concern

Table 4
DSM-IV criteria for major depressive disorder and reasons for further psychiatric evaluation

Major Depression	Indications for Further Psychiatric Evaluation
At least one of these *must* be present: Depressed mood Loss of interest or pleasure in most or all activities	Evidence of suicidal ideation, inability to care for self or dependent others, or aggressivity/homicidal ideation
Four or more of the following must be present: Insomnia or hypersomnia Change in appetite or weight Psychomotor retardation or agitation Low energy Poor concentration Thoughts of worthlessness or guilt Recurrent thoughts about death or suicide	Failure to respond to or is intolerant of initial treatment trial Patient or clinician interested in modalities requiring specialty expertise (psychotherapy or electroconvulsive therapy, transcranial magnetic stimulation) Psychotic symptoms present History of bipolar disorder or psychotic disorder Significant psychiatric comorbidity (anxiety disorders, substance use, cognitive disorder) Unclear diagnosis of depression

in this population is the risk for sexual side effects (decreased libido and difficulty with arousal and achieving orgasm). As depression can also affect a woman's sexual function, however, the risks of discontinuation of medication may outweigh the burden of these side effects. A switch to a different SSRI or another antidepressant class or the addition of bupropion (Wellbutrin), which acts on the dopaminergic system, may be helpful. As stated previously, estrogen can be helpful in treating perimenopausal depression and changes in sexual function as well. Conversely, several different SSRI antidepressants have been shown to be effective in treating perimenopausal vasomotor symptoms (**Box 3**).[38]

Serotonin and norepinephrine reuptake inhibitors, such as venlafaxine (Effexor) or duloxetine (Cymbalta) can be particularly helpful in patients with comorbid anxiety. Bupropion can be helpful when patients have low energy, but it can exacerbate anxiety and insomnia. Psychostimulants such as modafinil (Provigil) or methylphenidate (Ritalin) can sometimes be useful in these cases but have less evidence for efficacy. Tricyclic antidepressants and monoamine oxidase inhibitors are useful in treatment-resistant depression but often have more significant side effects, particularly in older patients. Electroconvulsive therapy is often very well tolerated, safe, and effective in these older patients who fail to respond to or do not tolerate medications. There is also growing evidence for the utility of transcranial magnetic stimulation in this group (**Box 4**).

Several forms of psychotherapy may be beneficial for patients with depression, including cognitive behavioral therapy, interpersonal therapy, and psychodynamic psychotherapy. A range of providers with psychotherapy training are available (social workers, psychologists, nurse practitioners, psychiatrists), but resources may be limited because of the patient's insurance, location, and financial situation.

In double-blind placebo-controlled trials, perimenopausal women receiving short-term 17β-estradiol transdermally had remission rates as high as 80%.[37,39] In other randomized controlled trials, when estrogen was given to postmenopausal women with depression, there were no significant improvements in symptoms[40] or the treatment was not superior to an SSRI agent.[36] So it seems that the low estrogen levels involved in the menopause transition is an important factor in the development of depression in some women but does fully explain the increased risk for depression in this population. Moreover, these data indicate a window of opportunity for estradiol's antidepressant effects, with women with perimenopausal but not postmenopausal depression responding to estrogen therapy (**Box 5**).

Menopause and cognition

Many women complain of changes in their cognitive function during the menopause transition, with the majority reporting worsening of memory. Verbal memory (word list learning and recall), which women generally excel at when compared with men,

---

Box 3
Evidence at a glance

SSRIs are the first choice: In a treatment study by Soares and colleagues,[36] the SSRI escitalopram proved superior to a combination of estrogen and progesterone in treating depression as well as other menopausal symptoms. Almost 75% of women on escitalopram achieved remission of depression compared with 25% of those on hormone replacement therapy. In this study, however, subjects' depressive symptoms did not necessarily begin during the menopause transition. Other treatment studies showing benefit of estrogen in treating depressive symptoms have focused solely on women with depression beginning during menopause.[37]

Box 4
Tips and tricks

Watch out for drug-drug interactions: In older women, with multiple medical comorbidities, citalopram or escitalopram are often preferred because they have fewer interactions with the metabolism of other medications.

Start low and go slow: Older women may be more prone to side effects of antidepressants; however, doses of antidepressants in the higher range may be necessary to achieve remission, particularly when comorbid anxiety is also present. So continue to adjust the dose as necessary while monitoring the patient every few weeks.

---

is often the type of complaint noted. Women may notice difficulty remembering names and other verbally told information. In addition, they may report other cognitive challenges, with more trouble organizing and planning or possibly with concentration. In one study of 205 menopausal women, 72% reported some subjective memory impairment.[41] Symptoms were more likely to be associated with perceived stress or depressive symptoms than perimenopausal stage, but overall, cognitive symptoms were more prevalent early in the menopause transition. Aside from being bothersome, these symptoms raise women's concerns regarding their risk for dementia; however, it remains unclear whether these symptoms correspond to an increased risk for more serious chronic issues.

The first cross-sectional study to measure cognitive change in association with menopause showed that women in early menopause, late menopause, and postmenopause did not vary in memory performance according to stage and did not have abnormalities in memory testing.[42] Overall, women who had initiated any form of hormone replacement therapy before their last period performed better on memory testing than those who started it after menopause. Longitudinal study of menopausal status and measured cognitive performance[8] showed no impairments in overall cognitive function, but women entering menopause failed to improve as much on repeated tests compared with premenopausal women (they would be expected to improve over time with practice on the same test) (**Box 6**).

An important question is whether women who have cognitive difficulties during the menopause transition are at greater risk for cognitive impairment later in life. Patients and their clinicians can be reassured, however, that for most women cognitive function is not likely to worsen in the postmenopause in any pattern other than that expected with normal aging. Although it is not likely that cognitive function returns to a woman's premenopausal baseline in postmenopause, she may adapt to and compensate for the symptoms with time.

A gradual decline in some cognitive functions is expected to occur with normal aging, beginning in midlife, around the age of 50 years. Decreases in processing speed

---

Box 5
Caution!

Use hormone replacement therapy with care: Estrogen can be helpful in treating depression in some perimenopausal women. Although estrogen is often recommended to treat hot flashes, women with depression with comorbid vasomotor symptoms are not more likely to respond to estrogen therapy.[37] Estrogen should be avoided in treating depressive symptoms in postmenopausal women, however, with lack of evidence for efficacy and increased risk of adverse events and side effects.

Box 6
Evidence at a glance

Again, timing may be key: The SWAN study[8] was a 4-year, multisite longitudinal study of cognitive function in women aged 42 to 52 years. Results showed that verbal memory and processing speed were improved with repeated testing in premenopausal, early perimenopausal, and postmenopausal women, but not in late perimenopausal women. Hormone use before the final menses was associated with better processing speed and verbal memory in all groups compared with current hormone use in postmenopause.

---

are often present, and sometimes mild changes in memory for newly learned information and executive function can also occur. However, some types of cognitive changes, collectively called mild cognitive impairment (MCI), are thought to be a manifestation of very early dementia. MCI and dementia are highly unlikely in people younger than 50 years, but risk increases significantly with age, with greater than 10% of the population older than 65 years at risk for developing dementia. (Those diagnosed with MCI have an increased risk of conversion to dementia like that in Alzheimer disease [AD], with approximately 10% developing dementia each year).[43] AD is by far the most common type of dementia, but other types of dementia can occur with varying presentations, including vascular dementia, Lewy body dementia, and frontotemporal dementia. AD often presents with impaired memory first, but other types of dementia can present with impaired language, behavioral changes, or motor abnormalities (**Box 7**).

In some individuals with MCI, dementia may never develop and cognition can even improve over time. Depression can also be present with MCI, and it can be difficult to discern whether the depression is causing the memory impairment, if a common pathologic process is causing depression and cognitive MCI, or if MCI puts one at risk of developing depression. Depression can also be an early manifestation of cognitive decline. In the unlikely situation that MCI presents in an individual younger than 50 years, it rarely represents a predementia syndrome, and search for another, possibly more treatable cause is important.

Box 7
Tips and tricks

Some cognitive changes are normal in aging

- More difficulty recalling newly learned lists, names, and other verbal information
- Slower rate of learning
- Decreased ability to perform newly learned complex tasks
- Shortened attention span

Some changes may be warning signs

- Loss of vocabulary or language skills
- Impaired reading comprehension
- Loss of older memories/fund of knowledge
- Inability to perform independent activities of daily living (shopping, handling finances, using transportation, using telephone, housekeeping, food preparation)
- Disorientation

Dementia is more common in women than in men, even after controlling for the effects of the female population's greater longevity. For this reason, many have focused on the role that estrogen plays in the risk for developing dementia. Estrogen interacts with both the cholinergic and serotonergic systems that are the main brain systems involved in normal cognitive functioning. In animal models, estrogen has positive effects on the cholinergic system, interacting with trophic factors for neuronal development and plasticity, with associated improved cognitive functioning.[44] Furthermore, studies have shown that estradiol can improve cognitive deficits produced by anticholinergic agents in normal postmenopausal women (**Box 8**).[45]

Evidence supports a significant role for estrogen in cognitive functioning. In premenopausal women, higher achievements in verbal memory performance occurred during phases of the menstrual cycle associated with high estrogen levels,[46] and hormone users in the SWAN sample had better cognitive performance in the perimenopause (although the same was not true for postmenopausal hormone use[8]). There was also early evidence in observational studies for a decreased risk of AD in women on hormone replacement therapy.[47] The relationship between estrogen and cognitive function has proved to be complicated, however, with varying effects with different formulations/combinations and when initiated during menopause, before the age of 65 years in postmenopause, and after the age of 65 years in the postmenopause. In several studies, estrogen alone in younger postmenopausal women showed some benefit to verbal memory but had neutral effects on older postmenopausal women.[48] CEE plus medroxyprogesterone acetate resulted in a negative change in the memory of younger and older postmenopausal women. Other formulations may be beneficial, with one study showing promise for the combination of estradiol valerate and dinogest in younger postmenopausal women[49] and another demonstrating a positive effect with cyclic oral estradiol and norethindrome in older postmenopausal women (**Box 9**).

Women experiencing a surgical menopause after hysterectomy and bilateral oophorectomy have also been a focus of study, because cognitive complaints are common in this subgroup and hormonal changes are certainly more abrupt and clearly defined. There is evidence that these women do develop impairments in verbal memory that can be prevented by administration of estrogen therapy.[46,50]

When a perimenopausal or postmenopausal woman presents with cognitive complaints, the practitioner is most often able to reassure the patient that these complaints are common and not necessarily progressive and may even improve over time. As in those with depressive symptoms, patients with cognitive impairment often present to primary care providers first and the gynecologist is in the position to evaluate for more serious issues and to provide education regarding prevention of chronic conditions such as dementia.

In 2001, the American Academy of Neurology (AAN) published practice guidelines for the early detection of memory problems (Petersen and colleagues, 2001). The

---

Box 8
Science revisited

Serotonin plays a role here too: There is ample evidence from animal studies showing that changes in serotonergic transmission can have effects on memory tasks. Administration of estradiol in ovariectomized rodents also does result in changes in serotonin levels and metabolism.[34] In humans, memory has repeatedly been shown to be impaired by tryptophan (TRP) depletion, a manipulation that results in rapid reduction of brain TRP and serotonin levels, and there is now some evidence that estrogen therapy may protect menopausal subjects from these effects.[34]

> **Box 9**
> **Evidence at a glance**
>
> *Is there a critical window?* The Women's Health Initiative Memory Study[51] demonstrated that MHT would not protect women from dementia as once thought and even showed an increased risk when used in older postmenopausal women. This study was limited to women between the ages of 65 and 79 years, however, and there is further evidence that hormone replacement therapy initiated earlier in the postmenopausal period may not present the same risk. More research is needed to determine whether a critical window exists when estrogen or combined MHT might protect cognitive function.

AAN workgroup of specialists identified the criteria for an MCI diagnosis (**Table 5**). Patients with MCI do not meet criteria for dementia (see **Table 5**), which involves impaired daily functioning.

The evaluation for MCI and dementia includes a thorough history provided by the patient and preferably a partner or family members in close contact with the patient. Medical history and review of systems aid in determining if any other medical illnesses could be contributing (particularly infectious illnesses or disorders of the cardiovascular, neurologic, or endocrine systems). A medication history is also particularly important because often analgesics, anticholinergics, psychotropic medications, and sedative-hypnotics can affect cognition. Family history to elicit information regarding family member with dementia; possibly early onset; before the age of 60 years; and other neurologic disorders is also important. Physical examination, including a basic neurologic examination and some cognitive assessment should also be completed.

The cognitive test most often used as a screen for cognitive impairment is the mini mental state exam (MMSE),[52] which takes approximately 7 minutes to complete. MMSE tests a broad range of cognitive functions including orientation, recall, attention, calculation, language manipulation, and constructional praxis (**Box 10**).

MMSE scores may be influenced by age and education, as well as language, motor, and visual impairments. Other cognitive tests are available for use in the office, such as the Montreal cognitive assessment test.[53] When a diagnosis of MCI is possible, however, a referral for more complete neuropsychological testing may be best. Initial

Table 5
Differentiation of MCI and dementia

MCI	Dementia (DSM-IV Criteria)
Memory complaint, preferably confirmed by an informant	Impairment in handling complex tasks
Objective memory impairment on standard neuropsychological batteries assessing memory (for age and education)	Impairment in reasoning ability
Normal general thinking and reasoning skills	Impaired spatial ability and orientation
Ability to perform normal daily activities	Impaired language
—	The cognitive symptoms must significantly interfere with the individual's work performance, usual social activities, or relationships with other people
—	This must represent a significant decline from a previous level of functioning

---

Box 10
MMSE Sample Items

Orientation to Time

"What is the date?"

Registration

"Listen carefully. I am going to say three words. You say them back after I stop.

Ready? Here they are…

APPLE (pause), PENNY (pause), TABLE (pause). Now repeat those words back to me." [Repeat up to 5 times, but score only the first trial.]

Naming

"What is this?" [Point to a pencil or pen.]

Reading

"Please read this and do what it says." [Show examinee the words on the stimulus form.]

CLOSE YOUR EYES

Reproduced by special permission of the Publisher, Psychological Assessment Resources, Inc., 16204 North Florida Avenue, Lutz, Florida 33549, from the Mini Mental State Examination, by Marshal Folstein and Susan Folstein, Copyright 1975, 1998, 2001 by Mini Mental LLC, Inc. Published 2001 by Psychological Assessment Resources, Inc. Further reproduction is prohibited without permission of PAR, Inc. The MMSE can be purchased from PAR, Inc. by calling (813) 968–3003.

---

laboratory work should include assessing thyrotropin and vitamin B_{12} levels to rule out potentially reversible causes of cognitive impairment (hypothyroidism and vitamin B_{12} deficiency). Brain imaging (computed tomography or preferably MRI) should be completed if MCI or dementia diagnosis is determined.

Once a diagnosis of MCI or dementia is made, these patients should often be referred to a neurologist or geriatric psychiatrist for further evaluation and/or treatment. Studies can be done to more clearly determine the risk for developing dementia in those with MCI (such as APOE allele, lumbar puncture with cerebrospinal fluid studies, functional imaging studies, and neuropsychological testing) and to clarify the type of dementia.

Medications are not clearly helpful in addressing these cognitive issues. Acetylcholinesterase inhibitors have been to shown to provide benefit for patients with early dementia but have not been shown to decrease the rate of progression to dementia in patients with MCI. As noted before, estrogen may be useful in some women, but its use is not recommended for this purpose. Antidepressant medications may result in improved cognition if comorbid depression is also present. Atomoxetine, the selective norepinephrine reuptake inhibitor often used to treat adult attention deficit disorder, has recently been shown to provide significant subjective improvement in memory and attention in perimenopausal and postmenopausal women presenting with midlife-onset subjective cognitive difficulties.[54] Similarly, stimulant medication may have a role in the treatment of subjective cognitive impairment, particularly for women with comorbid fatigue or impaired concentration, who are not showing evidence of objective impairment (**Box 11**).

There is some evidence that modifying lifestyle factors can decrease the risk for dementia and even cognitive decline associated with normal aging. Patients should be

> **Box 11**
> **Caution!**
>
> *Hormone replacement therapy for memory?* A trial of estrogen therapy or combined estrogen/ progesterone may prove beneficial for some types of cognitive complaints in some perimenopausal or early postmenopausal women. However, estrogen therapy has not been shown to be useful in treatment and prevention of cognitive decline in older postmenopausal women (>65 years old). Monitor patients on HRT often and be sure to thoroughly explain known risks and benefits to your patient.

encouraged to exercise regularly; to eat a nutritious diet, with adequate fruits, vegetables, and fish; to engage in regular social activities; and to participate in cognitive exercise (reading, crossword puzzles, etc.) Patients should also be encouraged to maintain good cardiovascular health, with treatment of hyperlipidemia, hypertension, and diabetes mellitus.

SUMMARY

The menopausal transition and postmenopausal years are associated with significant symptoms. Vasomotor symptoms and adverse mood often demonstrate improvement after a woman is postmenopausal, whereas sleep complaints, vaginal dryness/dyspareunia, and cognitive complaints tend to persist or worsen in association with aging. There is evidence that the changing hormone milieu, with significant changes in estrogen levels, can affect the brain systems involved in mood and cognition. Patients often present to their primary care provider with these symptoms first, and endocrinologists are in a position to identify more serious issues, provide education, begin treatment, and make appropriate referrals to when necessary. A better understanding of the nature of the risk for these common symptoms in menopausal women will aid in prevention, detection, and treatment.

REFERENCES

1. Dennerstein L, Dudley EC, Hopper JL, et al. A prospective population-based study of menopausal symptoms. Obstet Gynecol 2000;96:351–8.
2. Sherman S, Miller H, Nerukar L, et al. NIH State-of-the-Science Conference on Management of Menopause-Related Symptoms, March 21–25, 2005. Am J Med 2005;118(suppl 2):1–172.
3. Cohen L, Soares C, Vitonis A, et al. Risk for new onset of depression during the menopausal transition: the Harvard study of moods and cycles. Arch Gen Psychiatry 2006;63:386–90.
4. Guthrie JR, Dennerstein L, Taffe JR, et al. Health care-seeking for menopausal problems. Climacteric 2003;6:112–7.
5. Bromberger JT, Matthews KA, Schott LL, et al. Depressive symptoms during the menopausal transition: the Study of Women's Health Across the Nation (SWAN). J Affect Disord 2007;103:267–72.
6. Freeman EW, Sammel MD, Lin H, et al. Symptoms associated with menopausal transition and reproductive hormones in midlife women. Obstet Gynecol 2007; 110:230–40.
7. ACOG practice bulletin No. 141: management of menopausal symptoms. Obstet Gynecol 2014;123:202–16.

8. Greendale GA, Huang MH, Wight RG, et al. Effects of the menopause transition and hormone use on cognitive performance in midlife women. Neurology 2009; 72:1850–7.
9. Reed SD, Lampe JW, Qu C, et al. Premenopausal vasomotor symptoms in an ethnically diverse population. Menopause 2014;21:153–8.
10. Politi MC, Schleinitz MD, Col NF. Revisiting the duration of vasomotor symptoms of menopause: a meta-analysis. J Gen Intern Med 2008;23:1507–13.
11. Col NF, Guthrie JR, Politi M, et al. Duration of vasomotor symptoms in middle-aged women: a longitudinal study. Menopause 2009;16:453–7.
12. Gold EB, Colvin A, Avis N, et al. Longitudinal analysis of the association between vasomotor symptoms and race/ethnicity across the menopausal transition: Study of Women's Health Across the Nation. Am J Public Health 2006;96:1226–35.
13. Kligman L, Younus J. Management of hot flashes in women with breast cancer. Curr Oncol 2010;17:81–6.
14. Santoro N, Komi J. Prevalence and impact of vaginal symptoms among postmenopausal women. J Sex Med 2009;6:2133–42.
15. Pastore LM, Carter RA, Hulka BS, et al. Self-reported urogenital symptoms in postmenopausal women: Women's Health Initiative. Maturitas 2004;49: 292–303.
16. Henriksson L, Stjernquist M, Boquist L, et al. A one-year multicenter study of efficacy and safety of a continuous, low-dose, estradiol-releasing vaginal ring (Estring) in postmenopausal women with symptoms and signs of urogenital aging. Am J Obstet Gynecol 1996;174:85–92.
17. Leiblum S, Bachmann G, Kemmann E, et al. Vaginal atrophy in the postmenopausal woman. The importance of sexual activity and hormones. JAMA 1983; 249:2195–8.
18. Rioux JE, Devlin C, Gelfand MM, et al. 17beta-estradiol vaginal tablet versus conjugated equine estrogen vaginal cream to relieve menopausal atrophic vaginitis. Menopause 2000;7:156–61.
19. Hendrix SL, Cochrane BB, Nygaard IE, et al. Effects of estrogen with and without progestin on urinary incontinence. JAMA 2005;293:935–48.
20. Panjari M, Davis SR. Vaginal DHEA to treat menopause related atrophy: a review of the evidence. Maturitas 2011;70:22–5.
21. Zheng H, Harlow SD, Kravitz HM, et al. Actigraphy-defined measures of sleep and movement across the menstrual cycle in midlife menstruating women: Study of Women's Health Across the Nation sleep study. Menopause 2015;22(1):66–74.
22. Kravitz HM, Zhao X, Bromberger JT, et al. Sleep disturbance during the menopausal transition in a multi-ethnic community sample of women. Sleep 2008;31: 979–90.
23. Manber R, Armitage R. Sex, steroids, and sleep: a review. Sleep 1999;22:540–55.
24. Ohayon MM, Carskadon MA, Guilleminault C, et al. Meta-analysis of quantitative sleep parameters from childhood to old age in healthy individuals: developing normative sleep values across the human lifespan. Sleep 2004;27:1255–73.
25. Alexander JL, Neylan T, Kotz K, et al. Assessment and treatment for insomnia and fatigue in the symptomatic menopausal woman with psychiatric comorbidity. Expert Rev Neurother 2007;7:S139–55.
26. Kravitz HM, Joffe H. Sleep during the perimenopause: a SWAN story. Obstet Gynecol Clin North Am 2011;38:567–86.
27. Buysse DJ. Insomnia. JAMA 2013;309:706–16.
28. Earley CJ. Latest guidelines and advances for treatment of restless legs syndrome. J Clin Psychiatry 2014;75:e08.

29. Seedat S, Scott KM, Angermeyer MC, et al. Cross-national associations between gender and mental disorders in the World Health Organization World Mental Health Surveys. Arch Gen Psychiatry 2009;66:785–95.

30. Freeman EW, Sammel MD, Lin H, et al. Associations of hormones and menopausal status with depressed mood in women with no history of depression. Arch Gen Psychiatry 2006;63:375–82.

31. Schmidt PJ, Haq N, Rubinow DR. A longitudinal evaluation of the relationship between reproductive status and mood in perimenopausal women. Am J Psychiatry 2004;161:2238–44.

32. Kravitz HM, Schott LL, Joffe H, et al. Do anxiety symptoms predict major depressive disorder in midlife women? The Study of Women's Health Across the Nation (SWAN) Mental Health Study (MHS). Psychol Med 2014;44(12): 2593–602.

33. Freeman EW, Sammel MD, Lin H. Temporal associations of hot flashes and depression in the transition to menopause. Menopause 2009;16:728–34.

34. Amin Z, Canli T, Epperson CN. Effect of estrogen-serotonin interactions on mood and cognition. Behav Cogn Neurosci Rev 2005;4:43–58.

35. Schmidt PJ, Steinberg EM, Negro PP, et al. Pharmacologically induced hypogonadism and sexual function in healthy young women and men. Neuropsychopharmacology 2009;34:565–76.

36. Soares CN, Arsenio H, Joffe H, et al. Escitalopram versus ethinyl estradiol and norethindrone acetate for symptomatic peri- and postmenopausal women: impact on depression, vasomotor symptoms, sleep, and quality of life. Menopause 2006;13:780–6.

37. Schmidt PJ, Nieman L, Danaceau MA, et al. Estrogen replacement in perimenopause-related depression: a preliminary report. Am J Obstet Gynecol 2000;183:414–20.

38. Nelson HD, Vesco KK, Haney E, et al. Nonhormonal therapies for menopausal hot flashes: systematic review and meta-analysis. JAMA 2006;295:2057–71.

39. Soares CN, Almeida OP, Joffe H, et al. Efficacy of estradiol for the treatment of depressive disorders in perimenopausal women: a double-blind, randomized, placebo-controlled trial. Arch Gen Psychiatry 2001;58:529–34.

40. Morrison MF, Kallan MJ, Ten Have T, et al. Lack of efficacy of estradiol for depression in postmenopausal women: a randomized, controlled trial. Biol Psychiatry 2004;55:406–12.

41. Woods NF, Mitchell ES, Adams C. Memory functioning among midlife women: observations from the Seattle Midlife Women's Health Study. Menopause 2000;7: 257–65.

42. Henderson VW, Guthrie JR, Dudley EC, et al. Estrogen exposures and memory at midlife: a population-based study of women. Neurology 2003;60:1369–71.

43. Petersen RC, Stevens JC, Ganguli M, et al. Practice parameter: early detection of dementia: mild cognitive impairment (an evidence-based preview). Report of the Quality Standards Subcommittee of the American Academy of Neurology. Neurology 2001;56:1133–42.

44. Gibbs RB. Estrogen therapy and cognition: a review of the cholinergic hypothesis. Endocr Rec 2010;31:224–53.

45. Dumas J, Hancur-Bucci C, Naylor M, et al. Estradiol interacts with the cholinergic system to affect verbal memory in postmenopausal women: evidence for the critical period hypothesis. Hormones and Behavior 2008;53:159–69.

46. Phillips SM, Sherwin BB. Effects of estrogen on memory function in surgically menopausal women. Psychoneurodocrinology 1992;17:485–95.

47. Zandi PP, Carlson MC, Plassman BL, et al. Hormone replacement therapy and incidence if Alzheimer disease in older women: the Cache County Study. JAMA 2002;288:2123–9.
48. Maki P, Sundermann E. Hormone therapy and cognitive function. Hum Reprod Update 2009;15:667–81.
49. Linzmayer L, Semlitsch HV, Saletu B, et al. Double-blind, placebo-controlled psychometric studies on the effects of a combined estrogen-progestin regimen versus estrogen alone on performance, mood and personality of menopausal syndrome patients. Arzneimittelforschung 2001;51:238–45.
50. Phillips SM, Sherwin BB. Variations in memory function and sex steroid hormones across the menstrual cycle. Psychoneurodocrinology 1992;17:497–506.
51. Espeland MA, Rapp SR, Shumaker SA, et al. Women's Health Initiative Memory Study. Conjugated equine estrogens and global cognitive function in postmenopausal women: Women's Health Initiative Memory Study. JAMA 2004;291:2959–68.
52. Folstein MF, Folstein SE, McHugh PR. "Mini-mental state". A practical method for grading the cognitive state of patients for the clinician. J Psych Res 1975;12:189–98.
53. Nasreddine ZS, Philips NA, Bedirian V, et al. The Montreal Cognitive Assessment, MoCA: a brief screening tool for mild cognitive impairment. Journal of the American Geriatrics Society 2005;53:695–9.
54. Epperson CN, Pittman B, Czarkowski KA, et al. Impact of atomoxetine on subjective attention and memory difficulties in perimenopausal and postmenopausal women. Menopause 2011;18:542–8.

Bone Health and Osteoporosis

Beatrice C. Lupsa, MD*, Karl Insogna, MD

KEYWORDS

- Osteoporosis • Menopause • Fracture • Bone loss • Bone mineral density • DXA
- Calcium • Vitamin D

KEY POINTS

- Osteoporosis is characterized by low bone mass and microarchitectural deterioration of bone tissue leading to an increased risk of fragility fractures.
- Central dual-energy X-ray absorptiometry measurements are the gold standard for determining bone mineral density.
- A well-balanced diet containing adequate amounts of calcium and vitamin D, exercise, and smoking cessation are important to maintaining bone health as women age.
- Pharmacologic agents should be recommended in patients at high risk for fracture.

INTRODUCTION

Osteoporosis is the most common skeletal disease in humans. It is characterized by low bone mass and microarchitectural deterioration of the bone tissue, leading to decreased bone strength and increased risk of low-energy fractures, or so-called fragility fractures. Osteoporosis affects a large number of people of both sexes and all races and its prevalence increases with age. Osteoporosis is a risk factor for fracture just as hypertension is for stroke. The most common osteoporotic-related fractures are those of the vertebrae (spine), proximal femur (hip), and distal forearm (wrist).

This article focuses on postmenopausal bone health and osteoporosis. It provides guidance for providers of health care to women on proper screening, identification of secondary causes, and appropriate treatment of osteoporosis.

PATHOPHYSIOLOGY

The skeleton is one of the largest organ systems in the body. It consists of a mineralized matrix with a small but highly active cellular fraction. Bone is formed by

Disclosure: The authors have nothing to disclose.
Department of Internal Medicine, Yale Bone Center, Yale University School of Medicine, New Haven, CT, USA
* Corresponding author. 333 Cedar Street, FMP 107, P.O. Box 208020, New Haven, CT 06519.
E-mail address: beatrice.lupsa@yale.edu

osteoblasts, which are derived from marrow mesenchymal cells. Osteoblasts are also important for initiating resorption. Along with the osteocytes, they release receptor activator of nuclear factor kappa B ligand (RANKL) which is essential for osteoclastogenesis. In addition to RANKL, osteoblasts produce an inhibitor of osteoclastogenesis called osteoprotegerin (OPG). OPG is a soluble receptor for RANKL that binds this ligand and prevents interaction of RANKL with its cognate receptor, receptor activator of nuclear factor kappa B. Osteoclasts are derived from hematopoietic progenitors and are highly specialized cells involved in bone resorption. The principal stimulator of osteoclast formation is RANKL.

The osteoblasts and osteoclasts are involved in bone remodeling, which is a dynamic process by which old bone is removed from the skeleton and new bone is added. Remodeling can be activated by both systemic and local factors. Changes in mechanical force can activate remodeling to improve skeletal strength and to remove and repair the bone that has undergone microdamage. Systemic hormones influencing bone remodeling include parathyroid hormone (PTH), 1,25-dihydroxyvitamin D, calcitonin, growth hormone, glucocorticoids, thyroid hormones, gonadal hormones, and cytokines. Usually this cycle is tightly coupled and the amount of new bone formed by osteoblasts is equal to the amount resorbed by osteoclasts. Bone loss occurs when this balance is altered, resulting in greater bone removal than replacement. This imbalance occurs with menopause and advanced age.[1]

During the menopausal transition, serum estradiol levels decrease by 85% to 90% and serum estrone decreases by 65% to 75% relative to premenopausal values. With the onset of menopause and the decrease in estrogen levels, the rate of bone remodeling increases by 2-fold to 4-fold. There is a greater increase in bone resorption, resulting in an imbalance in bone remodeling. The imbalance in bone resorption leads to an accelerated phase of bone loss and an efflux of skeletal-derived calcium to the extracellular fluid. These changes lead to a negative total body calcium balance, which further aggravates the skeletal losses.[2]

At menopause, women undergo rapid trabecular bone loss, which usually continues for 5 to 8 years after the cessation of menses. Initially, about 20% to 30% of the trabecular bone and 5% to 10% of the cortical bone is lost. About 8 to 10 years after menopause, a second phase of bone loss becomes predominant in which both trabecular and cortical bone are lost at equal rates. The loss of bone tissue leads to deterioration in skeletal microarchitecture and an increase in fracture risk. Later in the course of menopause, age-related bone loss and accompanying changes in the material properties of bone exacerbate the bone loss associated with estrogen deficiency.

At the cellular level the increased number and activity of osteoclasts disrupts trabecular connectivity and increases cortical porosity. Resorption pits created as part of an accelerated bone remodeling cycle are incompletely filled because osteoblastic new bone formation does not keep pace with rates of bone resorption. Reduced bone density and bone quality compromise the mechanical weight-bearing properties of the skeleton and confer a predisposition to fractures.

Even though bone loss occurs as a consequence of the decrease in estrogen levels during menopause, several other disorders can lead to accelerated bone loss regardless of age and estrogen status. These secondary causes of osteoporosis include hyperparathyroidism, vitamin D deficiency, hypercortisolism, hyperthyroidism, plasma cell dyscrasias (eg, multiple myeloma and monoclonal gammopathy of undetermined significance), inflammatory diseases (eg, rheumatoid arthritis), gastrointestinal disorders (eg, chronic liver disease, celiac disease, and inflammatory bowel disease), chronic renal disease, renal calcium losses, and drugs (eg, steroids, antiepileptics, depot medroxyprogesterone acetate, anticoagulants, vitamin A, loop diuretics, and selective serotonin receptor uptake inhibitors).

DIAGNOSIS AND INITIAL EVALUATION
Measurement of Bone Mineral Density

Dual-energy X-ray absorptiometry
Dual-energy X-ray absorptiometry (DXA) measurement of the hip (femoral neck and to-tal hip) and spine is the preferred method of diagnosing osteoporosis, predicting future fracture risk, and monitoring patients (**Fig. 1**). Bone mineral density (BMD) measured by DXA at the one-third radius site can be used for diagnosis when the hip and/or spine cannot be measured. DXA measures bone mineral content (BMC) grams in and bone area (BA) in square centimeters. The areal BMD in grams per square centi-meter is calculated by dividing BMC by BA. The T-score, the value used for diagnosing osteoporosis, is calculated by subtracting the mean BMD of a young-adult reference population from the patient's BMD and dividing it by the standard deviation (SD) of the young-adult population. The Z-score, used to compare the patient's BMD with that of a population of peers, is calculated by subtracting the mean BMD of an age-matched, ethnicity-matched, and sex-matched reference population from the patient's BMD and dividing by the SD of the reference population.[3]

The BMD diagnosis of normal bone mass, osteopenia, and osteoporosis is based on the World Health Organization (WHO) diagnostic classification[4] (**Box 1**). This clas-sification should be used for postmenopausal women. A diagnosis of osteoporosis can also be made on a previous fragility fracture, even if the BMD is in the normal range. A fragility fracture denotes a fracture in adult life occurring spontaneously, or a fracture arising from trauma that, in a healthy individual, would not have resulted in a fracture.

In premenopausal women the WHO BMD diagnostic classification should not be applied. In this group, the diagnosis of osteoporosis should not be made from

A   **B**

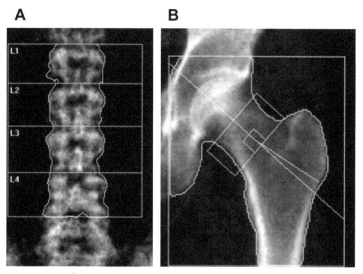

Fig. 1. Measurement of the bone density of the lumbar vertebrae and hip using DXA. (*A*) DXA of a normal lumbar spine L1 to L4. For clinical diagnosis of osteoporosis under almost all circumstances the bone density of all 4 vertebrae are used. (*B*) DXA of the left hip. For clinical diagnosis of osteoporosis, femoral neck and total hip are used.

Box 1
The WHO definitions based on BMD measurement at the spine, hip, or forearm by DXA devices

Normal:

BMD within 1 SD of a young normal adult (T-score equal to or greater than −1.0).

Low bone mass (osteopenia):

BMD between 1.0 and 2.5 SD less than that of a young normal adult (T-score between −1.0 and −2.5).

Osteoporosis:

BMD 2.5 SD or more less than that of a young normal adult (T-score at or less than −2.5). Patients in this group who have already experienced 1 or more fractures are deemed to have severe or established osteoporosis.

---

densitometric criteria alone. The International Society for Clinical Densitometry recommends that instead of T-scores ethnic or race-adjusted Z-scores should be used. Z-scores of −2.0 or lower are defined as either low BMD for chronologic age or less than the expected range for age, and those more than −2.0 as within the expected range for age.[3]

When using DXA to monitor change in BMD with time and therapy, the absolute BMD value (grams per square centimeter) should be used. Statistically significant change in BMD is calculated by 2.77 multiplied by precision at the site of measurement to provide least significant change. In an individual patient, an adequate interval of time (usually 18–24 months) is required between measurements to show significant change, unless larger changes in BMD are anticipated (eg, glucocorticoid treatment).[3] When using DXA to monitor change in BMD, it is important to use the same scanner and software because different manufacturers use different edge detection algorithms and different X-ray beam technologies.

Other technologies to measure bone mass

Other technologies, such as peripheral dual-energy X-ray absorptiometry, computed tomography–based absorptiometry, quantitative computed tomography (QCT), peripheral QCT, and quantitative ultrasonography densitometry, can be used to predict both site-specific and overall fracture risk. When performed according to accepted standards, these techniques are accurate and highly reproducible. However, T-scores from these technologies are not equivalent to T-scores derived from DXA and they cannot be used to diagnose osteoporosis based on the WHO classification.[3] Note that DXA is the only method that has been used in all osteoporosis treatment trials.

Assessment of Fracture Risk

All postmenopausal women should be evaluated clinically for osteoporosis risk in order to determine the need for BMD testing. Assessment of clinical risk factors that are independent of BMD is important for fracture prediction. Validated risk factors that are independent of BMD include advanced age, previous fracture, long-term glucocorticoid therapy, low body weight, family history of hip fracture, cigarette smoking, and excess alcohol intake.[5] In general, the more risk factors that are present, the greater the risk of fracture. Several of these risk factors have been included in the WHO 10-year fracture risk model (FRAX) available at http://www.sheffield.ac.uk/FRAX/. As validated by the WHO, these factors increase the risk for fractures independently of BMD, but can be combined with BMD measurements to assess an individual patient's risk of fracture. FRAX is based on data collected from large prospective observational studies but it has never been used as an end point in treatment trials.

Who Should be Screened for Osteoporosis?

The decision to perform bone density assessment should be individualized based on the patient's fracture risk profile. Measuring bone density is not indicated unless the results will influence the patient's treatment decision.

Most expert groups recommend that all women 65 years of age and older be screened routinely for osteoporosis regardless of clinical risk factors. Consideration should be given to screening younger postmenopausal women who have had a fracture or who have one or more risk factors for osteoporosis. Also, anyone being considered for pharmacologic therapy for osteoporosis, anyone being treated for osteoporosis (to monitor treatment effect), anyone not receiving therapy and in whom evidence of bone loss would lead to treatment, and all postmenopausal women discontinuing estrogen should be considered for bone density testing.[3,6,7]

Initial Evaluation

Initial evaluation includes a detailed history to assess for clinical risk factors for fracture and secondary causes of bone loss, a thorough physical examination, and basic laboratory tests.

The history should be focused on fragility fractures, height loss, medications associated with bone loss, smoking, alcohol intake, kidney stones, falls, and family history of osteoporosis and/or hip fracture. Patients should be evaluated for coexisting medical conditions that may contribute to bone loss, such as rheumatoid arthritis, hyperthyroidism, Cushing syndrome, hyperparathyroidism, multiple myeloma, inflammatory bowel disease, and celiac disease. Initial laboratory evaluation includes serum creatinine, calcium, phosphorus, magnesium, 25-hydroxyvitamin D, and liver function tests. If clinically indicated, a complete blood count, PTH, thyroid-stimulating hormone, serum protein electrophoresis, and 24-hour urine calcium and free cortisol should be measured. If kyphosis is identified or 2.5 cm (1 inch) or more height loss can be documented, radiographs of the thoracolumbar spine should be obtained to exclude the presence of vertebral compression fractures.

Bone turnover markers are emerging as promising tools in the management of osteoporosis, because they provide dynamic information regarding skeletal status. Commercial bone turnover marker assays, such as serum C-telopeptide and urine N-telopeptide are available for assessment of bone resorption. Serum bone-specific alkaline phosphatase, serum osteocalcin, or serum procollagen type 1 N-terminal propeptide are available for assessment of bone formation. Most of these markers have a circadian rhythm, peaking in the early morning, with a trough in the afternoon and evening. Sampling the fasting serum, early in the morning or using the first or second voided urine, is suggested to minimize variability.

TREATMENT
Nutrition

Bone health depends on a combination of mechanical load and adequate intake of macronutrients and micronutrients. The most important nutrients are calcium, vitamin D, and proteins.

Calcium is important for the bone formation phase of bone remodeling. An inadequate calcium intake can result in decreased calcium absorption and secondary hyperparathyroidism, which can cause increased bone resorption. With aging, the efficacy of intestinal calcium declines, thus adequate calcium intake is crucial in maintaining bone health. As noted earlier, vitamin D serves as the substrate for 1,25-dihydroxyvitamin D, which is a key regulator of intestinal calcium absorption. Recent meta-analyses of randomized controlled studies in postmenopausal women have shown that supplementation with calcium and vitamin D results in a reduced risk of fractures and a modest increase in BMD.[8]

The adequate intake of calcium and vitamin D, as well as the optimal levels of 25-dihydroxyvitamin D, have been controversial subjects for years. Recently the Institute of Medicine published recommendations regarding the dietary reference intakes on calcium and vitamin D. According to this report, the recommended calcium dietary allowance for women older than 50 years of age is 1200 mg per day. Although available data are inconclusive, some concerns remain about the safety of calcium supplements. Therefore, calcium supplements should be used only in patients who cannot achieve adequate dietary calcium intake. The recommended vitamin D dietary allowance is 600 IU per day for women age 50 to 70 years, and 800 IU per day for women older than 71 years of age. A serum 25-hydroxyvitamin D level of 20 ng/mL seems to be enough to protect most of the population from adverse skeletal outcomes such as fractures and falls.[8]

Data on the effect of protein intake on bone density are conflicting. Some studies suggest that higher protein intake may decrease the risk of hip fractures[9] and bone loss,[10] whereas others suggest that high protein intake may increase bone resorption and calcium excretion.[11] In general, available data suggest that an intake of 1.2 g/kg/day allows for normal calcium homeostasis.

Exercise

Physical activity has a modest antiresorptive effect but, in general, it has been associated with a decreased risk of hip fractures in older women[12] and decreased risk of falls by improving muscle strength, balance, mobility, and overall physical function. Women with osteoporosis (or seeking to prevent it) should exercise for at least 30 minutes 3 times per week. Any weight-bearing exercise regimen, including walking, jogging, tennis, and dancing, is acceptable. Non–weight-bearing exercises, such as swimming, can improve muscle strength, cardiovascular fitness, and coordination but they have less effect on BMD. A meta-analysis of 18 randomized trials on the exercise effect on BMD in postmenopausal women reports that aerobics, weight-bearing, and resistance exercises are effective of increasing BMD in the spine, whereas walking increases BMD at both spine and hip.[13]

Other Lifestyle Modifications

Smoking cessation should be stressed because smoking cigarettes is recognized as a risk factor for fractures and reduced BMD. Excess alcohol (3 or more drinks per day) is harmful to skeletal health and patients should be counseled on the importance of moderating alcohol intake.

Prevention of Falls

Most osteoporotic fractures occur as a result of a fall. Risk factors for falls include gait instability, visual impairment, weakness, cognitive impairment, vitamin D deficiency, home hazards, and treatment with medications such as benzodiazepines and other sedatives and antidepressants. Falls can be reduced by several interventions, such as initiation of an exercise regimen that improves gait, stability, and strength; avoidance of polypharmacy; vitamin D supplementation; vision assessment and correction; and the use of assistive devices. Hip protectors have not consistently been shown to decrease the risk of fractures.

Pharmacologic Treatment

Indication for treatment

The National Osteoporosis Foundation (NOF) has formulated treatment guidelines that have been widely promulgated in the United States. The NOF recommends treating postmenopausal women with a hip or vertebral (clinical or morphometric) fracture, postmenopausal women with osteoporosis at the femoral neck, total hip or spine (T-scores ≤ −2.5 by DXA) or with osteopenia at the femoral neck or spine (T-scores between −1.0 and −2.5), and a 10-year hip fracture probability greater than or equal to 3% or a 10-year major osteoporosis-related fracture probability greater than or equal to 20% based on the US-adapted WHO absolute fracture risk model (FRAX).[7] A suggested algorithm for diagnosis and management of postmenopausal osteoporosis is outlined in **Fig. 2**.

United States Food and Drug Administration–approved drugs for osteoporosis

Current US Food and Drug Administration (FDA)–approved drugs for the prevention and/or treatment of postmenopausal osteoporosis include bisphosphonates, estrogens, selective estrogen receptor modulators (SERMs), teriparatide, denosumab, and calcitonin (**Table 1**). All of these medications except teriparatide are classified as antiresorptive agents. As noted earlier, in estrogen-deficiency bone loss resorption outstrips formation, resulting in an increase in the numbers of excavated bone remodeling units that are not filled with new bone. Antiresorptive agents increase BMD in part by decreasing the rate of bone remodeling and allowing these open resorption pits to

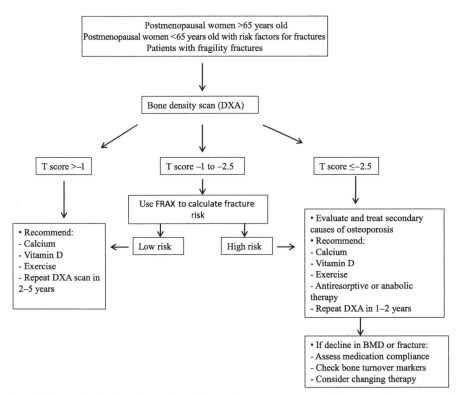

Fig. 2. Suggested algorithm for diagnosis and management of postmenopausal osteoporosis.

Table 1
Summary of fracture risk reduction of FDA-approved medications in postmenopausal osteoporosis

Drug	Vertebral Fracture	Hip Fracture	Nonvertebral Fracture
Alendronate	✔	✔	✔
Risedronate	✔	✔	✔
Ibandronate	✔	—	✔[a]
Zoledronic acid	✔	✔	✔
Estrogen	✔	✔	✔
Raloxifene	✔	—	—
Teriparatide	✔	—	✔
Denosumab	✔	✔	✔
Calcitonin	✔	—	—

[a] Effect shown in a post-hoc analysis.

be remodeled to a new bone. This so-called closure of the remodeling space explains most of the increase in BMD seen with these medications. There is additionally a change in extracellular matrix that occurs with antiresorptive therapy, which also contributes to their efficacy. Teriparatide is the only approved anabolic agent. It stimulates bone formation to a greater extent than bone resorption leading to increase in BMD. These medications have been shown to decrease fracture risk in patients who have had fragility fractures and/or osteoporosis by DXA. These drugs may also reduce fractures in patients with low bone mass (osteopenia) without fractures but the evidence is less strong.

Bisphosphonates Bisphosphonates are chemically stable derivatives of inorganic pyrophosphate. They have high affinity for calcium crystals and concentrate selectively in the bone, decreasing bone resorption. Bisphosphonates are preferentially incorporated into sites of active bone remodeling, which commonly occurs in conditions characterized by accelerated skeletal turnover. Bisphosphonates inhibit bone resorption by rapidly inhibiting the activity of osteoclasts. This abrupt reduction in the bone resorption eventually results in concomitant slowing of bone formation. This new steady state is reached 3 to 6 months after the exposure to these medications. Besides decreasing bone turnover, bisphosphonates maintain or improve trabecular and cortical architecture, and increase bone mineralization and BMD.[14,15] Recent studies suggest that bisphosphonates also function to limit osteoblast and osteocyte apoptosis.[16] The net effect of these actions is the decrease of the risk of fractures.

A key feature governing the clinical pharmacology of bisphosphonates is their bioavailability. Their intestinal absorption is poor (1%–5%) and they are rapidly cleared from the circulation. About half of the dose concentrates in the bone, whereas the other half is excreted unmetabolized in the urine. Skeletal uptake primarily depends on renal function, bone turnover, binding site availability, and bisphosphonate affinity for bone matrix.

Early non–nitrogen-containing bisphosphonates (etidronate, clodronate, and tiludronate) are considered first-generation bisphosphonates. They are now rarely used because of low potency and an increased risk of osteomalacia. Second-generation and third-generation bisphosphonates (alendronate, risedronate, ibandronate, pamidronate, and zoledronic acid) have nitrogen-containing R2 side chains. The nitrogen-containing bisphosphonates act primarily by inhibiting the enzyme farnesyl pyrophosphate (FPP) synthase in the mevalonate pathway (cholesterol biosynthetic pathway). Inhibition of FPP synthase disrupts protein prenylation, which creates cytoskeletal abnormalities in the osteoclast and promotes detachment of the osteoclast from the bone perimeter, ultimately leading to osteoclast apoptosis.[16,17]

Alendronate, risedronate, ibandronate, and zoledronic acid have been shown to improve BMD in postmenopausal women with underlying low bone density and to significantly decrease the risk of vertebral fractures. Alendronate, risedronate, and zoledronic acid have been proved to reduce the risk of hip and other nonvertebral fractures.[18–23]

Bisphosphonates are well tolerated when taken as prescribed. Side effects are few and rarely severe. The most common adverse effects include gastrointestinal problems such as esophagitis and esophageal ulcers with the oral preparations, and myalgia and arthralgia with both oral and intravenous (IV) bisphosphonates. Flu-like symptoms (arthralgia, myalgia, fever, headache) occur in about 30% of patients after the first dose of IV zoledronic acid. IV bisphosphonates have been associated with hypocalcemia. Serum calcium and 25-hydroxyvitamin D levels should be checked before initiating treatment. Adequate supplementation with calcium and vitamin D should be provided. Kidney function should be checked before initiating treatment and then periodically because bisphosphonates are generally not recommended for patients with creatinine clearance less than 30 to 35 mL/min. Other potential associations with bisphosphonate use include atrial fibrillation and esophageal cancer; however, a clear casual relationship has not been established.

Low-energy fractures of the femoral shaft (chalk stick fractures) have recently been observed in some patients on long-term bisphosphonate therapy, but the true prevalence is not known.[24] Atraumatic fractures can occur spontaneously in patients with osteoporosis, but there have been speculations that these atypical fractures are caused by skeletal fragility resulting from severely suppressed bone turnover. Patients on long-term alendronate (ie, >3 years) reporting femoral shaft or hip pain should undergo a bone scan or MRI to exclude the presence of an insufficiency fracture, which may be the harbinger for these atypical fractures.

Many articles have been published on the association of bisphosphonate therapy and the occurrence of osteonecrosis of the jaw (ONJ).[25] The incidence of ONJ is extremely low and it occurs primarily in patients with cancer treated with high-dose IV bisphosphonates.

There is currently no consensus on the length of bisphosphonate therapy. In the Fracture Intervention Trial Long-term Extension (FLEX), discontinuation of alendronate after 5 years of therapy resulted in a gradual decline in BMD and increase in biochemical markers of bone turnover, but no significant change in the risk of fracture (except for clinical vertebral fracture) compared with continuous therapy for 3 subsequent years.[26]

Based on data primarily from randomized controlled trials with oral bisphosphonates, Black and colleagues[27] suggested continuing the bisphosphonates beyond 3 to 5 years in patients who continue to have osteoporosis of the femoral neck (T-score ≤ -2.5) after 3 to 5 years of treatment and in patients with an existing vertebral fracture and a femoral neck T-score less than -2. These patients seem to be at the highest risk for vertebral fractures and therefore seem to benefit most from continuation of bisphosphonates. The evidence supporting the benefit of continuing treatment with zoledronic acid beyond 3 years is less conclusive.[28]

There are no data to support the appropriate length of drug holiday and it usually varies between 1 and 5 years. A decrease in BMD and/or increase in markers of bone turnover are indicators that can be used to evaluate the need for restarting treatment.

Estrogen therapy Estrogen therapy is approved by the FDA for the prevention of osteoporosis, and relief of vasomotor symptoms and vulvovaginal atrophy associated with menopause. However, given potential risks (eg, myocardial infarction, stroke, invasive breast cancer, pulmonary emboli, and deep vein thrombophlebitis) associated with hormonal therapy, especially when combined with a progestin, the FDA recommends that approved nonestrogen treatments should first be considered for treatment and prevention of osteoporosis. In the Women's Health Initiative, 5 years of combined estrogen and progestin therapy (Prempro) reduced the risk of clinical vertebral fractures and hip fractures by 34% and other osteoporotic fractures by 23%.[29]

Selective estrogen receptor modulators: raloxifene (brand name Evista) SERMs bind with high affinity to the estrogen receptor and have estrogen agonist and antagonist properties depending on the target organ. The only SERM approved for prevention and treatment of postmenopausal osteoporosis is raloxifene 60 mg orally once daily. Raloxifene has estrogenic activity in bone, thus preventing bone loss, improving BMD, and reducing the risk of fracture. In a 3-year trial, raloxifene reduces the risk of vertebral fractures by about 30% in patients with a prior vertebral fracture and by about 55% in patients without a prior vertebral fracture. Raloxifene does not reduce the risk of nonvertebral fractures.[30] It seems to reduce the risk of estrogen receptor–positive breast cancer, does not stimulate endometrial hyperplasia or vaginal bleeding, but it does increase the risk of venous thromboembolism.

Teriparatide (brand name Forteo) Recombinant human parathyroid hormone (1-34) (teriparatide) is approved for the treatment of postmenopausal osteoporosis in women who are at high risk for fracture. It is an anabolic agent administered by a daily subcutaneous injection at a dose of 20 μg for up to 2 years. In patients with osteoporosis, teriparatide was shown to decrease the risk of vertebral fractures by 65% and nonvertebral fractures by 53% after an average of 18 months of therapy.[31] Myalgias and arthralgias can occur with teriparatide use. Although hypercalciuria is common, it is usually not of concern because of the short duration of use. An exception is patients with calcium oxalate nephrolithiasis, in whom teriparatide should be used cautiously. Increase in serum calcium can occur transiently after the teriparatide injections, but persistent hypercalcemia is uncommon. Occasional hypotension or tachycardia can occur with the first few doses; the drug is therefore administered at bedtime. Because teriparatide increases the incidence of osteosarcoma in rats, patients at risk for osteosarcoma (eg, patients with Paget disease of bone and who have had skeletal radiation exposure) should not receive teriparatide. Bony metastases or history of skeletal malignancy are also considered contraindications for its use. The safety and efficacy of teriparatide have not been shown beyond 2 years of treatment.

Denosumab (brand name Prolia) Denosumab is a fully human monoclonal antibody to the RANKL. It reduces osteoclastogenesis, induces osteoclast apoptosis, decreases bone resorption, increases BMD, and reduces fracture risk. Denosumab is approved by the FDA for the treatment of postmenopausal women with osteoporosis at high risk for fracture or of patients who have failed or are intolerant of other available therapies. It is administered by subcutaneous injection at a dose of 60 mg every 6 months.

In the FREEDOM (Fracture Reduction Evaluation of Denosumab in Osteoporosis Every 6 Months) trial, 7868 postmenopausal women with osteoporosis were randomly assigned to subcutaneous denosumab or placebo for 3 years. Denosumab increases lumbar spine BMD by 9.2% and the total hip BMD by 4.0%. Biochemical markers of bone turnover were significantly reduced in patients taking denosumab. In the same trial, denosumab reduced the risk of vertebral fractures by 68%, the risk of hip fractures by 40%, and the risk of nonvertebral fractures by 20%.[32]

Available evidence suggests that denosumab is tolerated for up to 8 years.[33] Because denosumab is not cleared by the kidneys, it may offer a unique therapeutic option in patients with compromised renal function. Because of marked suppression of bone remodeling, concerns remain about increased risk of osteonecrosis of the jaw, atypical fractures, and delayed fracture healing. The most common adverse effects include musculoskeletal pain and increased risk of infections such as cellulitis and cystitis.

Calcitonin (brand names Miacalcin or Fortical) Salmon calcitonin (intranasal or injectable) is FDA approved for the treatment of osteoporosis in women who are at least 5 years postmenopausal. The intranasal preparation at a dose of 200 IU daily is almost exclusively used in clinical practice. Studies show that calcitonin reduces the risk of vertebral but not nonvertebral fractures.[34–36] It may have an analgesic effect in patients who have acute painful vertebral fractures, thus it could be used in the short term for pain management. Recent concerns have been raised about a possible association between intranasal calcitonin for osteoporosis and an increased overall risk in cancer rates, which may limit its long-term use.

Choice of antiosteoporotic therapy Cost, safety profile, and efficacy should be factored into the therapeutic decision. In patients with osteoporosis of the hip, drugs proved to have effect at this site should be used. Thus ibandronate, raloxifene, and calcitonin should not be used in this circumstance. Also, teriparatide has not been shown to decrease the risk of hip fractures. For most postmenopausal women with osteoporosis, oral bisphosphonates are considered first-line treatment. Intravenous bisphosphonates are alternatives for patients who cannot tolerate oral bisphosphonates because of gastrointestinal side effects. Teriparatide and denosumab are reserved for patients with severe osteoporosis and are not considered first-line medications.

Combination therapy Combination therapy, usually a bisphosphonate with a nonbisphosphonate, is not recommended. It can provide additional small increases in BMD compared with monotherapy; however, the effect on fracture rates is unknown. The added cost and potential side effects, such as oversuppression of bone turnover, should be weighed against potential benefits.

Monitoring response to treatment Several studies have shown poor compliance with osteoporosis medications. One year after initiating treatment of osteoporosis, about 45% patients do not refill the prescriptions. Thus, it is important to ask patients whether they are taking their medications and to encourage compliance with therapy. Sharing the bone density results with patients modestly increases the adherence to therapy.

Central DXA measurement of the spine and hip is the preferred method for serial assessment of the BMD. There is no consensus on the optimal frequency of monitoring and the preferred site to monitor. The NOF recommends that BMD assessments should be repeated every 2 years, but recognizes that testing more frequently may be warranted in certain clinical situations.[7] The frequency of measurements is, in part, determined by the precision of the machine and the anticipated bone loss.

A stable or increasing BMD is an acceptable response to therapy. A decrease in BMD if there is ongoing antiosteoporotic therapy is a cause for concern and should prompt further studies to exclude the presence of factors such as poor compliance, malabsorption, inadequate calcium and vitamin D intake, or diseases that could negatively affect the skeleton.

Measurement of the bone turnover markers may also help in evaluating the efficacy of therapy. A significant decrease in bone turnover with antiresorptive therapy or an increase in bone turnover with anabolic therapy provides evidence of compliance and drug efficacy.

SUMMARY

Osteoporosis is a major public health concern that is underdiagnosed and undertreated. Fragility fractures of the spine and hip can result in chronic pain, depression, disability, and death. Central DXA measurements are the gold standard for assessment of the BMD. Bone loss is an inevitable consequence of the decrease in estrogen levels during menopause, but additional risk factors for bone loss should be identified and treated. Pharmacologic agents in conjunction with a well-balanced diet, exercise, and smoking cessation should be recommended in all patients at high risk of fracture. Close attention should be paid to fall prevention.

REFERENCES

1. Bartl R, Frisch B. Osteoporosis: diagnosis, prevention, therapy. 2nd edition. Springer-Verlag (Berlin); 2009.
2. Khosla S, Atkinson EJ, Melton LJ 3rd, et al. Effects of age and estrogen status on serum parathyroid hormone levels and biochemical markers of bone turnover in women: a population-based study. J Clin Endocrinol Metab 1997;82(5):1522–7.
3. International Society for Clinical Densitometry Official Positions - Adult. 2013. Available at: www.iscd.org/official-positions/2013-iscd-official-positions-adult. Accessed December 9, 2014.
4. Kanis JA, Melton LJ, Christiansen C, et al. The diagnosis of osteoporosis. J Bone Miner Res 1994;9(8):1137–41.
5. Kanis JA, Borgstrom F, De Laet C, et al. Assessment of fracture risk. Osteoporos Int 2005;16(6):581–9.
6. US Preventive Services Task Force. Screening for osteoporosis recommendation statement. 2011. Available at: www.uspreventiveservicestaskforce.org/uspstf10/osteoporosis/osteors.htm. Accessed December 9, 2014.
7. National Ostoporosis Foundation. 2013 Clinician's guide to prevention and treatment of osteoporosis. Available at: http://nof/public/content/resource/913/files/580.pdf. Accessed December 9, 2014.
8. Ross CA, Taylor CL, Yaktine AL, et al. IOM report on calcium and vitamin D. Washington, DC: Institute of Medicine; 2010. Available at: http://www.iom.edu/vitaminD. Accessed December 9, 2014.
9. Wengreen HJ, Munger RG, West NA, et al. Dietary protein intake and risk of osteoporotic hip fracture in elderly residents of Utah. J Bone Miner Res 2004;19(4):537–45.
10. Hannan MT, Tucker KL, Dawson-Hughes B, et al. Effect of dietary protein on bone loss in elderly men and women: the Framingham Osteoporosis Study. J Bone Miner Res 2000;15(12):2504–12.
11. Kerstetter JE, O'Brien KO, Insogna KL. Dietary protein affects intestinal calcium absorption. Am J Clin Nutr 1998;68(4):859–65.
12. Gregg EW, Cauley JA, Seeley DG, et al. Physical activity and osteoporotic fracture risk in older women. Study of Osteoporotic Fractures Research Group. Ann Intern Med 1998;129(2):81–8.
13. Bonaiuti D, Shea B, Iovine R, et al. Exercise for preventing and treating osteoporosis in postmenopausal women. Cochrane Database Syst Rev 2002;(3):CD000333.

14. Rodan GA, Fleisch HA. Bisphosphonates: mechanisms of action. J Clin Invest 1996;97(12):2692–6.

15. Hughes DE, Wright KR, Uy HL, et al. Bisphosphonates promote apoptosis in murine osteoclasts in vitro and in vivo. J Bone Miner Res 1995;10(10):1478–87.

16. Russell RG. Bisphosphonates: mode of action and pharmacology. Pediatrics 2007;119(Suppl 2):S150–62.

17. Drake MT, Clarke BL, Khosla S. Bisphosphonates: mechanism of action and role in clinical practice. Mayo Clin Proc 2008;83(9):1032–45.

18. Black DM, Cummings SR, Karpf DB, et al. Randomised trial of effect of alendronate on risk of fracture in women with existing vertebral fractures. Fracture Intervention Trial Research Group. Lancet 1996;348(9041):1535–41.

19. Cummings SR, Black DM, Thompson DE, et al. Effect of alendronate on risk of fracture in women with low bone density but without vertebral fractures: results from the Fracture Intervention Trial. JAMA 1998;280(24):2077–82.

20. Harris ST, Watts NB, Genant HK, et al. Effects of risedronate treatment on vertebral and nonvertebral fractures in women with postmenopausal osteoporosis: a randomized controlled trial. Vertebral Efficacy With Risedronate Therapy (VERT) Study Group. JAMA 1999;282(14):1344–52.

21. McClung MR, Geusens P, Miller PD, et al. Effect of risedronate on the risk of hip fracture in elderly women. Hip Intervention Program Study Group. N Engl J Med 2001;344(5):333–40.

22. Chesnut IC, Skag A, Christiansen C, et al. Effects of oral ibandronate administered daily or intermittently on fracture risk in postmenopausal osteoporosis. J Bone Miner Res 2004;19(8):1241–9.

23. Black DM, Delmas PD, Eastell R, et al. Once-yearly zoledronic acid for treatment of postmenopausal osteoporosis. N Engl J Med 2007;356(18):1809–22.

24. Gedmintas L, Solomon DH, Kim SC. Bisphosphonates and risk of subtrochanteric, femoral shaft, and atypical femur fracture: a systematic review and meta-analysis. J Bone Miner Res 2013;28(8):1729–37.

25. Khosla S, Burr D, Cauley J, et al. Bisphosphonate-associated osteonecrosis of the jaw: report of a task force of the American Society for Bone and Mineral Research. J Bone Miner Res 2007;22(10):1479–91.

26. Black DM, Schwartz AV, Ensrud KE, et al. Effects of continuing or stopping alendronate after 5 years of treatment: the Fracture Intervention Trial Long-term Extension (FLEX): a randomized trial. JAMA 2006;296(24):2927–38.

27. Black DM, Bauer DC, Schwartz AV, et al. Continuing bisphosphonate treatment for osteoporosis–for whom and for how long? N Engl J Med 2012;366(22):2051–3.

28. Black DM, Reid IR, Boonen S, et al. The effect of 3 versus 6 years of zoledronic acid treatment of osteoporosis: a randomized extension to the HORIZON-Pivotal Fracture Trial (PFT). J Bone Miner Res 2012;27(2):243–54.

29. Rossouw JE, Anderson GL, Prentice RL, et al. Risks and benefits of estrogen plus progestin in healthy postmenopausal women: principal results From the Women's Health Initiative randomized controlled trial. JAMA 2002;288(3):321–33.

30. Ettinger B, Black DM, Mitlak BH, et al. Reduction of vertebral fracture risk in postmenopausal women with osteoporosis treated with raloxifene: results from a 3-year randomized clinical trial. Multiple Outcomes of Raloxifene Evaluation (MORE) Investigators. JAMA 1999;282(7):637–45.

31. Neer RM, Arnaud CD, Zanchetta JR, et al. Effect of parathyroid hormone (1-34) on fractures and bone mineral density in postmenopausal women with osteoporosis. N Engl J Med 2001;344(19):1434–41.

32. Cummings SR, San Martin J, McClung MR, et al. Denosumab for prevention of fractures in postmenopausal women with osteoporosis. N Engl J Med 2009; 361(8):756–65.

33. McClung MR, Lewiecki EM, Geller ML, et al. Effect of denosumab on bone mineral density and biochemical markers of bone turnover: 8-year results of a phase 2 clinical trial. Osteoporos Int 2013;24(1):227–35.

34. Chesnut CH 3rd, Silverman S, Andriano K, et al. A randomized trial of nasal spray salmon calcitonin in postmenopausal women with established osteoporosis: the prevent recurrence of osteoporotic fractures study. PROOF Study Group. Am J Med 2000;109(4):267–76.

35. Overgaard K, Hansen MA, Jensen SB, et al. Effect of salcatonin given intranasally on bone mass and fracture rates in established osteoporosis: a dose-response study. BMJ 1992;305(6853):556–61.

36. Civitelli R, Gonnelli S, Zacchei F, et al. Bone turnover in postmenopausal osteoporosis. Effect of calcitonin treatment. J Clin Invest 1988;82(4):1268–74.

Surgical Menopause

Maria Rodriguez, MD[a], Donna Shoupe, MD, MBA[b],*

KEYWORDS

- Menopause • Oophorectomy • Surgical menopause

KEY POINTS

- Compared with natural menopause, which is a gradual process, surgical menopause entails an abrupt withdrawal of estrogen, progesterone, and androgens.
- The sudden changes in hormones associated with surgical menopause are associated with more severe and prolonged menopausal symptoms.
- Long-term consequences of oophorectomy, particularly when it is performed before age 45 years, include increased risks for emotional, cognitive, and neurologic disease, as well as increased risks for cardiometabolic disorders and bone resorption.
- There is a survival benefit to retention of the ovaries up to age 65 years in women at low risk for ovarian cancer.

INTRODUCTION

Natural menopause is the permanent cessation of menstrual periods that is not brought on by any type of surgical procedure or medical treatment. Natural menopause occurs at a median age of 51 years and is the result of ovarian follicular depletion with concomitant declines in ovarian hormone secretion resulting in very low estrogen levels and high follicle-stimulating hormone concentrations. Undergoing natural menopause before 40 years of age is abnormal and is referred to as primary ovarian insufficiency or premature ovarian failure. Surgical removal of both ovaries before the natural age of menopause is called surgical menopause. Surgical removal of ovaries can be done at the time of hysterectomy or other pelvic surgery. The indications for surgical removal of ovaries can be for either inherent ovarian disorders or done as a preventive (prophylactic) measure. Weighing the risks and benefits for prophylactic oophorectomy and assessing the future risks associated with oophorectomy can now be based on a growing number of scientific studies.

This article reviews the implications and considerations that should be discussed with patients who are considering and/or undergoing surgical menopause, whether

Disclosure: The authors have nothing to disclose.
[a] Department of Obstetrics and Gynecology, Cedars-Sinai Medical Center, 8700 Beverly Boulevard, Suite 2622 South Tower, Los Angeles, CA 90048, USA; [b] Keck School of Medicine of University of Southern California, Los Angeles, CA 90033, USA
* Corresponding author.
E-mail address: donna.shoupe@med.usc.edu

Endocrinol Metab Clin N Am 44 (2015) 531–542
http://dx.doi.org/10.1016/j.ecl.2015.05.003
0889-8529/15/$ – see front matter © 2015 Elsevier Inc. All rights reserved.

it is medically indicated, such as risk-reducing prophylactic surgeries, underlying ovarian disorders, or pelvic adhesions that may preclude ovarian preservation at the time of surgery, or elective (prophylactic) oophorectomy at the time of hysterectomy for benign indications. These considerations include the effects of surgical menopause on menopausal symptoms, vaginal health, the cardiovascular system, the skeletal system and fracture risk, cognition and brain function, sexual function, and mortality.

CURRENT RECOMMENDATIONS IN LOW-RISK PREMENOPAUSAL PATIENTS

Hysterectomy is the second most common major surgical procedure, after cesarean section, performed on reproductive aged women in the United States.[1] Based on a 2005 nationwide study in the United States, unilateral or bilateral oophorectomy at the time of hysterectomy was reported to ensue in 68% of women undergoing abdominal hysterectomy, 60% of women undergoing laparoscopic hysterectomy, and 26% of women undergoing vaginal hysterectomy.[2] A more recent study estimated trends in the performance of oophorectomy using the New York State Department of Health Statewide Planning and Research Cooperative System. From 2001 to 2006 there was an 8% absolute decrease in the performance of oophorec-tomy at the time of benign hysterectomy for women of all ages and a 10.4% decrease in women aged younger than 55 years (for trend, $P<.001$).[3]

Although there are clear indications for oophorectomy in women with gynecologic malignancies, in the setting of benign disease, the indications and guidelines for decision making with regard to ovarian conservation or removal at the time of hyster-ectomy have recently changed, particularly for premenopausal patients. The most recent American College of Obstetrics and Gynecology (ACOG) recommendations are listed in **Table 1**. ACOG recommends that "strong consideration should be made

Table 1 ACOG Practice Bulletin #89 recommendations on elective and risk-reducing salpingo-oophorectomy	
Level A: good evidence	In women aged 50–79 y who have had hysterectomy, use of estrogen therapy has shown no increased risk of breast cancer or heart disease with up to 7.2 y of use
Level B: conflicting data	Bilateral salpingo-oophorectomy should be offered to women with BRCA1 and BRCA2 mutations after childbearing
Level C: consensus and expert opinion	Women with family histories suggestive of BRCA1 and BRCA2 mutations should be referred for genetic counseling and evaluation
	For women with an increased risk of ovarian cancer, risk-reducing salpingo-oophorectomy should include careful inspection of the peritoneal cavity, pelvic washings, removal of the fallopian tubes, and ligation of the ovarian vessels at the pelvic brim
	Strong consideration for retaining ovaries in premenopausal women who are not at increased genetic risk of ovarian cancer
	Given the risk of ovarian cancer in postmenopausal women, ovarian removal at the time of hysterectomy should be considered
	Women with endometriosis, pelvic inflammatory disease, or chronic pelvic pain have a higher risk of reoperation: the risk of subsequent ovarian surgery if the ovaries are retained should be weighed against the benefits of ovarian retention

Adapted from ACOG. ACOG practice bulletin no. 89: elective and risk-reducing salpingo-oophorec-tomy. Obstet Gynecol 2008;111(1):231; with permission.

for retaining normal ovaries in premenopausal women who are not at increased genetic risk of ovarian cancer." There is strong and growing evidence supporting poorer long-term health outcomes for women who undergo oophorectomy, particularly premenopausal women before the age of 50 years.[4]

INDICATIONS FOR OOPHORECTOMY IN HIGH-RISK PATIENTS

Women with gynecologic malignancies or metastatic cancer to the ovary of another primary source, such as gastrointestinal, have clear medical indications to undergo oophorectomy as part of their treatment and staging procedure. Inherited genetic mutations such as germline mutations in one of the breast cancer susceptibility genes (BRCA1 or BRCA2 gene mutations and Lynch syndrome or hereditary nonpolyposis colorectal cancer syndrome) have been identified to place women at increased risk of epithelial ovarian and fallopian tubal cancer. The lifetime risk of ovarian cancer is 39%, 11% to 17%, and 9% to 12% in women with BRCA1, BRCA2, and Lynch syndrome respectively.[5–7] This risk is significantly higher compared with the general population lifetime risk of 1.4%. These inherited syndromes account for approximately 15% of cases of epithelial ovarian and fallopian tube cancer.[5] Considering this dramatic increase in their risk of cancer, risk-reducing bilateral salpingectomy or salpingo-oophorectomy is recommended for women who carry these mutations, generally following their final childbirth.

Other indications for oophorectomy include benign ovarian neoplasms in cases in which lesser interventions, such as cystectomy, enucleation, or partial oophorectomy, is not technically possible. Oophorectomy is also performed on tubo-ovarian abscesses unresponsive to antibiotics, adnexal torsions with necrosis, or as definitive surgery for endometriosis to reduce the risk of reoperation for endometriosis.[8] In these scenarios the decision to proceed with oophorectomy should be made on a case-by-case basis and should always consider long-term health implications.

Procedures that remove or interrupt the fallopian tubes are alternatives to bilateral oophorectomy and are associated with reduced risk for ovarian cancer. Hysterectomy alone reduces the risk of ovarian cancer by 34%[8] and tubal ligation reduces the risk by a similar amount (34%).[9] Unilateral oophorectomy has had conflicting results in significantly reducing ovarian cancer risk.[10,11] Risk-reducing bilateral salpingectomy alone without oophorectomy at the time of hysterectomy/pelvic surgery is now standard of care in many locations.[12–14]

HORMONAL DIFFERENCES BETWEEN NATURAL MENOPAUSE AND SURGICAL MENOPAUSE

There are 2 important hormonal differences between surgical and natural menopause. Surgical menopause results in a sudden rather than gradual reduction in ovarian sex steroid production. Most importantly, surgical removal of the ovary also results in a complete absence of any steroid production compared with the intact postmenopausal ovary, which often retains a more limited production, particularly of testosterone.

Associated with the natural menopause is a transitional period known as the perimenopause. Changes in ovarian protein and steroid hormone production can often be detected 10 years before the final menstrual period.[15–17] This early stage of the perimenopause is marked by changes in menstrual flow and length of the cycle. The late stage of the perimenopause, which begins approximately 4 years before the final menstrual period, encompasses irregular menstrual cycles, declines in estradiol and testosterone, and often menopausal symptoms. The most common menopausal symptom, the hot flash, is reported by approximately 80% of perimenopausal and early postmenopausal women. Other symptoms include sleep and mood disturbances and vaginal dryness.[18] Laboratory abnormalities noticed with menopause include changes in lipid profiles as well as bone density.[19,20]

The cessation of menses in natural menopause is a result of ovarian follicular depletion and dramatic decreases in ovarian estradiol production. Serum androgen levels decline steeply in the early reproductive years but do not vary as a consequence of natural menopause and, for many postmenopausal women, the ovary seems to continue to be an ongoing site of testosterone production.[21–26] Importantly, testosterone stimulates bone and muscle formation and even small amounts of circulating testosterone seem to have a beneficial protective effect on bone loss and fracture risk.[27–32]

ADVERSE CONSEQUENCES OF SURGICAL MENOPAUSE
Menopausal Symptoms

In contrast with the normal menopausal transition associated with a natural menopause, surgical menopause is associated with an abrupt onset of symptoms. During the natural transition, there is a gradual decline in mean estradiol and, in some studies, mean testosterone, during the 40s and early 50s.[21–26] Although estradiol is eventually reduced to very low and often nondetectable levels, testosterone is only reduced by about 50% to 60%, ensuring that a cushion of androgen is available during the transition and throughout menopause. The sudden and complete loss of all ovarian steroids often results in the immediate postoperative appearance of hot flashes, which are often more severe than in women with natural menopause.[33] Many of the other menopausal symptoms appear earlier and are often more severe. These symptoms include vulvovaginal atrophy, mood changes, sleep disturbance, headaches, joint pain, dyspareunia, sexual problems, decreased libido, and decreased overall quality of life.[34–38] Use of hormone replacement may not entirely mitigate these symptoms.[39]

Cardiovascular Disease

Cardiovascular disease (CVD) continues to be the leading cause of mortality in women, specifically in those older than 65 years of age, accounting for more deaths in postmenopausal woman than cancer, chronic lower respiratory disease, and Alzheimer disease combined.[39–42] CVD, mainly coronary heart disease, is unusual in premenopausal women without other risk factors. Along with other risk factors that increase around the time of menopause, the decline in the natural hormone estrogen is associated with increased risk of heart disease.[43–45] Early menopause and surgical menopause are associated with increased risk of CVD.[45–55] Years since natural or surgical menopause has been directly related to thickness of plaque accumulation in carotid arteries.[56] Prior oophorectomy status is associated with increased lipid, lipoprotein, glucose, and insulin levels compared with women with hysterectomy alone,[48,57–60] and close monitoring of lipids following surgical menopause is recommended.[57]

There are large observational studies as well as a meta-analysis supporting the association between increased risk of CVD and premenopausal oophorectomy. Based on a meta-analysis of 18 studies, women who undergo surgical menopause are significantly more likely to develop CVD (relative risk [RR], 2.62; 95% confidence interval [CI], 2.05–3.35) compared with premenopausal age-matched women.[54] The Nurses Health Study reported that women who underwent bilateral oophorectomy without hormone therapy had an increased relative risk of fatal myocardial infarction (RR, 2.2; CI, 1.2–4.2)[49]; women with oophorectomy who had taken hormone therapy had no increased risk.

Although most studies report increased CVD risk in women following surgical menopause, there are several studies that refute these findings. Some make the mistake of adjusting the current rates of CVD events to current lipids or other CVD risk factors. Oophorectomy adversely affects these values and in part is responsible for the increased risk.[48,57–59,182] In the observational trial of the Women's Health Initiative, the investigators report that baseline CVD risk factors are worse in patients who had undergone prior hysterectomy/oophorectomy, and it is these risk factors, and not the oophorectomy, that are responsible for future CVD events. The obvious rebuttal to the conclusions of these articles is that the higher rate of myocardial infarction (MI), coronary artery bypass grafting/PTCA, stroke, angina, deep vein thrombosis, and congestive heart failure drawn at baseline for their study (but not at baseline before the hysterectomy/oophorectomy), as well as higher waist circumference, body mass index, blood pressure, and cholesterol in the participants with prior hysterectomy or oophorectomy, is solid evidence of an adverse CVD effect of the hysterectomy/oophorectomy that was done years before. An adverse effect of prior hysterectomy/oophorectomy is already present at baseline and this adverse effect persists throughout the trial.

Bone Loss, Osteoporosis, and Fracture Risk

The loss of sex steroids during the perimenopausal and menopausal periods results in accelerated bone loss. The earlier this loss occurs, the earlier the loss of bone and the lower the bone density later in life.[61] Bone loss has been reported to be as high as 20% during the 18 months following removal of both ovaries.[62] Oophorectomy before age 45 years has long been established as a risk factor for osteoporosis.[63] However, women undergoing bilateral oophorectomy even during menopausal years have an increased risk compared with women with intact ovaries.[62,64,65]

Overall, there is a growing body of evidence that bilateral oophorectomy, particularly before the natural menopause, is associated with greater bone loss and higher rates of osteoporosis and bone fractures.[52,66–72]

Cognition and central nervous system disease

Although the evidence for the effect of menopause on cognition has been conflicting, the data suggest an age-dependent neuroprotective effect of estrogen.[73] For women undergoing surgical menopause before the age of natural menopause, it seems that use of estrogen replacement up until the age of natural menopause may be particularly important. Many excellent studies have come from the Mayo Clinic Cohort of Oophorectomy and Aging. This group followed a large cohort of women for more than 25 years. The risk of cognitive impairment or dementia was increased in women who underwent oophorectomy before menopause compared with women who did not (HR, 1.46; 95% CI, 1.13–1.90). The largest increase was in women who underwent bilateral salpingo-oophorectomy (BSO) before 49 years of age and who were not treated with estrogen until at least 50 years of age (HR, 1.89; 95% CI, 1.27–2.83).[74]

In the Rancho Bernardo Study, older postmenopausal women, with a mean age of 74 years, were evaluated with memory testing. The women with prior bilateral oophorectomy performed significantly worse.[75] Although there was no significant difference in cognitive scores, women who had undergone hysterectomy were more likely to be using hormones at the time of cognitive testing than women who were naturally menopausal. In a similar British study, the lowest reading ability scores were in women who had hysterectomy or bilateral oophorectomy and were not taking estrogen therapy.[76]

Many other trials also support that the age at the time of surgical or natural menopause plays a critical factor in brain health and cognitive function.[77–81] Premature menopause, often defined as menopause at less than 40 years of age, has been associated with a decline of global cognition.[79] A significant decrease in global cognition has been related to younger age at bilateral oophorectomy in several large-scale studies.[80,81] One report found a significant increase in Alzheimer disease and neuritic plaques in women who had undergone surgical versus natural menopause. This association was not noted in women with natural menopause.[81] Use of estrogen or androgen therapy is reported to play a beneficial role in ameliorating these declines.[73,82,83]

The Mayo Clinic Cohort Study of Oophorectomy and Aging also reported on Parkinson disease with type of menopause and estrogen therapy.[84,85] Women with a history of hysterectomy without oophorectomy were at significantly increased risk of Parkinson disease (odds ratio [OR], 3.36; 95% CI, 1.05–10.77; $P = .04$) as well as women with menopause before age 47 years (OR, 2.18; 95% CI, 0.88–5.39; $P = .09$). For women who underwent bilateral oophorectomy before the onset of menopause, there was also an increased risk of parkinsonism (HR, 1.80; CI, 1.00–3.26; $P = .05$), and the risk increased with younger age at oophorectomy.[86]

Sexual function

As discussed earlier, surgical menopause results in an abrupt and complete loss of ovarian steroid production, resulting in significant decrease in estrogen, testosterone, and androstenedione. Within 1 to 2 years of surgery, the low levels of estrogen can precipitate vaginal atrophy and dryness, causing dyspareunia and making sexual function bothersome and less frequent.[27,87] By 5 years after premenopausal oophorectomy in BRCA mutation carriers, 54% of patients reported that sexual functioning was compromised.[38] In 2 cross-sectional studies, sexual function in women who had elected to have prophylactic salpingo-oophorectomy was compared with that of women who had chosen screening. Women who had surgery reported more vaginal dryness and dyspareunia and less pleasure and satisfaction during sexual activity.[34,39] Those women who had surgery and took hormone therapy experienced significantly less severe symptoms, but hormone replacement therapy (HRT) did not entirely mitigate vaginal dryness, pain with intercourse, and loss of interest in sex.[39]

Changes in the other ovarian steroids are also thought to play a role in sexual dysfunction. Circulating levels of testosterone and androstenedione are linked to direct positive impacts on libido.[88] The removal of the premenopausal ovary and the sudden and significant reductions in testosterone and androstenedione are thought to have a negative impact on sexual desire. During subsequent years, women with surgical menopause continue to have lower levels of testosterone than those with intact ovaries,[21–26,89] and continued impact on sexual function is also suspect.

In another study in high-risk women carrying mutations in the BRCA1 and BRCA2 genes who were undergoing prophylactic salpingo-oophorectomy, women who were premenopausal at the time of surgery experienced a decline in sexual functioning, including pleasure, desire, discomfort, and habit. Although these declines were mitigated by HRT, the symptoms did not return to presurgical levels.[37] A similar study in normal-risk women who underwent either vaginal or abdominal hysterectomy with BSO also reported significant unfavorable effects on sexual function that could not be reversed with estrogen replacement.[90] In a cross-sectional study of 2467 Europeans, a greater proportion of surgically menopausal women were reported to have low sexual desire compared with premenopausal or naturally menopausal women (OR, 1.4; CI, 1.1–1.9; $P = .02$).[91,92]

All-cause mortality

The link between premenopausal oophorectomy and increases in mortality has been one of the most important factors leading to reevaluation of the recommendations regarding the practice of prophylactic bilateral oophorectomy. Although an appreciation for the role of oophorectomy in reducing ovarian and, in some cases, breast cancer rates had been a driving force in favor of removal for many years, the more recent appreciation of serious life-threatening risks associated with premenopausal oophorectomy has led to a more balanced risk-benefit approach. For women with average risk of ovarian cancer, their benefit from prophylactic removal of both ovaries in the premenopausal years is low and generally overshadowed by increases in CVD and other serious diseases.

Theoretic concerns about increased mortality risk with oophorectomy have been verified by the Mayo Clinic Cohort Study of Oophorectomy and Aging and others. This study reported mortalities in women in their cohort who underwent prophylactic bilateral oophorectomy before age 45 years compared with referent women. Oophorectomized women had a significantly increased risk of mortality (HR, 1.67; CI, 1.16–2.40).[93] The increased mortality was primarily seen in those women who did not take estrogen up to the age of 45 years (HR, 1.25; CI, 1.25–2.98). These results are consistent with other studies showing that women with early natural menopause have an increased overall mortality.[94–99]

SUMMARY

There is a growing body of evidence that the loss of ovarian function before the time of natural menopause is associated with a host of negative consequences. Although estrogen treatment may ameliorate some of these consequences, surgical menopause is associated with increased risks of premature death, CVD, bone loss and osteoporosis, cognitive impairment or dementia, parkinsonism, sexual dysfunction, and increases in menopausal symptoms. When considering bilateral oophorectomy, these potential negative effects should be carefully weighed against potential benefits. Appropriate counseling and follow-up testing should also include attention to these issues.

REFERENCES

1. Centers for Disease Control and Prevention CDC 24/7: Saving lives. Protecting people. Available at: www.cdc.gov/reproductivehealth/data_stats/.
2. Jacoby VL, Vittinghoff WE, Nakagawa S, et al. Factors associated with undergoing bilateral salpingo-oophorectomy at the time of hysterectomy for benign conditions. Obstet Gynecol 2009;114(3):696–7.
3. Novetsky AP, Boyd LR, Curtin JP. Trends in bilateral oophorectomy at the time of hysterectomy for benign disease. Obstet Gynecol 2011;118(6):1280–6.
4. ACOG. ACOG practice bulletin no. 89. Elective and risk-reducing salpingo-oophorectomy. Obstet Gynecol 2008;111(1):231 [reaffirmed: 2014].
5. Antoniou A, Pharoah PD, Narod S, et al. Average risks of breast and ovarian cancer associated with BRCA1 or BRCA2 mutations detected in case series unselected for family history: a combined analysis of 22 studies. Am J Hum Genet 2003;72(5):1117–30.
6. Chen S, Parmigiani G. Meta-analysis of BRCA1 and BRCA2 penetrance. J Clin Oncol 2007;25(11):1329–33.
7. Cancer.Net. American Society of Clinical Oncology. Available at: www.cancer.net/cancer-types/lynch-syndrome.

8. Whittemore AS, Harris R, Itnyre J. Characteristics relating to ovarian cancer risk: collaborative analysis of 12 US case-control studies. II. Invasive epithelial ovarian cancers in white women. Collaborative Ovarian Cancer Group. Am J Epidemiol 1992;136:1184.

9. Cibula D, Widschwendter M, Majek O, et al. Tubal ligation and the risk of ovarian cancer: review and meta-analysis. Hum Reprod Update 2011;17:55.

10. Chiaffarino F, Parazzini F, Decarli A, et al. Hysterectomy with or without unilateral oophorectomy and risk of ovarian cancer. Gynecol Oncol 2005;97:318.

11. Beard CM, Hartmann LC, Atkinson EJ, et al. The epidemiology of ovarian cancer: a population-based study in Olmsted County, Minnesota. 1935–1991. Ann Epidemiol 2000;10:14.

12. Morelli M, Venturella R, Mocciaro R, et al. Prophylactic salpingectomy in premenopausal low-risk women for ovarian cancer: Primum non nocere. Gynecol Oncol 2013;129(3):448–51.

13. SGO clinical practice statement: salpingectomy for ovarian cancer prevention. 2013. Available at: https://www.sgo.org/clinical-practice/guidelines/sgo-clinical-practice-statement-salpingectomy-for-ovarian-cancer-prevention.

14. Greene MH, Mai PL, Schwartz PE. Does bilateral salpingectomy with ovarian retention warrant consideration as a temporary bridge to risk-reducing bilateral oophorectomy in BRCA1/2 mutation carriers? Am J Obstet Gynecol 2011;204:19.

15. Randolph JF Jr, Sowers MF, Gold EB, et al. Reproductive hormones in the early menopausal transition: relationship to ethnicity, body size, and menopausal status. J Clin Endocrinol Metab 2002;88(4):3760.

16. Burger H, Dudley EC, Chi J, et al. A prospective longitudinal study of serum testosterone, dehydroepiandrosterone sulfate, and sex hormone-binding globulin levels through the menopause transition. J Clin Endocrinol Metab 2000;85(8):6740.

17. Welt CK, McNichol DJ, Taylor AE, et al. Female reproductive aging is marked by decreased secretion of dimeric inhibin. J Clin Endocrinol Metab 1999;84(1):105–11.

18. Changes in vagina and vulva. Sexual health and menopause online, changes at midlife. Menopause Society. Available at: www.menopause.org/for-women/sexual-health-menopause-online/changes-in-the-vagina-and-vulva.

19. Carr MC, Kim KH, Zambon A, et al. Changes in LDL density across the menopausal transition. J Investig Med 2000;48(4):245–50.

20. Findelstein JS, Brockwell SE, Mehta V, et al. Bone mineral density changes during the menopause transition in a multiethnic cohort of women. J Clin Endocrinol Metab 2008;93(3):861–8.

21. Longcope C, Hunter R, Franz C. Steroid secretion by the postmenopausal ovary. Am J Obstet Gynecol 1980;138(5):564–8.

22. Fogle R, Stanczyk F, Zhang X, et al. Ovarian androgen production in postmenopausal women. J Clin Endocrinol Metab 2007;92:3040–3.

23. Meldrum D, Davidson B, Talaryn I, et al. Changes in circulating steroids with aging in postmenopausal women. Obstet Gynecol 1981;57:624–8.

24. Beavis ELG, Brown JB, Smith MA. Ovarian function after hysterectomy with conservation of the ovaries in premenopausal women. J Obstet Gynaecol Br Commonw 1969;76:969.

25. Davison SL, Bell R, Donath S, et al. Androgen levels in adult females: changes with age, menopause and oophorectomy. J Clin Endocrinol Metab 2005;90(7):3847–53.

26. Lasley BL, Santoro N, Randolf JF, et al. The relationship of circulating dehydroepi-androsterone, testosterone, and estradiol to stages of the menopausal transition and ethnicity. J Clin Endocrinol Metab 2002;87:3760–7.
27. Raisz LG, Wilta B, Artis A, et al. Comparison of the effects of estrogen alone and estrogen plus androgen on biochemical markers of bone formation and resorption in postmenopausal women. J Clin Endocrinol Metab 1996;81(1):37–42.
28. Longcope C, Baker RS, Hui SL, et al. Androgen and estrogen dynamics in women with vertebral crush fractures. Maturitas 1984;6(4):309–18.
29. Davidson BJ, Ross RK, Paganini-Hill A, et al. Total and free estrogens and andro-gens in postmenopausal women with hip fractures. J Clin Endocrinol Metab 1982; 54(1):115–20.
30. Cummings SR, Browner WS, Bauer D, et al. Endogenous hormones and the risk of hip and vertebral fractures among older women. Study of Osteoporotic Frac-tures Research Group. N Engl J Med 1998;339(1):733–8.
31. Ettinger BJ, Pressman A, Sklarin P, et al. Associations between low levels of serum estradiol, bone density and fractures among elderly women: the study of osteoporotic fractures. J Clin Endocrinol Metab 1998;83(7):2239–43.
32. Khosla SJ, Melton LJ 3rd, Atkinson EJ, et al. Relationship of serum sex steroid levels and bone turnover markers with bone mineral density in men and women: a key role for bioavailable estrogen. J Clin Endocrinol Metab 1998;83(7):2236–74.
33. Gallicchio L, Whiteman MK, Tomic D, et al. Type of menopause, patterns of hor-mone therapy use, and hot flashes. Fertil Steril 2006;85(5):1432–40.
34. Madalinska JB, Hollenstein J, Bleiker E, et al. Quality-of-life effects of prophylactic salpingo-oophorectomy versus gynecologic screening among women at increased risk of hereditary ovarian cancer. J Clin Oncol 2005;23(28):6890–8.
35. Fang CY, Cherry C, Devarajan K, et al. A prospective study of quality of life among women undergoing risk-reducing salpingo-oophorectomy versus gyne-cologic screening for ovarian cancer. Gynecol Oncol 2009;112(3):594–600.
36. Bachmann G, Mevadunsky NS. Diagnosis and treatment of atrophic vaginitis. Am Fam Physician 2000;16(10):3090–6.
37. Finch A, Metcalfe KA, Chiang JK, et al. The impact of prophylactic salpingo-oophorectomy on quality of life and psychological distress in women with a BRCA mutation. Gynecol Oncol 2011;121:163.
38. Elit L, Esplen MJ, Butler K, et al. Quality of life and psychosexual adjustment after prophylactic oophorectomy for a family history of ovarian cancer. Fam Cancer 2001;1(3–4):149–56.
39. Madalinska JB, van Beurden M, Bleiker EM, et al. The impact of hormone replacement therapy on menopausal symptoms in younger high-risk women after prophylactic salpingo-oophorectomy. J Clin Oncol 2006;24(22):3576–82.
40. Burge R, Dawon-Hughes B, Solomon DH, et al. Incidence and economic burden of osteoporosis-related fractures in the United States 2005–2015. J Bone Miner Res 2007;22(3):465–75.
41. Jemal A, Siegel R, Ward E, et al. Cancer statistics, 2008. CA Cancer J Clin 2008; 58:71–96.
42. American Heart Association Update. Heart disease and stroke statistics - 2008. Circulation 2008;117:e25–146.
43. Menopause and heart disease. American Heart Association. Life is why. Avail-able at: www.heart.org/HEARTORG/Conditions/More/MyHeartandStrokeNews/Menopause-and-heart-disease_UCM_448432_Article.jsp.
44. Rosano GM, Vitale C, Marazzi G, et al. Menopause and cardiovascular disease: the evidence. Climacteric 2007;10(Suppl 1):19–24.

45. Lobo RA. Surgical menopause and cardiovascular risks. Menopause 2007; 14(3Pt2):562–6.
46. Gordon T, Kannel WB, Hjortland MC, et al. Menopause and coronary heart disease. The Framingham Study. Ann Intern Med 1978;89(2):157–61.
47. Van der Schouw YT, van der Fraff Y, Steyerberg EW, et al. Age at menopause as a risk factor for cardiovascular mortality. Lancet 1996;347(9003):714–8.
48. Kritz-Silverstein D, Barrett-Connor E, Wingard DL. Hysterectomy, oophorectomy, and heart disease risk factors in older women. Am J Public Health 1997;87(4): 678–80.
49. Colditz GA, Willett WC, Stampfer JM, et al. Menopause and the risk of coronary heart disease in women. N Engl J Med 1987;316(18):1105–10.
50. Luoto R, Kaprio J, Reunanen A, et al. Cardiovascular morbidity in relation to ovarian function after hysterectomy. Obstet Gynecol 1995;85(4):515–22.
51. Rivera CM, Grossardt BR, Rhodes DJ, et al. Increased cardiovascular mortality after early bilateral oophorectomy. Menopause 2009;16(1):15–23.
52. Shuster L, Gostout B, Grossardt BR, et al. Prophylactic oophorectomy in premenopausal women and long term health – a review. Menopause Int 2008;14(3): 111–6.
53. De Kleijn MJ, van der Schouw YT, Verbeek AL, et al. Endogenous estrogen exposure and cardiovascular mortality risk in postmenopausal women. Am J Epidemiol 2002;155(4):339–45.
54. Atsma F, Barelelink ML, Grobbee DE, et al. Postmenopausal status and early menopause as independent risk factors for cardiovascular disease: a meta-analysis. Menopause 2006;13:265.
55. Hu FB, Grodstein F, Hennekens CH, et al. Age at natural menopause and risk of cardiovascular disease. Arch Intern Med 1999;159:1061.
56. Mack WJ, Slater CC, Xiang M, et al. Elevated subclinical atherosclerosis associated with oophorectomy related to time since menopause rather than type of menopause. Fertil Steril 2004;82(2):391–7.
57. Yoshida T, Takahashi K, Yamatani H, et al. Impact of surgical menopause on lipid and bone metabolism. Climacteric 2011;14(4):445–52.
58. Matthews KA, Meilahn E, Kuller LH, et al. Menopause and risk factors for coronary heart disease. N Engl J Med 1989;321(10):641–6.
59. Kannel WB, Hjortland MC, McNamara PM, et al. Menopause and risk of cardiovascular disease: the Framingham study. Ann Intern Med 1976;85(4):447–52.
60. Howard BV, Kuller L, Langer R, et al. Risk of cardiovascular disease by hysterectomy status, with and without oophorectomy. The Women's Health Initiative Observational Study. Circulation 2005;111:1462–70.
61. Gallagher JC. Effect of early menopause on bone mineral density and fractures. Menopause 2007;14:567–71.
62. Cann CE, Genant HK, Ettinger B, et al. Spinal mineral loss in oophorectomized women. Determination by quantitative computed tomography. JAMA 1980; 244(18):2056–9.
63. Pansini F, Bagni B, Bonaccorsi G, et al. Oophorectomy and spine bone density: evidence of a higher rate of bone loss in surgical-compared with spontaneous menopause. Menopause 1995;2(2):109–15.
64. Pansini F, Bagni B, Bonaccorsi G, et al. Oophorectomy and spine loss in surgical compared with spontaneous menopause. Menopause 1995;2:109–13.
65. Mucowski SJ, Mack WJ, Shoupe D, et al. The effect of prior oophorectomy on changes in bone mineral density and carotid artery intima-media thickness in postmenopausal women. Fertil Steril 2014;101(4):1117–22.

66. Paganini-Hill A, Ross RK, Gerkins VR, et al. Menopausal estrogen therapy and hip fractures. Ann Intern Med 1981;95(1):28–31.

67. Johansson C, Mellstrom D, Milsom I. Reproductive factors as predictors of bone density and fractures in women at the age of 70. Maturitas 1993;17(1):39–41.

68. Cohen JV, Chiel L, Boghossian L, et al. Non-cancer endpoints in BRCA1/2 carriers after risk-reducing salpingo-oophorectomy. Fam Cancer 2012;11(1):69–75.

69. Aitken JM, Hart DM, Anderson JB, et al. Osteoporosis after oophorectomy for non-malignant disease in premenopausal women. Br Med J 1973;2(5862): 235–328.

70. Tuppjrainen M, Kroger H, Honkanen R, et al. Risks of perimenopausal fractures – a prospective population-based study. Acta Obstet Gynecol Scand 1995;74(8): 624.

71. Challberg J, Ashcroft L, Lalloo F, et al. Menopausal symptoms and bone health in women undertaking risk reducing bilateral salpingo-oophorectomy: significant one health issues in those not taking HRT. Br J Cancer 2011;105(1):22–7.

72. Melton LJ 3rd, Khosta S, Malkasian GD, et al. Fracture risk after bilateral oophorectomy in elderly women. J Bone Miner Res 2003;18:900.

73. Rocca WA, Grossardt BR, Shuster LT. Oophorectomy, menopause, estrogen treatment, and cognitive aging: clinical evidence for a window of opportunity. Brain Res 2011;1379:188–98.

74. Rocca WA, Bower JH, Maraganore DM, et al. Increased risk of cognitive impairment or dementia in women who underwent oophorectomy before menopause. Neurology 2007;69(11):1074–83.

75. Kritz-Silverstein D, Barrett-Connor E. Hysterectomy, oophorectomy, and cognitive function in older women. J Am Geriatr Soc 2002;50:55–61.

76. Kok HS, Kuh D, Cooper R, et al. Cognitive function across the life course and the menopausal transition in a British birth cohort. Menopause 2006;13:19–27.

77. Nappi RE, Sinforiani E, Mauri M, et al. Memory functioning at menopause: impact of age in ovariectomized women. Gynecol Obstet Invest 1999;47:29–36.

78. Farrag AK, Khedr EM, Abdel-Aleem H, et al. Effect of surgical menopause on cognitive functions. Dement Geriatr Cogn Disord 2002;13:193–8.

79. Ryan J, Scali J, Carriere I, et al. Impact of a premature menopause on cognitive function in later life. BJOG 2014;121(13):1729–39.

80. Phung TK, Waltoft BL, Laursen TM, et al. Hysterectomy, oophorectomy, and risk of dementia: a nationwide historical cohort study. Gynecologic disorders. In: Papadakis MA, McPhee SJ, Rabow MW, editors. Current medical diagnosis and treatment. New York: McGraw-Hill; 2015.

81. Bove R, Secor E, Chibnik LB, et al. Age at surgical menopause influences cognitive decline and Alzheimer pathology in older women. Neurology 2014;82(3): 222–9.

82. Phillips SM, Sherwin BB. Effects of estrogen on memory function in surgically menopausal women. Psychoneuroendocrinology 1992;17:485–95.

83. Sherwin BB. Estrogen and/or androgen replacement therapy and cognitive functioning in surgically menopausal women. Psychoneuroendocrinology 1988;13: 345–57.

84. Rocca WA, Shuster LT, Grossardt BR, et al. Long-term effects of bilateral oophorectomy on brain aging: unanswered questions from the Mayo Clinic Cohort Study of Oophorectomy and Aging. Womens Health (Lond Engl) 2009;5(1):39–48.

85. Benedetti MD, Maraganore DM, Bower JH, et al. Hysterectomy, menopause and estrogen use preceding Parkinson's disease: an exploratory case-control study. Mov Disord 2001;16:16830–7.

86. Rocca WA, Bower JH, Maraganore DM, et al. Increased risk of parkinsonism in women who underwent oophorectomy before menopause. Neurology 2008;70: 200–9.
87. Robson M, Hensley M, Barakat R, et al. Quality of life in women at risk for ovarian cancer who have undergone risk-reducing oophorectomy. Gynecol Oncol 2003; 89(2):281–7.
88. Wahlin-Jacobsen S, Pedersen AT, Kristensen E, et al. Is there a correlation between androgens and sexual desire in women? J Sex Med 2015. http://dx.doi.org/10.1111/jsm.12774.
89. Sluijmer AV, Heineman MJ, DeJong FH, et al. Endocrine activity of the postmenopausal ovary: the effects of pituitary down-regulation and oophorectomy. J Clin Endocrinol Metab 1995;80(7):2163–7.
90. Celik H, Gurates B, Yavuz A, et al. The effect of hysterectomy and bilaterally salpingo-oophorectomy on sexual function in postmenopausal women. Maturitas 2009;61(4):358–63.
91. Dennerstein L, Koochaki P, Barton I, et al. Hypoactive sexual desire disorder in menopausal women: a survey of Western European women. J Sex Med 2006; 3(2):212–22.
92. Parker WH, Broder MS, Liu Z, et al. Ovarian conservation at the time of hysterectomy for benign disease. Obstet Gynecol 2005;106:219–26.
93. Rocca WA, Grossardt BR, de Andrade M, et al. Survival patterns after oophorectomy in premenopausal women: a population-based cohort study. Lancet Oncol 2006;7:821–8.
94. Mondul AM, Rodriguez C, Jacobs EJ, et al. Age at natural menopause and cause-specific mortality. Am J Epidemiol 2005;162:1089–97.
95. Ossewaarde ME, Bots ML, Verbeek AL, et al. Age at menopause, cause-specific mortality and total life expectancy. Epidemiology 2005;16:556–62.
96. Jacobsen BK, Heuch I, Kvale G. Age at natural menopause and all-cause mortality: a 37 year follow-up of 19,731 Norwegian women. Am J Epidemiol 2003;157: 923–9.
97. Snowden DA, Kane RI, Beeson WL, et al. Is early natural menopause a biologic marker of health and aging? Am J Public Health 1989;79:709–14.
98. Ciocca DR, Roig LM. Estrogen receptors in human non-target tissues. Biological and clinical implications. Endocr Rev 1995;16(1):32–65.
99. Allison MA, Manson JE, Langer RD, et al. Oophorectomy, hormone therapy, and subclinical coronary artery disease in women with hysterectomy: the Women's Health Initiative coronary artery calcium study. Menopause 2008;15(4 Pt 1): 639–47.

Premature Menopause

Saioa Torrealday, MD[a], Lubna Pal, MBBS, MRCOG, MS[b],*

KEYWORDS

- Premature menopause • Primary ovarian insufficiency • Premature ovarian failure
- Hypergonadotropic hypogonadism • Surgical menopause

KEY POINTS

- Women of reproductive age who experience loss of menstrual regularity for 3 or more consecutive months should have an evaluation for primary ovarian insufficiency (POI) at the time of the first visit.
- Two elevated levels of gonadotropins (>20 IU/L) with low estradiol levels on 2 occasions, at least 4 to 6 weeks apart, are consistent with a diagnosis of POI.
- Because of the potential detrimental long-term health implications of estrogen deprivation, prompt diagnosis and treatment by health care providers is of utmost importance.
- A multidisciplinary team approach is ideal for managing women diagnosed with POI, given the complexity and sensitive nature of the disorder.

INTRODUCTION

Cessation or loss of ovarian function before age 40 years is considered "premature," an age threshold that is 2 standard deviations below the mean estimated age of menopause (50 ± 4 years) seen in the reference population.[1] Premature menopause may be spontaneous or induced, for example, following chemotherapy, radiation, or surgical removal of the gonads.

Spontaneous premature menopause is not uncommon; it is estimated that approximately 0.3% to 1.1% of reproductive-age women experience menopause prematurely.[2] Among women younger than 40, the incidence increases with advancing age; premature menopause may be recognized in 0.01% of women younger than 20, 0.1% of those younger than 30, and approximately 1% of women younger than 40 years.[3] Premature menopause, primary ovarian insufficiency (POI), and premature ovarian failure (POF)

Disclosures: Dr Torrealday: None; Dr Pal: Consultant to Merck Pharmaceutical.
[a] Reproductive Endocrinology & Infertility, Department of Obstetrics & Gynecology, Womack Army Medical Center, 2817 Reilly Road, Fort Bragg, NC 28311, USA; [b] Division of Reproductive Endocrinology and Infertility, Department of Obstetrics, Gynecology and Reproductive Sciences, Yale University School of Medicine, 333 Cedar Street, New Haven, CT 06510, USA
* Corresponding author.
E-mail address: lubna.pal@yale.edu

Endocrinol Metab Clin N Am 44 (2015) 543–557
http://dx.doi.org/10.1016/j.ecl.2015.05.004
0889-8529/15/$ – see front matter © 2015 Elsevier Inc. All rights reserved.

endo.theclinics.com

are terms that are often used interchangeably. Given that premature cessation of ovarian function, either spontaneous or following iatrogenic insult other than castration, may not be "permanent," and keeping in perspective the negative connotation implied by the term "failure," POI has emerged in recent years as the preferred terminology. Spontaneous premature menopause is henceforth referred to as POI.

SYMPTOMS

By definition, cessation of menstrual function for longer than 1 year in an appropriate clinical setting defines menopause; however, shorter durations of amenorrhea are equally meaningful in the context of POI. Although primary amenorrhea may be the presenting symptom in up to 10% of cases, in most cases POI manifests after attainment of normal pubertal development and after the establishment of regular menses.[4] Occasionally, secondary amenorrhea following a pregnancy or cessation of hormonal contraceptive regimen may be the first presenting sign of POI. Persistent elevation in circulating gonadotropins with concomitant hypoestrogenemia is the endocrine hallmark of ovarian failure. Documented elevation in circulating gonadotropins along with low estradiol levels detectable on 2 occasions, at least 4 to 6 weeks apart, is required before labeling a reproductive-age woman with the diagnosis of POI in the context of infrequent or absent menses.[4–7]

Menstrual irregularities may also be accompanied with constant or intermittent hypoestrogenic symptoms that define the menopausal syndrome, such as hot flashes, night sweats, emotional lability, vaginal dryness, or sleep disturbances. Notable, however, is the absence of menopausal symptoms in the setting of primary amenorrhea; namely, these symptoms are uncommon in those who were never exposed to estrogen.[8] Concerns relating to subfertility may be yet another presenting symptom. The clinical presentation of POI can thus vary from woman to woman.

DIAGNOSTIC EVALUATION AND TESTS

A thorough review of the woman's medical history, including family history, may offer critical insights leading to the diagnosis. Of particular relevance are details regarding menstrual history, including age at menarche and pattern of menses. Any prior medication or treatment that may have caused gonadal impairment must be documented. In addition, the history should focus on the presence or absence of nonreproductive endocrinopathies, including hypothyroidism, hypoadrenalism, and hypoparathyroidism. Furthermore, any family history of POI, mental retardation, particularly in male progeny (see fragile X mental retardation 1 [FMR1] in the section Differential Diagnoses), or chromosomal abnormalities should be noted.

Diagnosis of POI is commonly delayed despite a manifest clinical picture, partly because of the relative infrequency of this entity. Furthermore, POI is often misdiagnosed and improperly managed because of lack of familiarity with this disorder by health care providers. Thus, the first challenge is to arrive at the diagnosis in a timely fashion. Definitive diagnostic criteria have not been delineated. The challenge lies in deciding how long to wait before initiating investigations into the loss of menstrual regularity in a young woman. Loss of regular menses for more than 3 consecutive months merits further investigation, and POI should be considered among the differential diagnoses.

Physical Evaluation

Careful attention should be placed on the presence or absence of secondary sex characteristics, particularly in the setting of primary amenorrhea. Although most patients are without obvious physical stigmata, particular focus should be placed on identifying clinical features suggestive of an underlying pathogenic mechanism, for example, characteristics of Turner syndrome (short stature, shield chest, low hairline), ptosis, and features of autoimmunity (thyroid enlargement, skin pigmentation, or vitiligo). The estrogenic state of the external genitalia and presence or absence of genital atrophy should also be recorded during the course of a pelvic examination.

Tests

There are several tests that are warranted in the initial evaluation of a woman who presents with POI symptoms (**Table 1**). Pregnancy must be considered in any reproductive-age woman presenting with amenorrhea and, if applicable, excluded with either a urine or serum human chorionic gonadotropin level. Common endocrinopathies that are associated with menstrual dysfunction, such as hypothyroidism and hyperprolactinemia, should be screened for thorough measurements of thyroid-stimulating hormone (TSH) and prolactin levels. Diagnosis of POI requires evidence of persisting hypergonadotropic hypogonadism, established through assessment of circulating levels of the pituitary gonadotropin, follicle-stimulating hormone (FSH), and serum estradiol (E2). Elevated FSH levels (>20 mIU/mL) concomitant with hypoestrogenism (E2 <30 pg/mL), should be confirmed by documentation of persistent hypergonadotropic hypogonadism on repeat testing in 4 to 6 weeks. Although the progestin-challenge test is commonly used to assess whether the uterus has been adequately exposed to estrogen in the initial evaluation of secondary amenorrhea, results of this study may be misleading. A subset of women with POI will have intermittent resumption of ovarian function resulting in a positive progestin-challenge test,

Table 1
Diagnostic considerations for primary ovarian insufficiency

Test	Rationale
Human chorionic gonadotropin	Exclude pregnancy
Follicle-stimulating hormone Luteinizing hormone Estradiol	Assess hypothalamic pituitary ovarian axis
Anti-Mullerian hormone Inhibin B Antral follicle count	Measure ovarian reserve Assess likelihood for spontaneous resumption of menses/ovarian function
Fasting prolactin	Exclude hyperprolactinemia
Karyotype FMR1 premutation	Assess for genetic etiology
Thyroid-stimulating hormone Antithyroid peroxidase antibodies	Evaluate for thyroid disease
21-Hydroxylase antibody Antiadrenal antibodies Morning cortisol level	Screen for adrenal insufficiency
Calcium Magnesium Phosphorus Parathyroid hormone	Screen for parathyroid disease
Fasting glucose	Screen for diabetes mellitus
25-Hydroxyvitamin D Dual-energy x-ray absorptiometry scan	Assess skeletal health

thus providing a false sense of reassurance and subsequently leading to a delay in the diagnosis.[9,10]

Peptide factors of ovarian origin, such as inhibin B and anti-Mullerian hormone, may be informative in corroborating suspicion of POI; these biomarkers become undetectable in peripheral circulation well before the increase in FSH or onset of amenorrhea occurs.[11,12]

Although not a requisite for diagnosing POI, a transvaginal ultrasonogram may offer clarifying information regarding the number of residual antral follicles ($\leq$10 mm) within the ovaries. A low or absent antral follicle count offers supportive evidence for POI, whereas evidence of residual visible follicles may offer some reassurance regarding the possibility of spontaneous resumption of ovarian function. Furthermore, the presence of small, streak ovaries may suggest Turner syndrome or mosaic karyotypes. Ovarian enlargement caused by lymphocytic oophoritis or a steroidogenic enzyme defect may serve to further guide evaluation and management.

Although chromosomal abnormalities are relatively rare in women with secondary amenorrhea (13%) compared with those presenting with primary amenorrhea (50%), a karyotype should be considered for all women diagnosed with POI.[4,13] Some researchers suggest that karyotypic analyses could be restricted to those with onset of POI at age less than 30 years, whereas others stress that the informative yield is relevant for all diagnosed with POI given the unique health concerns that relate to specific genotypes (eg, risk for aortic dissection in women with Turner syndrome and risk for gonadal malignancy for Y chromosome–bearing gonads). Similarly, testing for fragile X (FMR1) gene mutations should be considered. The FMR1 results will be informative not just regarding the pathophysiology of POI, but will also provide relevance for the immediate family and may affect a couple's decision to seek fertility treatment.[14]

Screening for autoimmune disorders must be considered in the setting of POI. Thyroid disease is by far the most commonly associated autoimmune disorder, and TSH assessment is a pertinent screen for thyroid function. Screening for antithyroid (thyroid peroxidase and antithyroglobulin) antibodies should be considered. Addison disease affects 3% of women diagnosed with POI, and this risk is particularly relevant in those screening positive for antiadrenal (specifically, anti–21-hydroxylase) antibodies. A morning (8 AM) serum cortisol level is a common screening test for adequacy of adrenal function, with further consideration for corticotropin stimulation testing as needed.[15] Type I diabetes mellitus affects approximately 2.5% of women with POI, so assessment of fasting glucose and insulin levels is recommended.[15]

Skeletal fragility is a recognized long-term sequela to POI. Therefore, the earlier in life that POI occurs, the higher the likelihood of presenting with lower bone density in later years. A baseline bone mineral density assessment should be considered once the diagnosis of POI has been established, particularly for those with a family history of skeletal compromise (such as history of osteoporosis or hip fracture) if hormone replacement has not been initiated.[9] Timely initiation of preventive strategies may mitigate the progressive bone loss that follows cessation of ovarian function. Delay in diagnosis and evaluation may thus be contributory to lifetime fracture risk.

DIFFERENTIAL DIAGNOSIS

Female reproductive biology is earmarked for eventual senescence from inception. Women are endowed with their maximum lifetime number of ovarian follicles while still in utero; beyond 20 weeks intrauterine gestation, the process of progressive follicular atresia is evident.[16] At puberty, a time of achieving reproductive competence, only a small subset of follicles remain from the initial cohort, and the processes of progressive atresia and follicular depletion continue until near exhaustion of the ovarian gamete repertoire, a state synonymous with menopause.[6,17] Mechanistically, a truncated reproductive life span may occur secondary to an intrinsically reduced inherited complement of oocytes, an accelerated rate of follicular atresia, or a combination of these processes.

Spontaneous Primary Ovarian Insufficiency

More than 90% of POI cases are idiopathic, with no clear detectable cause; an identifiable contributor, however, may be evident in a subset of women.[8,18] Familiarity with scenarios that predispose one to the risk for POI allows for early detection and timely initiation of interventions that may help mitigate the myriad sequelae of POI (**Box 1**).

X Chromosome Abnormalities

Turner syndrome, the phenotype associated with complete or partial monosomy X in females, is the most common genetic anomaly encountered in women with POI.[8] The pathogenesis of Turner syndrome is complex; however, it is believed that POI results

---

Box 1
Etiology of premature menopause

Spontaneous

Idiopathic (90%)

Genetic

    Turner syndrome (45XO) or mosaic Turner (45X/46XX)

    Trisomy X (47XXX or mosaic)

    Galactosemia (galactose-1-phosphate uridyltransferase deficiency)

    Autoimmune polyglandular syndrome (types 1 and 2)

    Follicle-stimulating hormone receptor mutations

    17α-Hydroxylase deficiency

    Aromatase deficiency

    Blepharophimosis, ptosis, epicanthus inversus syndrome

    Bloom syndrome

    Ataxia telangiectasia

    Fanconi anemia

Autoimmune

Infection

    Mumps oophoritis

    Tuberculosis, malaria, varicella, and shigella

Induced

Chemotherapy

Radiation

Pelvic vessel embolization

Oophorectomy

from mutations on the X chromosome in loci that regulate germ cell development and viability.[19] Although primary amenorrhea is the classic presentation associated with Turner syndrome, a small percentage (3%–5%) of these cases, primarily those with mosaic XX/XO genotype, may exhibit normal secondary sexual development, experience spontaneous menses, and even achieve a pregnancy before the onset of POI.[10] Timely detection of XO/mosaic Turner genotypes is also of vital importance because of the severe comorbidities, primarily aortic dissection, that merit prompt evaluation.[20]

FMR1 premutation carriers are recognized to be at risk for POI. Women with POI should therefore be screened for fragile X premutations to help elucidate a potential contributory mechanism for premature ovarian compromise, and to guide family counseling given potential health implications for both present and future generations. Fragile X syndrome is the most common cause of familial mental retardation; an inherited triplet repeat mutation in the X-linked FMR1 underlies the disorder, although the exact mechanisms whereby FMR1 premutation may disrupt the oocytes repertoire remain elusive.[21] Normal CGG repeats in the untranslated region of the FMR1 gene number less than 40. Repeat lengths between 55 and 200 are termed premutations, whereas more than 200 repeats are considered a full mutation.[21] Only premutation carriers have been found to have an increased risk of POI, whereas full-mutation carriers and their noncarrier siblings seem to have the same risk seen in the general population.[22] Premutations of the FMR1 gene are present in as many as 14% to 20% of women with familial POI and are found in up to 6% of women with isolated POI.[22,23] A family history of fragile X syndrome, unexplained mental retardation, POI, tremor/ataxia syndrome, or a child with developmental delays may be the first suggestion of fragile X premutation carriage as a cause for POI. Although impaired fertility in the setting of POI is real, the ovarian compromise may not be absolute in a subset; spontaneous ovulation and even pregnancy are described in almost 10% of women with POI.[8] This latter probability is of particular relevance for FMR1 premutation carriers given that spontaneous expansion of the triple repeat number can occur in the offspring, thus increasing the likelihood of fragile X syndrome in those inheriting the full mutation. Genetic counseling is recommended for women with POI who are identified as FMR1 premutation carriers.

Uncommon Genetic Disorders Associated with Primary Ovarian Insufficiency

Y chromosome–related gonadal dysgenesis is a relatively uncommon genetic variation encountered in young women presenting with primary amenorrhea and features of POI.[8] Given that Y chromosome bearing dysgenetic gonads are associated with a substantial risk for future neoplasms with malignant potential (eg, germ cell tumor such as gonadoblastoma, dysgerminoma, yolk sac tumor, or choriocarcinoma), bilateral gonadectomy should be offered without delay following establishment of the diagnosis.

Galactosemia, an autosomal recessive genetic disorder, results from mutations in galactose 1-phosphate uridyl transferase (GALT), the enzyme that converts galactose to glucose.[21,24] Classic homozygous mutations have no GALT enzyme activity; failure to metabolize galactose to glucose results in intracellular accumulation of toxic galactose metabolites with ensuing cell damage.[21,25,26] Clinically these patients present with symptoms of mental retardation, liver failure, and renal insufficiency.[6] Ovarian damage has been attributed to the toxic accumulation of galactose, or one of its metabolites, on follicular structures during early fetal life.[26] Thus, women affected with GALT will often develop POI early in life and commonly present with primary amenorrhea.

Blepharophimosis, ptosis, epicanthus inversus syndrome (BPES) is a rare autosomal dominant disorder characterized by a typical phenotype (small palpebral fissures, ptosis, and epicanthus inversus).[21] Two forms of BPES exist. In type I, infertility in the form of ovarian failure is an adjunct to the condition and is sex-linked (only females affected), whereas in type II, only facial abnormalities are present.[21] A mutation in FOXL2, a gene found in the eyelids and in granulosa cells, is of pathophysiologic relevance.[6] In animal studies, BPES results in an arrest in granulosa cell differentiation, early activation of primordial follicles, and subsequent oocyte apoptosis.[27]

FSH receptor mutations are inherited in an autosomal recessive pattern and have also been described in association with POI.[6]

Autoimmunity

In excess of 20% of women with POI manifest features of an autoimmune disease, which may commence before the ovarian dysfunction becomes apparent.[28] Circulating antiovarian antibodies are commonly detected in this group, with different studies reporting detection rates ranging from 10% to 69% in women with POI. Despite this association, testing for antiovarian antibodies is of poor prognostic relevance and is seldom undertaken in the setting of POI.[29,30] In addition, the assays and interpretation of antiovarian antibodies are highly variable. Therefore, testing for antiovarian antibodies is not recommended.

Autoimmune thyroiditis and hypothyroidism may be seen in almost one-fourth of women with POI.[15] Family and personal histories of thyroid disease should be cues to pursue directed testing in the setting of clinical suspicion for POI.

Autoimmune adrenalitis is possibly the most clinically meaningful autoimmune disorder cosegregating with POI, as resulting adrenal insufficiency can be life threatening. Indeed, compromised adrenal function may be evident in up to 3% of women with POI.[8,15]

Type 1 diabetes mellitus and hypoparathyroidism may be seen in approximately 2.5% of cases of POI.[7,15] Other associated autoimmune disorders include myasthenia gravis, Crohn disease, vitiligo, and pernicious anemia.

Autoimmune polyglandular syndrome (APS) types 1 and 2 are autosomal recessive disorders associated with POI. Commonly presenting in childhood or early adolescence, APS type 1 is characterized by hypoparathyroidism, Addison disease, and mucocutaneous candidiasis.[8] APS type 2, also known as Schmidt syndrome, is more common than type 1 and typically presents in the third and fourth decade of life. APS type 2 consists of Addison disease and either insulin-dependent diabetes mellitus or thyroid autoimmune disease.[8] POI in the form of primary amenorrhea may be seen in 60% of patients with APS type 1, whereas occurrence of POI in patients with APS type 2 is variable.[7,29] It is estimated that 10% of patients with Addison disease develop POI between 5 and 14 years before the onset of adrenal dysfunction.[6,31]

Autoimmune lymphocytic oophoritis is an uncommon cause of POI attributable to steroidogenic cell autoimmunity. The oophoritis is characterized primarily by an infiltrate of macrophages, natural killer cells, T lymphocytes, plasma cells, and B lymphocytes within the ovaries.[32] This condition is often associated with adrenal insufficiency; testing for adrenal antibodies using an indirect immunofluorescence assay can identify the 4% of women with spontaneous POI who have steroidogenic cell autoimmunity.[33] Vigilant monitoring for symptoms and signs of adrenal insufficiency is warranted in women with POI testing positive for antiadrenal antibodies, given the potentially life-threatening hazard of this entity.

Infection

Infections have been implicated to cause POI, although a direct cause-and-effect relationship has not been clearly established to explain the association. Infections that have been associated with POI include mumps oophoritis, tuberculosis, malaria, varicella, and shigella.[11,34] Complete remission and return of normal ovarian function ensues in most women following the infectious insult. An infectious cause of POI should be a consideration on an individual case basis, based on the patient's presentation and associated risk factors (eg, travel, exposure, immunization).

Iatrogenic

Surgical premature menopause

Approximately 1 in 9 women aged 35 to 45 years has undergone a hysterectomy, with 40% of them undergoing bilateral oophorectomy at the time of surgery.[35,36] Surgical menopause is distinct from its natural counterpart, as much in its abruptness as in the severity of associated symptomatology. A precipitous drop in serum levels of ovarian sex steroids following gonadal extirpation underlies the severity of symptoms following surgical gonadal loss. Beyond the burden of menopausal symptoms, surgical menopause is linked with serious long-term health consequences including all-cause premature death, cardiovascular disease, cognitive deterioration, and osteoporosis.[36] Adverse outcomes can be prevented or improved with initiation of estrogen therapy; however, not all of the long-term risks of surgical menopause may be eliminated. The decision to perform oophorectomy for benign disease in premenopausal years should thus not be taken lightly.

Chemotherapy and radiation

Chemotherapy and pelvic radiation are well-recognized culprits of ovarian dysfunction. Due to a combination of advancements in diagnostic and screening techniques allowing cancer detection at earlier stages, and increasingly effective treatment options, there has been a significant improvement in overall survival rates among reproductive age women diagnosed with cancer. Consequently, more women with a previous cancer diagnosis are now dealing with the repercussion of their gonadotoxic treatments as they advance in age. Premature menopause is commonly encountered in cancer survivors with concerns and sequelae that are distinct from those recognized with spontaneous POI. The gonadotoxic effects of chemotherapy and radiotherapy vary according to the dose, duration, agent administered, and age of the patient at the time of treatment.[11] Anthracyclines and alkylating agents, which are the backbone of many cancer therapies, are particularly toxic to the ovaries, although the detrimental effects of combination chemotherapies can also be significant.[10] Younger patients are more resistant to the oophorotoxic effects of these treatments, although inevitably even the gonads of young patients take a detrimental hit.[6] Direct radiation to the pelvis for treatment accelerates atresia in ovarian follicles. Despite pelvic shielding, it remains difficult to protect ovarian function, which is highly sensitive to radiation. Surgical transposition of the ovaries outside the pelvis, well away from the radiation field, is effective at minimizing radiation exposure.[10] Following cancer therapy, ovarian failure may be relatively immediate or may follow a more insidious course. The effect may also be transient, with unpredictably spontaneous recovery occurring after months to years.

TREATMENT

Hypoestrogenemia of POI is not only premature but, in many circumstances, fairly abrupt. Menopausal symptoms such as hot flashes, night sweats, and dyspareunia relating to vaginal atrophy are commonly encountered in women with POI, and may be of profound severity, particularly when POI sets in suddenly. Despite a hesitation to use hormone replacement on the part of patients and physicians alike in the post-Women's Health Initiative era, estrogen therapy remains the most efficacious, and safe, approach for symptom control in this young cohort. Early initiation of estrogen therapy in chronologically young women with POI not only offers symptom control and improved quality of life, but additionally offers benefit against chronic health concerns that this otherwise prematurely hypoestrogenic population is at risk for developing (eg, skeletal fragility and, possibly, cardiovascular disease).[11]

An absence of evidence-based guidelines regarding the ideal hormone replacement strategy for young women with POI poses a clear management challenge. Symptomatic control in this young population may require the use of relatively higher doses of estrogen to achieve symptom benefit in comparison with the older and naturally menopausal populations. Clinicians can choose from several available therapeutic options for systemic estrogen replacement including oral, transdermal (topical gels, sprays, patches), and vaginal formulations. Transdermal estradiol in a daily dose of 100 µg, oral estradiol in a dose of 1 to 2 mg/d, or conjugated estrogen at a dose of 0.625–1.25 mg daily are commonly used in symptom management for women with POI.[8,37]

Dose equivalents for common estrogen formulations are as follows: 1 mg micronized 17β-estradiol = 50 µg/d transdermal 17β-estradiol = 0.625 mg conjugated equine estrogens.[38,39]

Consideration should be made for adding progesterone to estrogen therapy in all women with a uterus to minimize untoward risk of endometrial disorder that is well recognized with the use of unopposed estrogen (eg, endometrial hyperplasia or adenocarcinoma). Both natural progesterone and synthetic progestins are available in an array of formulations (oral tablets, vaginal creams and pessaries, intramuscular and subcutaneous injection, and intrauterine devices) and regimens (continuous, sequential, cyclic). Oral or vaginal micronized progesterone 100 mg daily or 200 mg daily for 10–12 days each month, or medroxyprogesterone acetate 10 mg daily for 10 days each month, are commonly prescribed progesterone regimens for estrogen users.[4] The cyclic hormone regimen is likely to induce regular withdrawal bleeding, a phenomenon that may assure the young woman with a sense of normalcy in comparison with her peers. Alternatively, the levonorgestrel-releasing intrauterine device can be used for endometrial protection with the added benefit of being a contraceptive method. Newer progesterone therapies such as progesterone vaginal gel (Crinone 4%) or tablet (Endometrin 100 mg) have not been studied for use in POI patients. However, extrapolating data from postmenopausal studies, both progesterone gel (cyclically or twice weekly) and progesterone capsules (every other day) were protective against endometrial hyperplasia. Therefore, it is likely that these modalities may also be used in POI patients.

Combined hormonal contraceptive options (pills, vaginal ring or patch) offer an alternative and, in many cases, a psychologically preferable management option for symptom control in young women diagnosed with POI. With periodic surveillance and reassessments, hormone use may be safely continued in this group until the woman reaches approximately 50 years of age, or the average age of menopause, at which time reassessment should be offered and a decision on whether to continue with the hormone regimen should be individualized.

Whereas the efficacy of nonhormonal treatment options, such as serotonin and norepinephrine reuptake inhibitors and GABAergic agents, against menopausal symptoms is well described in populations of women undergoing iatrogenic premature menopause, such as in survivors of breast cancer, effective use of these alternative agents for women with POI remains essentially unexplored.

ADDITIONAL MANAGEMENT CONSIDERATIONS

The sensitive nature of the diagnosis warrants careful attention to the setting and word selection used when the patient is informed of the diagnosis. As a strategy to help mitigate the patient from feeling overwhelmed, a newly diagnosed patient may benefit from the breadth of implications being addressed at a subsequent visit. A potential for spontaneous remission must additionally be underscored, particularly in young women. The formation of a multidisciplinary team to address both the emotional and physical needs of a patient is often crucial given the complexity of the diagnosis.[39] A multidisciplinary approach is ideal, with professionals from various disciplines and specialties participating to address the myriad requisites of the affected population (psychological support, fertility management, evaluation and management of coexisting endocrinopathies, prevention and management of chronic health sequelae). Individualized needs of the afflicted family may additionally merit attention and should not be discounted.[40]

Psychological Well-Being

Rapid and unanticipated truncation in the reproductive life span, symptoms of hypoestrogenism, fear of aging, and the realization of her fertility prognosis underlie, to varying degrees, the psychological havoc that is well described in women diagnosed with POI. The condition has been associated with higher than average levels of depression, anxiety, and psychological distress.[41] Many women experience severe emotional anguish and desire guidance on how to cope with the emotional sequelae; few, however seek help, an aspect that underscores a need for heightened sensitivity among physicians. Loss of reproductive capability is a major upsetting element, regardless of the patient's parity status. Frequent follow-up visits are recommended to allow assessment of how the individual is coping and to address unmet needs. Professional counseling and support groups should be advocated, and made accessible, for any woman stepping into menopause prematurely.

Reproductive Concerns

While fertility is compromised, infertility in the setting of POI may not be absolute. Resumption of ovarian activity, although it may only be intermittent, occurs in approximately 50% of these women.[9] Up to 25% of women with POI may spontaneously ovulate, and 5% to 10% will conceive and deliver.[4,9,42] Women for whom fertility is a priority should seek medical assistance from a reproductive endocrinologist. Assisted conception by in vitro fertilization (IVF) using donor gametes or embryos, or adoption, may be an alternative for patients who elect to pursue parenthood. Of relevance is the choice of egg donor, as sisters of women with POI may not be the ideal egg donors given the familial risk for ovarian compromise. Pregnancy in women with XO or mosaic XX/XO karyotype holds unique risks, and may be particularly hazardous given the risk for common cardiac abnormalities seen in this population. There is particular concern for structural abnormalities of the aortic root, which may rupture during pregnancy. These patients need a baseline echocardiogram with repeat imaging every 5 years.[19]

The commonly encountered endocrinopathies associated with POI, such as thyroid disorders, adrenal insufficiency and diabetes mellitus, require close surveillance and management during pregnancy and the postpartum period. Consultation with a perinatologist may be of value in women with POI and underlying comorbidities from complications that may arise during pregnancy. Those screening positive for FMR1 premutation are at risk for conceiving a male infant with fragile X mental retardation; preconception genetic counseling is therefore suggested. Use of IVF with preimplantation genetic diagnosis may be an option for families at risk of passing known genetic mutations, although the success of IVF with the patient's own eggs in the setting of POI remains poor.[43] Recently, short-term treatment with dehydroepiandrosterone, an adrenal steroid available as an oral supplement, has been suggested to offer some hope in improving the biology of any residual gametes in the ovaries of young women diagnosed with POI.[44–46]

Despite the recognized reproductive compromise, women diagnosed with POI remain at risk for unplanned conception, given that spontaneous resumption of follicular activity is not uncommon. Contraceptive strategies are thus recommended for those wishing to avoid pregnancy. Anecdotal failures are reported in users of combined oral contraceptive pills (OCP); although the exact mechanism is unknown, the elevated gonadotropin levels seen in POI may not be completely suppressed by the hormone content in the relatively low-dose OCP, resulting in occasional ovulation. Barrier contraceptives and intrauterine contraceptive devices offer the most reliable alternatives.

Sexuality: Role for Androgen Therapy?

The adrenal glands and ovaries represent the main source of circulating androgens in women. Women with POI have significantly lower levels of free and total testosterone than regular menstruating women of similar age; this phenomenon is even more apparent following surgical menopause.[4,42,47,48] Improved sexual function and overall sense of well-being are described with the addition of androgen to estrogen-based hormonal regimens.[49] Although data are limited, androgen replacement may be of consideration in the certain women who remain symptomatic despite use of estrogen-based hormone therapy of adequate dose and duration.[50]

Genetic Counseling

Women with POI who are found to have an abnormal karyotype and those harboring the FMR1 premutation should be offered genetic counseling. Not only might these diagnoses affect the patient's health, they may also have important health implications for the patients' relatives and potential offspring. A genetic counselor can effectively convey this information to patients and family members.

Skeletal Health

Early estrogen withdrawal and coexisting morbidities, particularly thyroid disease and diabetes, place women with POI at risk for early onset osteoporosis and bone fractures in comparison with their peers. Bone mineral density screening allows quantification of the individual risk, and women should be educated on the importance of bone health maintenance. No clear recommendations have been established on the amount of calcium and vitamin D that should be consumed by women with POI. Intake of 1200 mg of elemental calcium (from dietary and supplementation sources) per day and maintenance of adequate vitamin D (serum 25-hydroxyvitamin D >30 ng/mL) is recommended by the North American Menopause Society for perimenopausal and postmenopausal women.[51] These same standards would likely apply to the population of women with POI. In women with inadequate exposure to the sun, intake of 800 to 1000 IU of vitamin D per day may be of benefit.[51] In addition, women should be encouraged to participate in weight-bearing exercise on a regular basis. Bisphosphonate therapy is cautioned against in young women for whom pregnancy is possible, owing to the uncertain fetal affects secondary to the long half-life of these medications.[52]

Cardiovascular Health

Endothelial dysfunction is a known sequela to hypoestrogenemia, and is recognized as an initiating process for atherogenesis.[53] Impaired endothelial function is evident in women with POI, and within a month following bilateral oophorectomy.[54] Conversely, a reversal of the phenomenon is observed within a few months of initiating estrogen therapy, in the context of an otherwise healthy vasculature.[54,55] Given that emerging data suggest that estrogen therapy when initiated early in the process of menopause may retard the onset of atherogenesis, timely initiation of estrogen replacement in women with POI may additionally hold long-term cardiovascular benefit for this population that is otherwise weighed down by the burden of increased lifetime risk for chronic diseases.

Associated Disorders

Women with POI should be screened yearly for autoimmune thyroid disease with a TSH level. Yearly screening of antiadrenal antibodies should be considered, as women with adrenal autoimmunity have a 50% risk of developing adrenal insufficiency.[56] A positive test for adrenal antibodies should be further evaluated annually with the use of a corticotropin stimulation test. Patients should be educated on the warning signs and symptoms of adrenal insufficiency (such as weight loss, fatigue, disorientation, skin discoloration, and nausea) given the severity of the disease and its potential lethal consequences.

SUMMARY

Beyond the psychological devastation and the symptomatic havoc that dominate the "now" lie long-term health implications of the relatively swift and sometimes dramatic loss of ovarian function seen with POI. Whether spontaneously or induced, premature menopause renders a woman deficient in ovarian endocrine and reproductive function well before the natural age of menopause. Early estrogen deprivation as occurs in women with POI holds myriad implications, both short-term and long-term, for the physical and psychological well-being of this population. A multidisciplinary approach is needed to meet the unique physical, emotional, and psychological challenges that follow early loss of ovarian function. The first step is to achieve a heightened level of awareness for the symptomatology and the commonality of POI, and to remain cognizant of the physical and psychological burden that may follow surgical menopause. Once the diagnosis of premature menopause has been established, hormone replacement therapy remains the mainstay for symptom control and prevention of long-term sequelae.

REFERENCES

1. van Noord PA, Dubas JS, Dorland M, et al. Age at natural menopause n a population-based screening cohort: the role of menarche, fecundity, and lifestyle factors. Fertil Steril 1997;68(1):95–102.
2. Luborsky JL, Meyer P, Sowers MF, et al. Premature menopause in a multi-ethnic population study of the menopause transition. Hum Reprod 2003;18:199–206.
3. Coulam CB, Adamson SC, Annegers JF. Incidence of premature ovarian failure. Obstet Gynecol 1986;67(4):604–6.
4. Reber RW. Premature ovarian failure. Obstet Gynecol 2009;113(6):1355–63.

5. Albright F, Smith PH, Fraser R. A syndrome characterized by primary ovarian insufficiency and decreased stature. Am J Med Sci 1942;204:625–48.
6. Welt CK. Primary ovarian insufficiency: a more accurate term for premature ovarian failure. Clin Endocrinol 2008;68:499–509.
7. Lebovic DI, Naz R. Premature ovarian failure: think 'autoimmune disorder'. Sex Reprod Menopause 2004;4:230–3.
8. Kodaman PH. Early menopause: primary ovarian insufficiency and surgical menopause. Semin Reprod Med 2010;8(5):360–9.
9. Reber RW, Connolly HV. Clinical features of young women with hypergonadotropic amenorrhea. Fertil Steril 1990;53:804–10.
10. Cox L, Liu JH. Primary ovarian insufficiency: an update. Int J Womens Health 2014;5:235–43.
11. Panay N, Kalu E. Management of premature ovarian failure. Best Pract Res Clin Obstet Gynaecol 2009;23(1):129–40.
12. Broekmans FJ, Kwee J, Hendricks DJ, et al. A systemic review of tests predicting ovarian reserve and IVF outcome. Hum Reprod Update 2006;12(6):685–718.
13. Rebar RW, Erickson GF, Yen SS. Idiopathic premature ovarian failure: clinical and endocrine characteristics. Fertil Steril 1982;37(1):35–41.
14. Wittenberger MD, Hagerman RJ, Sherman SL, et al. The FMR-1 premutation and reproduction. Fertil Steril 2007;87(3):456–65.
15. Kim TJ, Anasti JN, Flack MR, et al. Routine endocrine screening for patients with karyotypically normal spontaneous premature ovarian failure. Obstet Gynecol 1997;89(5 Pt 1):777–9.
16. Baker TG. A quantitative and cytological study of germ cells in human ovaries. Proc R Soc Lond B Biol Sci 1963;153:417–33.
17. Faddy MJ. Follicle dynamics during ovarian ageing. Mol Cell Endocrinol 2000;163:43–8.
18. Pouresmaeili F, Fazeli Z. Premature ovarian failure: a critical condition in the reproductive potential with various genetic causes. Int J Fertil Steril 2014;8(1):1–12.
19. Laml T, Preyer O, Wmek W, et al. Genetic disorders in premature ovarian failure. Hum Reprod Update 2002;8(4):483–91.
20. Practice Committee of American Society for Reproductive Medicine. Increased maternal cardiovascular mortality associated with pregnancy in women with Turner syndrome. Fertil Steril 2005;83(4):1074–5.
21. Beck-Peccoz P, Persani L. Premature ovarian failure. Orphanet J Rare Dis 2006;1:1–5.
22. Sherman SL. Premature ovarian failure in the fragile X syndrome. Am J Med Genet 2000;97(3):189–94.
23. Sullivan SD, Welt C, Sherman S. FMR1 and the continuum of primary ovarian insufficiency. Semin Reprod Med 2011;29:299–307.
24. Beutler E, Baluda ML, Sturgeon P, et al. A new genetic abnormality resulting in galactose-1-phosphate uridyltransferase deficiency. Lancet 1965;1:353–5.
25. Segal S, Berry GT. Disorders of galactose metabolism. In: Scriver CR, Beaudent AL, Sly WS, et al, editors. The metabolic and molecular bases of inherited disease. New York: McGraw-Hill, Inc; 2000. p. 967–1000.
26. Levy HL, Driscoll SG, Porensky RS, et al. Ovarian failure in galactosemia. N Engl J Med 1984;310:50.
27. Uhlenhaut NH, Treier M. Foxl2 function in ovarian development. Mol Genet Metab 2006;88:225–34.

28. LaBarbara AR, Miller MM, Ober C, et al. Autoimmune etiology in premature ovarian failure. Am J Reprod Immunol Microbiol 1988;16(3):115–22.

29. Anasti JN. Premature ovarian failure: an update. Fertil Steril 1998;70(1):1–15.

30. Silva CA, Yamakami LY, Aikawa NE, et al. Autoimmune primary ovarian insufficiency. Autoimmun Rev 2014;13(4-5):427–30.

31. Hoek A, Schoemaker J, Drexhage HA. Premature ovarian failure and ovarian autoimmunity. Endocr Rev 1997;18:107–34.

32. Sedmak DD, Hart WR, Tubbs RR. Autoimmune oophoritis: a histopathologic study of involved ovaries with immunologic characterization of the mononuclear cell infiltrate. Int J Gynecol Pathol 1987;6:73–81.

33. Bakalov VK, Anasti JN, Calis KA, et al. Autoimmune oophoritis as a mechanism of follicular dysfunction in women with 46,XX spontaneous premature ovarian failure. Fertil Steril 2005;84(4):958–65.

34. Kokcu A. Premature ovarian failure from current perspective. Gynecol Endocrinol 2010;26(8):555–62.

35. Keshavarz H, Hillis SD, Kieke BA, et al. Hysterectomy surveillance—United States, 1994-1999. Surveillance summaries, July 12, 2002. MMWR Morb Mortal Wkly Rep 2002;51:1–8.

36. Shuster LT, Rhodes DJ, Gostout BS, et al. Premature menopause or early menopause: long-term health consequences. Maturitas 2010;65:161–6.

37. Nelson LM. Clinical practice: primary ovarian insufficiency. N Engl J Med 2009; 360(6):606–14.

38. Chetkowski RJ, Meldrum DR, Steingold KA, et al. Biologic effects of transdermal estradiol. N Engl J Med 1986;314(25):1615–20.

39. Mashchak CA, Lobo RA, Dozono-Takano R, et al. Comparison of pharmacodynamics properties of various estrogen formulations. Am J Obstet Gynecol 1982;144(5):511–8.

40. Groff AA, Covington SN, Halverson LR, et al. Assessing the emotional needs of women with spontaneous premature ovarian failure. Fertil Steril 2005;83(6):1734–41.

41. Van der Stefe JG, Groen H, van Zadelhoff SJ, et al. Decreased androgen concentrations and diminished general and sexual well-being in women with premature ovarian failure. Menopause 2008;15(1):23–31.

42. Nelson L, Anasti JN, Kimzey LM, et al. Development of luteinized graafian follicles in patients with karyotypically normal spontaneous premature ovarian failure. J Clin Endocrinol Metab 1994;79:1470–5.

43. Sermon K, Seneca S, De Rycke M, et al. PGD in the lab for triplet repeat diseases—myotonic dystrophy, Huntington's disease, and. Fragile X syndrome. Mol Cell Endocrinol 2001;183(Suppl 1):577–85.

44. Yimaz N, Uygur D, Inal H, et al. Dehydroepiandrosterone supplementation improves predictive markers for diminished ovarian reserve: serum AMH, inhibin B and antral follicle count. Eur J Obstet Gynecol Reprod Biol 2013;169(2): 257–60.

45. Fouany MR, Sharara FI. Is there a role for DHEA supplementation in women with diminished ovarian reserve? J Assist Reprod Genet 2013;30(9):1239–44.

46. Narkwichean A, Maalouf W, Campbell B, et al. Efficacy of dehydroepiandrosterone to improve ovarian response in women with diminished ovarian reserve: a meta-analysis. Reprod Biol Endocrinol 2013;11:44–52.

47. Gleicher N, Kim A, Weghofer A, et al. Hypoandrogenism in association with diminished functional ovarian reserve. Hum Reprod 2013;28(4):1084–91.

48. Elias AN, Pandian MR, Rojas FJ. Serum levels of androstenedione, testosterone and dehydroepiandrosterone sulfate in patients with premature ovarian failure

compared to age-matched menstruating controls. Gynecol Obstet Invest 1997; 43:47–8.

49. Davis SR. Testosterone influences libido and well being in women. Trends Endocrinol Metab 2001;12:33–7.

50. Kalantaridou SN, Davis SR, Nelson LM. Premature ovarian failure. Endocrinol Metab Clin North Am 1998;27(4):989–1006.

51. North American Menopause Society. The role of calcium in peri and postmenopausal women: 2006 position statement of the North American Menopause Society. Menopause 2006;13(6):862–77.

52. Vujovic S, Brincat M, Erel T, et al. EMAS position statement: managing women with premature ovarian failure. Maturitas 2010;67:91–3.

53. Ross R. Atherosclerosis—an inflammatory disease. N Engl J Med 1999;340(2): 115–26.

54. Virdis A, Ghiadoni L, Pinto S, et al. Mechanisms responsible for endothelial dysfunction associated with acute estrogen deprivation in normotensive women. Circulation 2000;101(19):2258–63.

55. Kalantaridou SN, Naka NN, Papnikolaou E, et al. Impaired endothelial function in young women with premature ovarian failure: normalization with hormone therapy. J Clin Endocrinol Metab 2004;89(8):3907–13.

56. Betterle C, Volpato M, Rees Smith B, et al. Adrenal cortex and steroid 21-hydroxylase autoantibodies in adult patients with organ-specific autoimmune disease: markers of low progression to clinical Addison's disease. J Clin Endocrinol Metab 1997;82(3):932–8.

Menopause and the Heart

Chileshe Nkonde-Price, MD[a], Jeffrey R. Bender, MD[b],*

KEYWORDS

- Menopause • Heart • Hormone replacement therapy • Cardiovascular risk

KEY POINTS

- HRT is not currently recommended solely to prevent future heart attacks in perimenopausal or postmenopausal women.
- For perimenopausal, recently perimenopausal, or even more than a decade postmenopausal women with life-disrupting vasomotor and urogenital symptoms, topical estrogens should be first considered, followed by hormone patches with the lowest effective estrogen dose possible.
- Treatment should be maintained for the shortest duration possible.
- For women who are a decade or the more after the menopause and are no longer troubled by symptoms, HRT should be discontinued.
- Whether HRT increases risk for the conditions already prevalent in older women, such as heart attacks, strokes and breast cancer, remains unclear, and is still under investigation.

INTRODUCTION

Cardiovascular disease (CVD), including coronary artery disease (CAD), peripheral arterial disease, cerebrovascular disease, and congestive heart failure, is the leading cause of death in US women. Premenopausal women are relatively protected against CVD, compared with age-matched men. However, this gender gap narrows at menopause, the incidence of CVD in women increasing sharply and continuing to increase with advancing age. This long-standing observation led to a belief that ovarian steroid hormones and, in particular, estrogens, are cardioprotective. Large databases of women taking hormone replacement therapy (HRT) for a variety of postmenopausal symptoms were retrospectively evaluated for CVD incidence. These analyses supported the aforementioned belief, as did a series of observational studies. However,

Disclosures: Dr Bender is a consultant for Merck; Dr Nkonda-Price: None.
The authors have nothing to disclose.
[a] Penn Heart and Vascular Center for Women's Cardiovascular Health, Perelman School of Medicine, University of Pennsylvania, Philadelphia, PA 19104, USA; [b] Section of Cardiovascular Medicine, Yale Cardiovascular Research Center, Raymond and Beverly Sackler Cardiovascular Laboratory, Yale University School of Medicine, 300 George Street, Room 773G, New Haven, CT 06511, USA
* Corresponding author.
E-mail address: jeffrey.bender@yale.edu

Endocrinol Metab Clin N Am 44 (2015) 559–564
http://dx.doi.org/10.1016/j.ecl.2015.05.005
0889-8529/15/$ – see front matter © 2015 Elsevier Inc. All rights reserved.

endo.theclinics.com

those data generally have not been supported by randomized clinical trials (RCTs). The discordance is surprising also in light of the beneficial effects of estrogen on the vascular endothelium at the cellular and molecular levels and on blood vessels in animal CVD models. This conundrum has been a confusing and still controversial area in women's health. In this article, the observational studies and RCTs are reviewed, the gaps and perhaps weaknesses of these trials are described, the ongoing studies intended to fill these gaps are mentioned, and recommended approaches to hormone therapy (HT) in postmenopausal women are commented on.

OBSERVATIONAL STUDIES

Numerous large-scale observational studies, most commonly performed to assess benefits of multiyear HRT use in a variety of clinical conditions, included CVD in their assessment. From these studies, there were 2 consistent observations: (1) women lacking endogenous estrogen have a greater CVD risk than those with functioning ovaries and (2) HRT reduces CVD incidence and prevalence in postmenopausal women. The NHS (Nurses Health Study) was the largest of these studies.

Nurses Health Study

The NHS was a large, prospective cohort study investigating the relationship between HT and a variety of clinical conditions, including breast cancer, gall bladder disease, and, most notably for this review, CVD.[1] The study, beginning in 1976, surveyed all registered nurses aged 30 to 55 years in 11 states. A total of 122,000 nurses responded to questionnaires providing information on hormone use, the presence of cardiovascular risk factors, and the development of CVD. Participants were surveyed every 2 years over a 4-year follow-up period, with a high degree of continued participation (93% follow-up). Although some concern grew regarding an increased incidence of breast cancer, HT users appeared to have a significantly reduced risk of CVD. Criticism of the NHS included a potential selection bias, women choosing HT possibly being healthier with more favorable CVD risk profiles than non–hormone users.

RANDOMIZED CLINICAL TRIALS

To address the healthy women bias, and to perform studies in a prospective fashion, several RCTs were designed. These RCTs included CVD surrogate marker studies, secondary prevention trials, and primary prevention trials. The PEPI (Postmenopausal Estrogen/Progestin Intervention) trial randomized 875 women, aged 45 to 64 years, analyzing the effect of HT on low-density lipoprotein (LDL), high-density lipoprotein (HDL), and fibrinogen, among other clinical parameters (eg, bone density). In 1995, study conclusions included that HT improved CVD risk, given observed reductions in LDL, fibrinogen, and increases in HDL levels. PEPI thus was consistent with the aforementioned observational studies. RCTs addressing CVD events were then initiated. The 2 most influential have been HERS (Heart and Estrogen/Progestin Replacement Study) and WHI (Women's Health Initiative), which ran concurrently.

HERS: a Secondary Prevention Trial

HERS was a multicenter, randomized, blind, placebo-controlled secondary prevention trial.[2] Secondary prevention refers to reduction of coronary events in individuals with established CAD, defined as myocardial infarction (MI), coronary artery bypass surgery or percutaneous coronary intervention, or angiographic evidence of at least a 50% occlusion of 1 or more major coronary arteries. A total of 2763 postmenopausal women with an intact uterus were randomized to either combined estrogen/progestin therapy or placebo. Postmenopausal was defined as age at least 55 years without natural menses for at least 5 years, or no natural menses for at least 1 year and serum follicle-stimulating hormone (FSH) levels greater than 40 IU/L, or documented bilateral oophorectomy, or reported bilateral oophorectomy with FSH level greater than 40 IU/L and estradiol level less than 92 pmol/L (25 pg/mL). The age range of participants was 44 to 79 years, with a mean of 67 years. All received a baseline clinical examination, electrocardiogram (EKG), and measurement of fasting lipid levels. Compliance was addressed by frequent clinical visits, with EKG and lipid profile analyses performed yearly. The primary outcome assessed was nonfatal MI or CAD-related death. Secondary outcomes included coronary revascularization, unstable angina, congestive heart failure, resuscitated cardiac arrest, stroke or transient ischemic attack, peripheral arterial disease, and all-cause mortality. Overall, there was no significant reduction in any of the primary or secondary outcomes achieved in the HRT arm. However, within this composite null effect, a statistically significant time trend was noted. There were more CAD events within the first year of HRT, and fewer events in years 4 and beyond. The absence of protection overall, and the increased CVD risk within 1 year, led to significant cardiovascular concerns regarding HRT use in postmenopausal women. Thus, HERS was the first in a wave of negative studies, triggering conclusions regarding a lack of support for HRT use in cardiovascular prevention. The time trend did cause speculation regarding differential early and late biological vascular effects of estrogen. Questions arose concerning pro-thrombotic early, and antiatherogenic late, effects. Adding weight to the HERS conclusions, the study had a robust trial design and enrolled women with a CVD risk profile similar to the National Health and Nutrition Examination Survey III database, encompassing a random sample of postmenopausal US women with known heart disease. Despite the potential to generalize the HERS results, the study population did not address whether HT would be cardioprotective in postmenopausal women without established CVD. It was acknowledged that primary prevention trials were needed.

WHI: a Primary Prevention Trial

The WHI was a large, National Institutes of Health–sponsored, multicenter, randomized, double-blind, placebo-controlled trial investigating strategies for preventing chronic diseases in postmenopausal women.[3] The wide range of chronic diseases included gallbladder disease, dementia, kidney stones, diabetes, colon cancer, breast cancer, osteoporotic fractures, venous thromboembolic disease, stroke, and heart disease. With regard to CVD, this was a primary prevention trial, because 27,000 healthy postmenopausal women had no evidence of CVD at the time of enrollment. The trial was intended to provide the definitive conclusion with regard to HT and cardiovascular risk. Postmenopausal was defined as the absence of vaginal bleeding for 6 months (12 months for younger women, age 50–54 years), documented oophorectomy, or previous use of postmenopausal HRT. The enrollee age range was 50-79 years, with a mean of 63 years, and an average of 12.5 years after menopause. Two arms consisted of combined (estrogen plus progestin) HRT or placebo in women with an intact uterus, and estrogen replacement therapy alone or placebo in women after hysterectomy. Assessed primary outcomes were nonfatal MI, CAD death, and the development of invasive breast cancer. A global health index, combining the incidence of all primary and secondary outcomes, was generated. The planned study duration was 8.5 years, but the combined HRT arm was terminated at 5 years because the global health index was significantly higher (worse) in the treatment group. Regarding CVD, there was an increase (0.07%) in cardiovascular events in those taking hormone (both combined and estrogen alone regimens). Thus, it was concluded that HRT does not confer a cardiovascular risk benefit in healthy postmenopausal women and may increase risk. As with HERS, there was a time trend, with a greater number of CV events among hormone users in the first year, and fewer in years 4 and beyond. The WHI gained huge worldwide attention and led to a defined change in clinical practice, that of avoiding HRT in postmenopausal women, in the context of CVD.

Sorting Through the Conundrum

Since the 2002 publication of the WHI results, clinicians and scientists have reviewed the RCTs with a critical eye, attempting to explain the discordance between a logical hypothesis, many observational studies, and the more recent clinical trials. As noted earlier, the average WHI enrollment age was 63 years, 11 to 12 years older than the age at which HRT is commonly prescribed in clinical practice. In general, women enrolled in observational studies were newly menopausal. As these timing questions arose, WHI investigators reviewed the data, assessing CVD risk of HT by age decades (50–59, 60–69, 70–79 years). This secondary analysis was published in 2007. Those who were youngest had the lowest risk of coronary heart disease. Hazard ratios were highest for those in the oldest age group, and HT appeared protective in the youngest age group. Definitive conclusions could not be made about the latter, because the study was statistically underpowered to show cardiovascular protection in those within the menopausal transition group. There was also a WHI ancillary study published in 2007, using coronary artery calcium (CAC) scoring as a surrogate marker for atherosclerosis, in the 50-year to 59-year age group. Those in the estrogen treatment group had lower CAC scores than placebo control, suggesting a potential protective effect on plaque burden. Consistent with these trends, a meta-analysis of more than 39,000 women enrolled in 23 clinical trials concluded that HRT reduces coronary heart disease risk in women younger than 60 years, but not in older women. Thus, although the WHI trial was initially considered unfavorable with regard to HT and CVD, and the prescriptions for those specific hormones used in the WHI decreased by 66% in the year after the trial, those ancillary and secondary analyses supported the notion that timing of intervention and patient selection are critical in balancing HRT risks and benefits.

More recently, a long-term RCT, the Danish Osteoporosis Prevention Study, was completed.[4] A total of 1006 recently menopausal (as determined by medical and surgical history and FSH levels, mean age 49.7 years) healthy women were randomized to either HRT or no treatment, and followed for 12 to 16 years. Analysis included cumulative hazard ratios for mortality, heart failure, and MI. There were significantly favorable hazard ratios in the estrogen only (posthysterectomy) and estrogen plus progestin groups, supporting a cardiovascular primary prevention benefit for HRT when started in recently menopausal women.

RECENTLY COMPLETED TRIALS

Because of the very low cardiovascular event rates in women in those younger age groups mentioned earlier, and the fact that 16-year randomized HRT clinical trials are not common, further documentation of a favorable HRT treatment window will most likely be obtained with trials in which progressive CVD, rather than clinical event rates, are determined. There are 2 recent such clinical trials, KEEPS (Kronos Early Estrogen Prevention Study) and ELITE (Early Versus Late Intervention Trial with Estrogen).

The Kronos Early Estrogen Prevention Study

KEEPS was a multicenter, randomized, placebo-controlled US trial, following 720 healthy women for 4 years, assessing the presence and progression of subclinical atherosclerosis.[5] Enrollees were 42 to 58 years old, and within 36 months of their last menstrual cycle. They were randomized to 0.45 mg of conjugated equine estrogens, 0.05 mg weekly transdermal estradiol (both in combination with cyclic, oral micronized progesterone, 200 mg for 12 days each month), or placebo. Assessment included progression of carotid intimal medial thickness (CIMT) by ultrasonography, and accrual of CAC by computed tomography (CT) scan, as primary end point correlates of complex atherosclerosis, with progression. A variety of ancillary studies, evaluating intermediate cardiovascular metabolic, cognitive, and bone effects are still being analyzed. At the 4-year time point, mean CIMT and CAC scores were similar across all groups. Lipid levels improved in the HT group, as did insulin sensitivity (in the transdermal estrogen group). Thus, the profile of at least some risk factors and markers of atherosclerosis was better with HRT, although cardiovascular disease, by imaging, was not.

Early Versus Late Intervention Trial with Estrogen

ELITE is a single-center, randomized placebo-controlled US trial sponsored by the National Institute of Aging.[6] It was designed to compare the effects of estrogen on the progression of early atherosclerosis in 2 groups of healthy postmenopausal women: those within 6 years of menopause and those at least 10 years after menopause. Enrollees are receiving either 17-β estradiol (Estrace) or placebo (with vaginal progesterone or placebo, for the last 10 days of each month, if an intact uterus is present). As with KEEPS, primary analytical end points were CIMT by ultrasonography and atherosclerosis by cardiac CT. A total of 643 women were enrolled, with a treatment duration of 5 years. Although the results have not yet been published, Dr Howard Hodis, the senior investigator on this study, reported positive findings at the American Heart Association Scientific Sessions in November, 2104. These positive findings included a reduction in progression of vascular disease in the HRT groups, but only if HT was initiated within the first 6 years. This finding reinforces the timing hypothesis that has evolved since subset analysis of the WHI data and of more recent RCTs (**Table 1**).

Recommendations

CVD remains the number 1 cause of death in US postmenopausal women. Long-standing beliefs regarding cardioprotective effects of estrogen have been strongly

Table 1
Effect of HT on CVD incidence is summarized by 3 clinical study results

	Science Revisited		
	CAD	Stroke	VTE
NHS	↓	Not accessed	Not accessed
HERS	↔	↔	↑
WHI	↑	↑	↑↑

A 0.07% increase in coronary events was detected in the WHI HT arm, although a trend toward protective (fewer events) was noted in the youngest (50–59 year) age group.

Abbreviations: ↑, increased incidence on HT; ↓, decreased incidence on HT; ↔, no difference; VTE, venous thromboembolic disease.

challenged. Conclusions are now drawn from a continuum of studies, including retrospective database analyses, observational studies, and primary and secondary prevention RCTs. After conclusion and even publication of some of these studies, secondary data analyses were performed, in attempts to define a favorable age of treatment initiation. There are 2 parallel relevant contexts and conclusions. The first relates to any current recommendation of postmenopausal HRT specifically for CVD prevention. Given the ongoing concerns, it is not within the current standard of cardiovascular care for postmenopausal women. However, statistically significant data in support of HRT use, within a specific age window, are accumulating. We remain speculative and cautiously optimistic, in light of those favorable statistical trends in women treated within the menopausal transition. We await the publication of complete results of recent clinical trials, designed specifically to assess benefit, within this age group and beyond, with great anticipation.

In addition to addressing the standard of care for CVD prevention, it is also critical to assess cardiovascular risk when HRT is deemed necessary to treat menopausal vasomotor and estrogen-deficient urogenital symptoms or beneficial to reduce menopausal bone loss and osteoporotic fractures. The International Menopause Society (IMS) reinforces that HRT is the most effective therapy for the aforementioned postmenopausal symptoms. However, it acknowledges that CVD risk is the principle risk concern of postmenopausal HRT use. If symptoms are lifestyle limiting, the IMS endorses HRT use when started during the menopausal transition, given the timing issues described earlier. Decision regarding initiating treatment beyond the age of 60 years, or continuing use past that age, when started earlier, must be individualized per patient, using conservative risk-benefit assessments, including all standard cardiovascular risks. If deemed necessary and within acceptable risk, the lowest hormone doses, effective to maintain quality of life, should be used.

REFERENCES

1. Stampfer MJ, Willett WC, Colditz GA, et al. A prospective study of postmenopausal estrogen therapy and coronary heart disease. N Engl J Med 1985;313:1044–9.
2. Hulley S, Grady D, Bush T, et al. Randomized trial of estrogen plus progestin for secondary prevention of coronary heart disease in postmenopausal women. Heart and Estrogen/progestin Replacement Study (HERS) Research Group. JAMA 1998; 280:605–13.
3. Rossouw J, Anderson G. Risks and benefits of estrogen plus progestin in healthy postmenopausal women: principal results from the Women's Health Initiative randomized controlled trial. JAMA 2002;291:1701–12.
4. Schierbeck LL, Rejnmark L, Tfteng CL, et al. Effect of hormone replacement therapy on cardiovascular events in recently postmenopausal women: randomised trial. BMJ 2012;345:e6409.
5. Harman S, Black D, Naftolin F, et al. Arterial imaging outcomes and cardiovascular risk factors in recently menopausal women. Ann Intern Med 2014;161:249–60.
6. Hodis HN, Mack WJ, Shoupe D, et al. Methods and baseline cardiovascular data from the Early versus Late Intervention Trial with Estradiol testing the menopausal hormone timing hypothesis. Menopause 2015;22:391–401.

Menopausal Hormone Therapy: Current Considerations

Cynthia A. Stuenkel, MD

KEYWORDS

- Menopausal hormone therapy • Estrogen • Progestogen
- Selective estrogen receptor modulator • Bazedoxifene • Ospemifene

KEY POINTS

- Menopausal hormone therapy (MHT) is the most effective method to improve vasomotor and vaginal symptoms associated with the menopause; for carefully selected women, benefits exceed risks.
- Optimal candidates for MHT include women younger than age 60 or within 10 years of menopause, without contraindications, and without increased risk of cardiovascular disease or breast cancer.
- Individualization is a key factor when formulating a treatment plan for relief of menopausal symptoms.
- Currently available choices of MHT allow for tailoring therapy to integrate personal preference, consideration of varying risk profiles, and individual treatment requirements.
- The decision to use MHT should be revisited at least annually or whenever a change in the patient's medical status, treatment priorities, or personal preferences occurs.

Practicing evidence-based medicine, in the realm of menopausal hormone therapy (MHT), is an ever-evolving challenge, and one that requires an ongoing awareness of emerging scientific findings and updated recommendations. In this article, a practical approach to navigating the use of MHT and available options are presented.

MENOPAUSAL HORMONE THERAPY: THE STATE OF THE EVIDENCE

For many years, menopausal medicine was more eminence-based than evidence-based.[1] Women were encouraged to use MHT to stay *Feminine Forever* (the title of a 1966 bestseller,[2] which was very persuasive, but received mixed reviews).[3] Eventually, small clinical trials confirmed symptom relief by various MHT preparations; others showed benefit on bone density measurements and lipid determinations.[4]

The author has nothing to disclose.
Department of Medicine, University of California, San Diego, School of Medicine, 6376 Castejon Drive, La Jolla, CA 92037, USA
E-mail address: castuenkel@ucsd.edu

Endocrinol Metab Clin N Am 44 (2015) 565–585
http://dx.doi.org/10.1016/j.ecl.2015.05.006
0889-8529/15/$ – see front matter © 2015 Elsevier Inc. All rights reserved.

During the 1980s, impressive evidence from several prospective cohort and case-control studies began to accumulate, and with few exceptions, consistently described reduction of coronary heart disease (CHD) and osteoporotic fractures in women who used MHT. In 1992, in response to mounting supportive data from studies examining surrogate endpoints and accompanying enthusiasm of the medical community, the American College of Physicians recommended MHT for postmenopausal women, particularly those with history of CHD or at risk for CHD, primarily for cardioprotection and osteoporosis prevention.[5] Breast cancer was a recognized risk, but the overwhelming cardiovascular benefit seemed to outweigh concerns.

Randomized clinical outcome trials (RCT) lagged decades behind clinical practice. The Postmenopausal Estrogen and Progestogen Intervention (PEPI) trial,[6] funded by the National Institutes of Health and published in 1995, evaluated effects of commonly prescribed MHT preparations on surrogate cardiovascular disease (CVD) risk factors and endometrial safety (**Table 1**). The results were reassuring and consistent with the anticipated benefits, but the trial was too small and too short to assess the effects of MHT on hard clinical endpoints, such as heart attack, stroke, blood clots, osteoporotic fractures, and breast cancer risk.

Although a lightning rod for more than a decade of controversy, the subsequent landmark Women's Health Initiative (WHI) trials have provided the best available RCT evidence for assessing risks and benefits of MHT. Conceived in the late 1980s as an effort to confirm the validity of prevailing practice recommendations at the time to prescribe MHT for prevention of CHD, osteoporosis, and possibly cognitive decline, the WHI was designed to evaluate the preventive benefits of conjugated equine estrogens (CEE) and medroxyprogesterone acetate (MPA), the most commonly prescribed drugs in America in postmenopausal women ages 50 to 79.[7] CHD was the primary outcome, with breast cancer as the primary safety outcome (see **Table 1**). The WHI was not designed to evaluate symptom relief because this had previously been shown in many adequately powered RCTs.[4] Furthermore, women who had severe vasomotor symptoms (VMS) were intentionally excluded from the WHI, because investigators hoped to minimize dropout of highly symptomatic women assigned to placebo therapy.

In 2002, the initial results of the WHI combined estrogen plus progestin (E + P) MHT trial were prematurely announced after 5.6 years (rather than 8.5 as planned), because MHT-related risks (CHD, stroke, breast cancer, and venous thromboembolic events [VTE]) were noted to exceed preventive benefits (reduced fractures, reduced colon cancer) (see **Table 1**).[7] In response to the unanticipated negative results of the WHI E + P trial, prescriptions for MHT declined by 70%.[11] In early 2003, the US Food and Drug Administration (FDA) required package labeling changes for all MHT products, with the assumption that risks and benefits were similar.

The initial results of the 7.2-year WHI conjugated equine estrogen (CEE-alone) trial, published in 2004, differed from the combination trial in several ways (see **Table 1**).[8] With CEE-alone, there was no overall increase in CHD or breast cancer, while fractures were reduced, as anticipated.[8] In women ages 50 to 59, the risk of CHD, although not statistically different from rates in older age groups, suggested a trend consistent with observational studies showing that CEE use may offer CHD benefit.

In the intervening decade, since the WHI results were initially reported, continued participant follow-up and outcome analyses have accentuated the divergent findings between the WHI CEE-alone and the WHI E + P clinical trials[12] (**Box 1**, **Table 2**). Furthermore, when data were stratified by participant age and years since menopause, the effect of timing of initiation of MHT on clinical outcomes, particularly CHD and breast cancer, was brought into sharper focus.[13,17] Most recently, the

Table 1
Landmark clinical trials of menopausal hormone therapy in healthy postmenopausal women

Trial (y)	Treatment Arms	Duration (y)	N	Age (Mean) (y)	Years Since Menopause	Defined Outcomes/MHT Effects
PEPI 1995[6]	Placebo CEE 0.625 mg/d CEE 0.625 mg/d; MPA 10 mg 12 d/m CEE 0.625 mg/d; MPA 2.5 mg/d CEE 0.625 mg/d; MP 200 mg 12 d/m	3	875	45–64 (56.1)	<10	HDL, BP, glucose & insulin, fibrinogen HDL ↑ by CEE or CEE/MP > CEE/MPA > PBO BP not significantly different by treatment groups Fasting glucose ↓ in all active treatment groups 2-h postprandial ↑ with all MHT; MPA > MP Fibrinogen ↓ in all active treatment groups CEE ↑ endometrial hyperplasia 10%/y All combined MHT prevented hyperplasia
WHI 2002[7]	Placebo CEE 0.625 mg/d; MPA 2.5 mg/d	5.6	16, 608	50–79 (63.3)	<10 to >20	CHD (efficacy) and breast cancer (safety) ↑ CHD in first year, ↑ stroke, VTE, breast cancer ↓ Colon cancer, fractures, diabetes
WHI 2004[8]	Placebo CEE 0.625 mg/d	7.2	10, 739	50–79 (63.6)	<10 to >20	CHD (efficacy) and breast cancer (safety) ↑ Stroke and DVT ↓ Fractures and diabetes
KEEPS 2014[9]	Placebo CEE 0.45 mg/d; MP 200 mg 12 d/m T-E$_2$ 50 μg/d; MP 200 mg 12 d/m	4	727	42–58 (52.7)	>0.5 to <3	CIMT and CAC progression No effect of either regimen
ELITE 2015[10] (preliminary)	Placebo 17B-E$_2$ 1 mg po/d; ± MP gels 4% (45mg) pv 10d/m	12	643 271 372	 (55.4) (65.4)	>0.5 <6 ≥10	CIMT and CAC progression CIMT ↓; no effect on CAC No effect on CIMT or CAC

Abbreviations: CAC, coronary artery calcium score; CEE, conjugated equine estrogens; CHD, coronary heart disease; CIMT, carotid intima-media thickness; d, day; DVT, deep vein thrombosis; E$_2$, estradiol; ELITE, Early versus Late Intervention Trial with Estradiol; h, hour; KEEPS, Kronos Early Estrogen Prevention Study; m, month; MP, micronized progesterone; MPA, medroxyprogesterone acetate; PBO, placebo; PEPI, Postmenopausal Estrogen and Progestogen Intervention trial; po, per os (oral); pv, per vagina; T, transdermal; VTE, venous thromboembolic event; WHI, Women's Health Initiative trials.

Box 1
The Women's Health Initiative clinical trials: lessons learned

*Effects of unopposed CEE differ from combined MHT for several outcomes (see **Table 2**).[12]*

- *Cardiovascular outcomes* reflect a woman's age and time since menopause at the time of MHT initiation with increasing risks of CHD and stroke with increasing age and time since menopause.[13]

  o With *combined MHT*, there was no difference in relative risk of CHD by age, although when examined by time since menopause, there was a trend for increasing risk with advancing duration from less than 10 years to greater than 20 years ($P = .08$).[12]

  o With *CEE*, there was some evidence of CHD benefit in women ages 50 to 59:

    ▪ During the intervention phase, the risk of CHD trended lower in younger women ($P = .08$)[12]

    ▪ Trends by age for total MI ($P = .02$), revascularization ($P = .06$), composite outcomes (MI, CHD death, CABG, PCI, and angina), and CAC[14] provide some evidence for benefit in women younger than age 60 and thus the timing hypothesis.

    ▪ In cumulative 13-y follow-up, the risk of total MI was lower in younger women (hazard ratio [HR] 0.60 in women ages 50 to 59; P for trend by age = .007)[12]

- *Breast cancer risk* varied by type of MHT, timing of exposure, and duration of therapy

  o *Combined* Estrogen Progestogen Therapy increased breast cancer risk and breast cancer mortality[15]

    ▪ Early reports from the combined therapy arm of WHI suggested that postmenopausal women naïve to MHT could anticipate a 5-year window without increased risk of breast cancer.[16]

    ▪ Later reports suggested that women who started MHT within 3 to 5 y of menopause might be at greater risk than those with a longer gap time between menopause and initiation of therapy.[17]

    ▪ EPT duration greater than 5 y in women ages 50 to 59 is associated with persistent risk in 13-y cumulative follow-up: HR 1.34 (confidence interval 1.03–1.75); 9 added cases/10,000 PY[12]; cancers detected were more advanced with greater chance for spread.[15]

  o *CEE alone* did not increase breast cancer risk and reduced breast cancer mortality.[18]

    ▪ In 13-y cumulative follow-up, breast cancer risk was significantly decreased overall; in women ages 50–59, HR 0.76 (0.52–1.11), and 7 fewer cases/10,000 PY.[12]

---

results of 13 years of cumulative follow-up of enrollees of the WHI hormone trials reconfirms MHT-related risks and benefits during the intervention phase (see **Table 2**).[12]

Questions still remain regarding CHD preventive benefits of MHT. Recently, 2 small RCTs specifically designed to evaluate effects of MHT, when initiated early in menopause, on surrogate markers (carotid intima-media thickness [CIMT] and coronary artery calcium [CAC]) of atherosclerosis progression have reported inconsistent findings (see **Table 1**). The first, the Kronos Early Estrogen Prevention Study (KEEPS), compared oral CEE with transdermal estradiol (E_2) versus placebo, and reported no evidence of benefit of oral CEE or transdermal E_2 on atherosclerosis progression when started in healthy women early after onset of menopause[9]; those assigned to estrogen (both oral CEE and transdermal E_2) additionally received cyclic oral micronized progesterone for 12 days each month. Preliminary findings for the second trial, the Early versus Late Intervention Trial with Estrogen (ELITE) that compared oral E_2 with placebo, in contrast, showed that change in CIMT was less when oral E_2 was started within 6 years of menopause rather than after 10 years[10]; women with a uterus who

Table 2
Women's Health Initiative: risks and benefits of menopausal hormone therapy for women ages 50 to 59

Outcome	CEE + MPA Difference/ 10,000 PY	P for Trend by Age	CEE-Alone Difference/ 10,000 PY	P for Trend by Age
Primary end points				
CHD	+5	.81	−11	.08
Invasive breast cancer	+6	.68	−5	.89
Other end points in global index				
Stroke	+5	.50	−1	.77
Pulmonary embolism	+6	.61	+4	.28
Colorectal cancer	−1	.66	−3	.02
Endometrial cancer	0	.81	NA	NA
Hip fracture	−3	.38	+3	.33
All-cause mortality	−10	.20	−11	.04
Selected secondary end points				
Total MI	+4	.55	−11	.02
CABG or PCI	0	.67	−17	.06
Deep vein thrombosis	+10	.58	+5	.93
Vertebral fracture	−6	.02	−4	.20
Diabetes	−11	.10	−26	.99

Abbreviations: CABG, coronary artery bypass graft; CEE, conjugated equine estrogens; MI, myocardial infarction; MPA, medroxyprogesterone acetate; NA, not applicable because woman had hysterectomy; PCI, percutaneous coronary intervention; PY, person-years.

Data from Manson JE, Chlebowski RT, Stefanick ML, et al. Menopausal hormone therapy and health outcomes during the intervention and extended poststopping phases of the Women's Health Initiative randomized trials. JAMA 2013;310:1353–68.

were assigned to estrogen also received vaginal progesterone gel for 10 days of each month. Detailed publications based on results for both KEEPS and ELITE are awaited.

MENOPAUSAL HORMONE THERAPY—CURRENT CONSIDERATIONS

Today, the pendulum of MHT favor has moved beyond the center of the fulcrum and back into positive territory. Formal treatment indications (relief of menopausal symptoms and prevention of osteoporosis) remain (**Box 2**). Practice has changed, however, to reflect the lessons learned from continued follow-up of WHI participants and outcome analyses (**Box 3**). Experts now agree that MHT is a reasonable choice for relief for menopausal symptoms in carefully selected women, primarily those younger than age 60 or less than 10 years since menopause, who do not have contraindications and are not at an innately elevated risk for CVD or breast cancer.[19,20] Given the consistency of recent clinical guidelines (**Table 3**),[21–27] MHT for menopausal symptom relief is certainly a viable option (see **Box 2**). The role of MHT solely for the prevention of osteoporosis, however, remains controversial,[28,29] but may be an option for some women (see **Box 2**). Perhaps the most important clinical shift is from the one-size-fits-all perspective, popular during the second half of the last century, to the current emphasis on individualization of MHT. Now, personal preference, baseline risk profile, and characteristics of MHT based on hormone type, dose, and route of administration are factored into this important decision.[21,24]

> **Box 2**
> **Treatment indications for menopausal hormone therapy according to US product package labeling**
>
> 1. Treatment of moderate to severe VMS due to menopause
>
>   Use of estrogen alone, or in combination with a progestin, should be with the lowest effective dose and for the shortest duration consistent with treatment goals and risks for the individual woman. Postmenopausal women should be re-evaluated periodically as clinically appropriate to determine if treatment is still necessary.
>
> 2. Treatment of moderate to severe symptoms of vulvar and vaginal atrophy due to menopause
>
>   When prescribing solely for the treatment of moderate to severe symptoms of vulvar and vaginal atrophy due to menopause, topical vaginal products should be considered.
>
> 3. Treatment of hypoestrogenism due to hypogonadism, castration, or primary ovarian failure
>
>   Adjust dosage, upward or downward, according to severity of symptoms and response of the patient. For maintenance, adjust dosage to lowest level that will provide effective control (see Premature Menopause by Saioa Torrealday and Lubna Pal).
>
> 4. Prevention of postmenopausal osteoporosis
>
>   When prescribing solely for the prevention of postmenopausal osteoporosis, therapy should only be considered for women at significant risk of osteoporosis and nonestrogen medication should be carefully considered.

CONTEMPORARY APPROACH TO THE PATIENT
Engage Your Patient and Individualize Her Care

With full acknowledgment of the time required to embark on this complex conversation, attention to the following key points contributes to the success of shared decision-making and safety of MHT.

How bothered is she by her symptoms?

Clinical trials evaluating the effectiveness of MHT in reducing VMS use FDA-mandated criteria based on specific number and severity of moderate-to-severe hot flashes per day or per week. In clinical practice, however, the fundamental question relates to the patient's quality of life. Whether hot flashes are the main bother, or even a source of embarrassment in the workplace, or sleep deprivation, due to repeated awakenings relating to night sweats, is taking its toll, or emotional lability, resulting from a combination of the aforementioned happenings, is the issue, it is ultimately the patient, rather than any arbitrary cutoff, who determines the degree of bother and her readiness to consider prescription therapy for symptom relief.

What does she want?

Currently, there are many options for menopausal symptom control. General measures are straightforward and sensible and considered safe for all women. Several nonhormonal prescription therapies with proven efficacy are also available for consideration by symptomatic women for whom risks of MHT are deemed to outweigh potential for MHT-related benefit or who choose not to take MHT (see Menopausal Symptoms and Their Management by Nanette Santoro, C. Neill Epperson, and Sarah B. Mathews and Complementary and Alternative Approaches to Menopause by Maida Taylor). Although MHT is the most effective treatment for menopause symptoms and is available in many preparations, dose ranges, and routes of administration (**Table 4**), personal fears might limit a patient's willingness to consider a trial of MHT.[30,31]

Box 3
Practice changes following the Women's Health Initiative and resulting questions for future study

Clinical Changes	Remaining Questions
• Initiation of hormone therapy limited to women	• How can we best identify appropriate candidates for MHT?
○ Less than age 60 y or	
○ Within 10 y of menopause	
• Starting with doses half those studied in the WHI has become the standard of care	• Are lower doses safer?
	• Will women experience anticipated benefits beyond symptom relief (such as fracture reduction) with lower doses?
• FDA-approved biochemically identical hormone preparations— oral preparations, patches, gels, and emulsions—are prescribed in increasing numbers	• Do they have a better benefit/risk profile as some observational studies suggest?
• Alternatives to MPA for uterine protection used more frequently include	• Will long-term endometrial safety be demonstrated?
○ Micronized progesterone	
○ Combination therapy with BZA	
○ Levonorgestrel IUD[a]	
○ Long-cycle progestogens with endometrial monitoring	
• Recommended duration of combined MHT limited to a few (3–5) y to minimize breast cancer risk	• How to reconcile with the 'timing hypothesis'— possible CHD benefits if estrogen started early and continued?
	• How to determine when to stop therapy?
	• What is the best way to monitor after stopping combined MHT for persistent breast cancer risk?

[a] Not approved in the United States for endometrial protection with estrogen therapy in post-menopausal women.

Table 3
Recommendation statements for treatment of menopause symptoms

Organization	Date
Overall symptoms:	
Endocrine Society Clinical Practice Guideline: Treating Menopause Symptoms	2015[21]
ACOG Practice Bulletin No. 141: Management of Menopausal Symptoms	2014[22]
Managing Menopause: Canadian Recommendations	2014[23]
North American Menopause Society Hormone Therapy Position Statement	2012[24]
American Association of Clinical Endocrinologists Medical Guidelines	2011[25]
Vaginal symptoms:	
Management of symptomatic VVA: Position Statement of the NAMS	2013[26]
IMS Recommendations for management of postmenopausal vaginal atrophy	2010[27]

Abbreviations: ACOG, American College of Obstetricians and Gynecology; IMS, International Menopause Society; NAMS, North American Menopause Society; VVA, vulvovaginal atrophy.

Table 4
Commonly prescribed menopausal hormone therapy preparations and doses

	Dosages	
Preparations	Starting Dose/d	Dose Range
Systemic estrogen therapy		
Oral		
Conjugated equine estrogens	0.3 mg oral	0.3, 0.45, 0.625, 0.9, 1.25 mg
Micronized 17-β-estradiol	0.5 mg oral	0.5, 1.0, 2.0 mg
Transdermal		
17-β-estradiol patch	25 μg	0.025, 0.0375, 0.05, 0.075, 0.10 mg (0.014 mg for bone effects)
Estradiol gel	0.25 mg	0.25, 0.5, 0.75, 1.0, 1.5 mg
Estradiol spray	1.53 mg/spray	—
Vaginal ring (systemic effects)		
Estradiol acetate	0.05 mg	0.05, 0.10 mg (every 90 d)
Progestogen therapy		
Oral		
Medroxyprogesterone acetate	2.5 mg	2.5, 5.0, 10 mg
Micronized progesterone	100 mg	100, 200 mg
Combination estrogen/progestin products		
Oral		
CEE with daily MPA	0.3 or 0.45 mg with 1.5 mg	0.625 mg with 2.5 or 5.0 mg
CEE with cyclic MPA	0.625 mg with 5.0 mg/d × 2 wk	MPA 10 mg/d × 2 wk
17-β E$_2$ with norethindrone acetate	0.5 mg/d with 0.1 mg/d	1 mg/d with 0.5 mg/d
17-β E$_2$ with drospirenone	0.5 mg with 0.25 mg	1 mg/d with 0.5 mg/d
Transdermal		
17-β-E$_2$ with norethindrone acetate	0.05 mg with 0.14 mg	0.05 with 0.25 mg
17-β-E$_2$ with levonorgestrel	0.045 mg with 0.015 mg	—
Vaginal estrogen therapy		
Vaginal creams		
Conjugated equine estrogens Start	0.5–2 g/d for 1–2 wk	Then, 0.5 g/d just 2–3×/wk
17-β-estradiol	Start 2–4 g/d for 1–2 wk	Then, 1 g/d just 2–3×/wk
Vaginal rings		
17-β-estradiol	7.5 μg/d	Change every 90 d
Vaginal tablets		
Estradiol hemihydrate	Start 10 μg/d for 2 wk	Then, 10 μg/d for 1–2×/wk

Realistically, she may have been influenced by media personalities, the women in her book club or carpool, or Internet "experts" as to the specific therapy she wants. Establishing each symptomatic woman's preference early in the conversation helps establish trust and direct identification of an optimal therapeutic strategy.

Will therapy be safe?

Several steps contribute to evaluating the appropriateness of MHT for the patient. In addition to evaluating her personal medical profile (detailed in later discussion), quality of evidence for safety and efficacy varies by product.

For example, the popularity of compounded bioidentical hormone therapy (BHT) has succeeded despite a vacuum of evidence for efficacy or safety.[32] This industry has grown since the flight from traditional MHT following initial publication of the WHI. Compounded pharmacies are regulated directly by state agencies rather than the FDA. The primary concerns about BHT are linked to lack of RCT evidence of claims that these products are superior (or even comparable) to FDA-approved preparations. Package labeling outlining risks of MHT are not consistently distributed. Lack of manufacturing standards and quality control of purity and potency are added concerns. Finally, there is no scientific basis for the recommendation for BHT practitioners to conduct salivary hormone testing to establish initial dosing or monitor ongoing therapy. Because of these limitations and safety concerns, compounded BHT use has been discouraged by leading medical societies.[21,24,33]

The desire for biochemically identical MHT, however, can be optimally addressed by using FDA-approved MHT formulations that have undergone stringent scrutiny as regards manufacturing standards and quality control of purity and potency of the ingredients; oral and transdermal 17-β-estradiol (pills, patches, gels, sprays, and emulsions) and oral or vaginally applied micronized progesterone are all examples of FDA-approved MHT formulations that are biochemically identical to the natural ovarian hormones of reproductive years (see **Table 4**).

Choose Your Patients (for Whom You Recommend Menopausal Hormone Therapy) Wisely

Consider age, time since menopause, medical history, baseline cardiovascular health, and breast cancer risk.

Limit initiation of hormone therapy to women younger than 60 years of age or less than 10 years past onset of menopause

Findings from the WHI are convincing that, for the most part, MHT initiation in younger women close to menopause yields safer benefit/risk outcomes.[12] Rates of stroke increase after age 60, and total myocardial infarction (MI) and all-cause mortality, are significantly higher in women more remote from menopause (>20 years past) than in younger (<10 years past) women.[12,13]

Review contraindications to menopausal hormone therapy

Package labeling for MHT includes contraindications and cautions (**Box 4**). In general, nonhormonal therapies should be preferentially recommended for women with contraindications for MHT, with few exceptions. As written in the recent Endocrine Society Clinical Guidelines, "As the impact of severe menopausal symptoms on quality of life may be substantial, however, there are instances in which a woman with a history of coronary heart disease or breast cancer, for example, will choose to accept a degree of risk that might be considered to outweigh the benefits of MHT. An accepted philosophy is that a fully informed patient should be empowered to make a decision that best balances benefits to that individual when weighed against potential risks."[21]

Box 4
Cautions for use of menopausal hormone therapy per US product package labeling

Contraindications

- Undiagnosed abnormal genital bleeding
- Known, suspected, or history of breast cancer
- Known or suspected estrogen-dependent neoplasia
- Active DVT, PE, or a history of these conditions
- Active arterial thromboembolic disease (for example, stroke and MI), or a history of these conditions
- Known anaphylactic reaction or angioedema with product
- Known liver impairment or disease
- Known protein C, protein S, or antithrombin deficiency, or other known thrombophilic disorders
- Known or suspected pregnancy

Warnings and precautions

- Estrogens increase the risk of gallbladder disease
- Discontinue estrogen if severe hypercalcemia, loss of vision, severe hypertriglyceridemia, or cholestatic jaundice occurs
- Monitor thyroid function in women on thyroid replacement therapy

Abbreviations: DVT, deep vein thrombosis; MI, myocardial infarction; PE, pulmonary embolism.

Document the risk/benefit discussion specific to each patient in the medical record along with the treatment decision and plans for follow-up.

Assess cardiovascular risk

As the prevalence of obesity, diabetes, and cardiovascular risk increases in younger women, assessment of individual CVD risks before initiating MHT is increasingly relevant. Total 10-year cardiovascular risk can be calculated with the 2013 American College of Cardiology/American Heart Association Risk Calculator,[34] and then according to one paradigm, the risk estimate can be used to suggest the best approach to menopausal symptom relief.[35] For women at greater than 10% 10-year risk (usually implying a history of CVD or risk equivalent), options other than MHT may be safer. For those with a 10-year risk of 5% to 10%, transdermal estrogen therapy should be preferred (see later discussion). For those with less than 5% total 5-year CVD risk, choice of therapy to address menopausal symptoms depends on patient preference and other health factors.[21,35] In 2014, the American Stroke Association also released guidelines specifically for identifying women at increased risk of stroke.[36] Although stroke risk associated with MHT is small in women younger than age 60 or less than 10 years since menopause, those with specific stroke risks, such as pre-existing hypertension or migraine with aura, might be best served by transdermal rather than oral estrogen therapies.

Assess breast cancer risk

Breast cancer, from a woman's perspective, is a feared potential risk of MHT[30,31]; therefore, measures to quantify and clarify baseline risk will help direct choice of therapy while alleviating undue concerns. Breast cancer risk can be estimated using the National Cancer Institute (NCI)-Breast Cancer Risk Equation (http://www.cancer.gov/bcrisktool/) or the International Breast cancer Intervention Study risk calculator,[37] although neither method is ideal for assessing individual risk.[38] Elements of the patient's history, including one or more first-degree relatives with breast cancer, presence of susceptibility genes such as BRCA1 or BRCA2, and personal history of breast biopsy with atypia, are considered meaningful for risk quantification. Breast density, as reported on mammography reports, may be incorporated into future risk algorithms. Increased breast density renders mammograms difficult to interpret, and epidemiologic data support a link between increased breast density and breast cancer.[39] Moreover, some studies suggested that women with very dense breasts have a higher risk of breast cancer when using MHT.[40,41]

Personal breast cancer risk assessment also provides an opportunity, if women are found to be at elevated breast cancer risk, to discuss recommendations for use of the selective estrogen receptor modulators (SERMs), tamoxifen and raloxifene, and the aromatase inhibitor, exemestane, for breast cancer prevention (**Table 5**). The US Preventive Services Task Force recommends discussing preventive strategies in postmenopausal women with 5-year risk of 3% or higher, as calculated using the NCI breast cancer risk tool,[38] whereas the American Society of Clinical Oncologists recommends a discussion about chemoprevention with women who have a 5-year risk of 1.66% or more,[42] comparable with the enrollment criteria in the breast cancer prevention trials. As these chemopreventive agents can actually worsen VMS, nonhormonal prescription therapies such as selective serotonin reuptake inhibitors/serotonin and norepinephrine reuptake inhibitors or gabapentin should be considered for women with bothersome hot flushes who are deemed at an increased risk for breast cancer (see Menopause and Cancers by Mark H. Einstein, Nanci F. Levine, and Nicole S. Nevadunsky).

Table 5
Selective estrogen receptor modulators

Agent	Daily Dose (mg)	Approved Indications	Comments
Bazedoxifene[a] with CEE	20	Treatment of VMS	Alternative to progestogen for endometrial protection
	0.45	Prevention of osteoporosis	At 1 y, no increase of breast density
Ospemifene	60	Dyspareunia due to menopause	Systemic therapy also improves vaginal dryness and female sexual function; contraindications same as MHT
Raloxifene	60	Prevention and treatment of osteoporosis	Modest fracture benefit vs bisphosphonates. Prevents vertebral fractures; increases VMS
		Prevention of breast cancer	Marginally less effective than tamoxifen with better safety profile; no endometrial effects; increases VTE
Tamoxifen	20	Prevention of breast cancer	Reduces invasive ER + breast cancer > raloxifene
		Adjuvant breast cancer therapy	Increases VTE, endometrial cancer, cataracts

[a] Bazedoxifene is available as a single agent for osteoporosis prevention and treatment in some countries outside the United States with clinical effectiveness similar to raloxifene.

Consolidate benefit/risk assessment

As it can be daunting to conduct several risk assessments and then present findings succinctly to each patient, the North American Menopause Society (NAMS) has created an online application precisely for this purpose. *MenoPro* can be obtained free of charge from the Apple store. In 3 to 4 minutes, it provides a summary that can be given (e-mail or print) to the patient and includes links to NAMS' patient information materials.[35] This resource helps ensure a complete baseline evaluation of women considering MHT and provides information about options, dosing, and side effects.

Consider Lower Doses

Most current recommendations suggest starting treatment with approximately half the estrogen dose studied in the WHI (see **Table 4**). This practice seems reasonable and is consistent with the "lowest dose for the shortest time" adage suggested in the wake of the WHI. Several trials have shown that lower doses of estrogen improve VMS, but may not be as effective at completely eliminating symptoms.[43] Lower doses may also require longer duration of therapy for full benefit to manifest.[44] These limitations are acceptable for many women, especially when coupled with expectations (although not yet proven in RCT) for improved safety with the use of lower-dose MHT regimens. For those whose symptoms are not adequately treated with lower-dose formulations, MHT doses can be slowly (every few months) titrated upward until symptom relief is achieved.

Exceptions to the "lower dose, shortest time" approach include women with premature or early menopause whether due to surgical oophorectomy or primary ovarian insufficiency; younger women, and particularly those rendered surgically menopausal, require higher estrogen doses for symptom control.[21,24] Although discussed in detail elsewhere (see Surgical Menopause by Maria Rodriguez and Donna Shoupe), a straightforward approach is to consider starting MHT at a higher initial dose than would be used for the naturally and age-appropriate menopausal population (eg, 100 μg transdermal E_2 is an appropriate dose consideration for an otherwise healthy prematurely menopausal woman accustomed to higher endogenous E_2 levels). As these women age and approach the usual age of natural menopause, the MHT dose can be progressively reduced. The decision regarding duration of MHT use can be periodically reassessed at and beyond age 50.

The risk reduction potential with lowering of hormone dose in MHT regimens is recognized, but the magnitude of risk reduction using lower MHT doses is not entirely clear. In the Nurses' Health Study, CEE 0.3 mg daily did not increase stroke risk compared with CEE 0.625 mg, which was associated with a 1.5-fold increased risk.[45] In other observational studies, no differences by estrogen dose were noted in CVD outcomes.[46,47]

The 14-μg transdermal E_2 patch maintains E_2 levels within the normal postmenopausal range (<20 pg/mL), and in 2 trials of women older than age 60, during 2 years of therapy, spinal bone mineral density was observed to increase with this low-dose regimen.[48,49] In these and two 12-week trials conducted in younger women, ages 53 to 57, VMS improved,[49,50] as did vaginal symptoms[51,52] and signs.[52–54] Breast density did not increase with this ultra-low-dose E_2 regimen,[49,55] and although endometrial effects seemed minimal, clinical trial evidence was inadequate to reassure regarding long-term safety of unopposed estrogen even at this very low dose.[49,53]

Consider Transdermal Therapies

Although clinical trials with surrogate endpoints demonstrate that transdermal therapies are metabolically more benign (ie, less adverse effects on clotting parameters, blood pressure, triglycerides, C-reactive protein, and sex hormone and thyroid binding globulins) compared with oral estrogen therapies, no RCT with outcomes such as MI, stroke, or VTE have compared transdermal versus oral MHT therapies. Oral versus transdermal E_2 effects on surrogate CVD outcomes (CIMT and CAC) were compared in KEEPS; the trial results showed no difference by treatment (including placebo), but in retrospect, may have been underpowered.[9] Lower risk of MI with transdermal E_2 has been reported in one observational study.[47] Another study described a lower risk of stroke with transdermal E_2 at a dose less than or equal to 50 μg compared with higher doses or with oral therapy.[56]

Several observational studies suggest that transdermal E_2 may not increase VTE risk in contrast to oral estrogens, and that progesterone has a lower VTE risk than progestogens such as MPA.[4,21,57] Transdermal estrogen may be the preferred preparation for women at risk of VTE.[21,58] Whether concurrent statin therapy attenuates the increased VTE risk of oral MHT has been suggested by findings in one observational study,[59] but this has not been confirmed in an RCT.

Keep Progestogens in Perspective

The combined E + P arm of the WHI confirmed that daily CEE 0.625 mg in combination with daily MPA 2.5 mg prevented endometrial cancer during 5 years of MHT use, and during the 13-year cumulative follow-up period, endometrial cancer risk was significantly reduced.[12] In contrast, after more than 5 years of therapy, sequential regimens may be associated with a 2-fold increased risk of endometrial cancer.[4] Although micronized progesterone effectively prevented endometrial hyperplasia in the 3-year PEPI trial,[6] in observational studies beyond 5 years, micronized progesterone therapy was associated with a 2-fold increased endometrial cancer risk.[60] Whether this represents a compliance issue with progesterone therapy or effectiveness of the preparation has not been ascertained.

The endometrial protective benefit of MPA has been overshadowed by increased breast cancer risk that was evident during the intervention phase and persisted during the cumulative follow-up of the WHI.[12] Both the type of progestogen and the duration of exposure have been suggested to be of relevance for MHT-related breast cancer risk; breast cancer risk may be less with micronized progesterone than with MPA,[61] although data are limited, and at least in observational studies, long-term use of progesterone has also been associated with increased breast cancer risk.[61]

The overall findings from the WHI hormone trials of more benefit and less harm with CEE-alone, compared with the E + P regimen, have led clinicians to experiment with MHT regimens in an effort to reduce progestogen exposure without jeopardizing endometrial safety. The NAMS cautions, however, that evidence of endometrial safety is insufficient to recommend infrequent or long cycle progestin dosing regimens (ie, 12–14 days every 3–6 months), or routine use of vaginally administered progesterone formulations (although this was used in the ELITE trial but endometrial effects have not yet been published),[10] or use of low-dose estrogen without a progestogen.[24]

The levonorgestrel-releasing intrauterine system, a long-acting contraceptive strategy, is increasingly being used as an approach to ensure focal (endometrial) delivery of a potent progestin in menopausal women using systemic estrogen for symptom control. Although this approach has been shown to be effective and acceptable,[62–64] the levonorgestrel intrauterine system is not approved in the United States for use in postmenopausal women. Of note, the levornorgestrel intrauterine device (IUD) minimizes systemic progestogen absorption, but increased blood levels do occur, and an increase in breast cancer has been reported.[65]

Endometrial surveillance (annual endometrial ultrasound or biopsy) is recommended in those who elect not to use progestogens,[21,24] and for women being managed on long-cycle progestin regimens; prompt evaluation of any unanticipated vaginal bleeding must be considered regardless of MHT use, hormone dose, or regimen.[21,24]

Combination Therapy with Conjugated Equine Estrogens and Bazedoxifene

Some women do not tolerate progestogens and complain of mood disturbances, ongoing breast discomfort, or displeasure with vaginal bleeding. Risk for endometrial hyperplasia and endometrial cancer attributable to use of unopposed estrogen for symptom management is a real concern for estrogen users who are poorly compliant with recommended progestogen regimens due to progesterone or progestin related side effects.

In 2013, the FDA approved a combination formulation incorporating CEE 0.45 mg with a SERM, bazedoxifene (BZA) 20 mg, as an oral once per day regimen. A series of clinical trials (SMART [Selective estrogens, Menopause, And Response to Therapy] trials) have evaluated efficacy of CEE + BZA for relief of VMS, vaginal symptoms, and for bone preservation.[66,67] The CEE/BZA combination was superior to placebo and comparable to CEE 0.45 mg with MPA 1.5 mg for the relief of common menopausal symptoms. On measures of bone preservation, CEE/BZA was intermediate in effectiveness between placebo and the MHT comparator.[68] Overall, in symptomatic postmenopausal women with a uterus, the magnitude of benefit against common menopausal symptoms with CEE/BZA is similar to that seen with traditional oral MHT.

However, in contrast to traditional MHT, in trials up to 2 years in duration, CEE/BZA seems to have a neutral effect on the breast and protects against endometrial hyperplasia and endometrial cancer without causing bleeding; amenorrhea rate with CEE/BZA use over a period of 1 year was comparable to placebo without evidence of endometrial stimulation.[68] Although the safety profile of CEE/BZA has been reassuring, clinical trials thus far have not been adequately powered to fully assess the effects of this combination on risks of CHD, stroke, VTE, breast cancer, and fracture.

The CEE/BZA preparation seems best suited to women who prefer and are without contraindications to oral estrogen or SERM therapies, and those who wish to avoid symptomatic and potentially adverse effects of progestogen therapies.

Plan to Limit the Duration of Menopausal Hormone Therapy (with Some Caveats)

Current recommendations for duration of therapy are primarily based on the length of treatment in the WHI hormonal trials.[12] As such, recommendations for duration of E + P combination MHT are classified between 3 to 5 years to minimize breast cancer risk. For women with hysterectomy taking unopposed estrogen, a longer duration of ~7 years is reasonable, although in the WHI, stroke risk, while small, persisted.[12] As women age, baseline risks for CVD increase, such that risks of stroke, VTE, and CHD in response to MHT, at an acceptable level when therapy was initiated (ie, a time when the woman was younger), might later exceed the perceived benefit. For women with primary ovarian insufficiency or surgical menopause, continuation of treatment until the anticipated time of natural menopause is recommended (see Premature Menopause by Saioa Torrealday and Lubna Pal).

Caveats for extended use of MHT have been offered by several expert groups.[21,22,24] Extended use of MHT seems reasonable because recent observational studies inform that menopausal VMS may last a decade or even longer. According to NAMS, "Provided that the lowest effective dose is used, that the woman is well aware of the potential benefits and risks, and that there is clinical supervision, extending HT use for an individual woman's treatment goals is acceptable if in her own opinion, benefits for symptom relief outweigh risks."[24] NAMS also allows for extended use in a woman with established reduction in bone mass for whom alternate therapies are not appropriate or cause unacceptable side effects.[24] In their 2014 practice recommendations, American College of Obstetricians and Gynecology (ACOG) allows that MHT need not be arbitrarily discontinued in women at age 65 who need systemic therapy to manage VMS.[22] The 2015 Endocrine Society Clinical Guidelines also include provisions for extended therapy following adequate counseling.[21]

Recognize and Treat Genitourinary Symptoms of Menopause

An essential recommendation is to directly ask the patient about vaginal and urinary symptoms, because many women are embarrassed and reluctant to initiate this discussion.[27] In an effort to emphasize broader adverse effects of menopause beyond vaginal atrophy, new terminology, Genitourinary Syndrome of Menopause (GSM), has been introduced and is now preferred by many groups.[69]

Vaginal estrogen therapies
Low-dose vaginal estrogen therapy is effective for the treatment of vaginal symptoms with some evidence of additive benefit against recurrent urinary tract infections and dysuria.[26] Local vaginal therapy is likely associated with fewer risks than systemic MHT.[70]

Several vaginal preparations are available, including vaginal creams, tablets, and a silastic ring that releases E_2 locally over a 3-month period (see **Table 4**). Of these, the 10-μg E_2 tablet and the 7.5-μg vaginal ring result in the least amount of systemic estrogen absorption.[71] When low-dose vaginal estrogen therapies are used according to labeling, it is unlikely that endometrial stimulation will occur, and progestogen therapy is therefore not routinely recommended for women using only vaginal estrogen therapy.[21,26] Clinical trial safety data, however, are limited to 1 year of unopposed low-dose vaginal estrogen use, and any vaginal bleeding (even spotting) should be promptly reported and investigated. Cost, accessibility, and individual preferences should dictate the choice of treatment formulation for managing GSM.

Ospemifene therapy
Systemic SERM therapy is also available for treating dyspareunia due to menopause. Oral ospemifene, 60 mg daily, improves dyspareunia, vaginal dryness, and female sexual function.[72] In safety studies up to 1 year, vaginal bleeding was comparable to placebo, and endometrial thickness increased (-0.81 mm in placebo vs 0.07 mm with treatment [$P<.001$]), with one case of endometrial hyperplasia, and no endometrial cancers. Hemorrhagic stroke and DVT occurred at rates of 1.45 events per 1000 women. Contraindications are similar to those with oral estrogen therapies. Outcomes in women with breast cancer have not been evaluated. Ospemifene seems well suited for women who prefer oral therapy rather than vaginal estrogens, and who are without contraindications.

Revisiting the Decision to Continue Menopausal Hormone Therapy

Once a decision to initiate MHT for symptom control is made, one or more trials of dose titration may be required before identifying the lowest estrogen dose that effectively mitigates symptom burden. Changes in dosage and preparation may be necessary to adequately relieve symptoms and minimize side effects, such as breast tenderness, vaginal bleeding, weight gain, bloating, and headache. Once a patient has decided to continue with therapy and is taking a stable dose of MHT, recommended follow-up varies between 6 months and a year, depending on the patient's wishes and concurrent health concerns. During these visits, a few essential monitoring points should be addressed because changing clinical profile might necessitate treatment change (**Box 5**).

Box 5
Patient monitoring during menopausal hormone therapy administration

- Review efficacy of prescribed MHT, because intensity and frequency of VMS usually diminish with age, and dose reductions are possible.

- If symptoms worsen or do not improve on oral therapy, a trial of transdermal therapy is merited. If still not effective, it is reasonable to measure serum E_2 to assess absorption; remember to distinguish menopausal VMS from other rare causes of flushing and spells.

- Monitor breast symptoms and schedule annual mammography. Breast tenderness can improve with change in progestogen or reduction in estrogen dose. A change to the CEE/BZA combination might improve symptoms.

- Query about bleeding. Depending on the specific preparations, the schedule of MHT prescribed, and the time since menopause when therapy was initiated, bleeding often resolves by the end of the first year when the endometrium becomes atrophic.[73] Unscheduled bleeding thereafter should be promptly investigated to rule out uterine pathologic abnormality.

- Ask about vaginal symptoms and recurrent urinary tract infections, because these can develop years after menopause and despite low-dose systemic MHT.[26]

- Note emerging medical concerns, because development of new health issues may alter the advisability of continuing hormone therapy or merit a change in therapy.

- Review risks and benefits of prolonged ($\geq$5 years) therapy and discuss the patient's desire to continue (or stop) MHT.

What to Do After Stopping Menopausal Hormone Therapy?

Whether women using hormone therapy should stop MHT "cold turkey" or whether MHT cessation should follow a gradual taper off therapy is an individual choice because clinical trials have not shown one approach to be superior to another.[21] Depending on the duration of MHT use and coexisting medical concerns, monitoring after discontinuation of MHT is recommended (**Box 6**). If, after a few months, the patient finds her VMS to be intolerable, a discussion should follow regarding the risks of

---

Box 6
Points for follow-up after discontinuing systemic menopausal hormone therapy

- VMS might recur. In the WHI, VMS resumed in half of the women with baseline VMS after MHT was discontinued.[74] The patient will need to determine how bothersome her symptoms are and whether they need to be re-treated.

- Bone loss will resume when MHT is discontinued, although an increase in fractures was not demonstrated in the 13-y cumulative follow-up of the WHI.[12] Depending on the patient's age and risk for osteoporosis, bone mineral density measurement may be indicated as well as consideration of osteoporosis therapy.

- Breast cancer risk, with combined MHT in the WHI, persisted for at least 7 years after 5 years of combined MHT.[12] Continued surveillance with mammography seems prudent. Persistence of breast cancer risk has also been reported in observational studies.[61]

- Vaginal and urinary symptoms may begin or resume when systemic MHT is discontinued. Vaginal estrogen therapies can be initiated (or continued) regardless of age or duration of systemic therapies.

- Metabolic changes after discontinuation of oral MHT could include increase in fasting glucose, serum calcium, total and low-density lipoprotein cholesterol, and decreased thyroid stimulating hormone.[75]

restarting MHT or considering a nonhormonal prescription therapy for symptom relief (see Alternative Approaches to Menopause by Maida Taylor). Individual preference coupled with the patient's age and health status should be factored into the therapeutic decision.

SUMMARY

The past decade has witnessed an amazing progress in the understanding of MHT and in the choice of treatment modalities that are available to address the symptom burden of menopause. The art of menopause management lies in adopting a *tailored* approach to each individual patient's needs, mindful that menopausal symptom relief is just one segment along her path to healthy aging. Summary points include the following:

- Relief of vasomotor and vaginal symptoms remains the primary indication for hormone therapy.
  - Focus initiating MHT in younger women close in time to menopause when baseline risks are low.
  - Symptom relief can be achieved with lower doses but more time may be required to achieve effectiveness.
  - Type of hormone therapy and duration of use will be dictated by individual symptoms, risk profile, and personal preference.
  - The need for ongoing MHT should be revisited at least annually.
- Stay abreast of current research findings because much is yet to be learned.

REFERENCES

1. Isaacs D, Fitzgerald D. Seven alternatives to evidence-based medicine. Oncologist 2001;6:390–1.
2. Wilson RA. Feminine forever. New York; Philadelphia: M. Evans and Co., Inc; J.B. Lippincott Co; 1966.
3. Huss KS. Estrogen therapy (The book forum). JAMA 1966;197:196.
4. Santen RJ, Allred DC, Ardoin SP, et al. Postmenopausal hormone therapy. An endocrine society scientific statement. J Clin Endocrinol Metab 2010;95(Suppl 1):S1–66.
5. Grady D, Rubin SM, Petitti DB, et al. Hormone therapy to prevent disease and prolong life in postmenopausal women. Ann Intern Med 1992;117:1016–37.
6. Effects of estrogen or estrogen/progestin regimens on heart disease risk factors in postmenopausal women. The Postmenopausal Estrogen/Progestin Interventions (PEPI) Trial. The Writing Group for the PEPI Trial. JAMA 1995;273:199–208.
7. Rossouw JE, Anderson GL, Writing Group for the Women's Health Initiative, et al. Risks and benefits of estrogen plus progestin in healthy postmenopausal women. JAMA 2002;288:321–33.
8. Anderson GL, Limacher M, The Women's Health Initiative Steering Committee, et al. Effects of conjugated equine estrogen in postmenopausal women with hysterectomy. The Women's Health Initiative Randomized Controlled Trial. JAMA 2004;291:1701–12.
9. Harman SM, Black DM, Naftolin F, et al. Arterial imaging outcomes and cardiovascular risk factors in recently menopausal women. Ann Intern Med 2014;161: 249–60.
10. Hodis HN, Mack WJ, Shoupe D, et al. Testing the menopausal hormone therapy timing hypothesis: the Early versus Late Intervention Trial with Estradiol. American

Heart Association Annual Meeting. Abstract Oral Session, Number 13283. Chicago, Illinois, November 18, 2014.

11. Tsai SA, Stefanick ML, Stafford RS. Trends in menopausal hormone therapy use of US office-based physicians, 2000–2009. Menopause 2011;18:385–92.

12. Manson JE, Chlebowski RT, Stefanick ML, et al. Menopausal hormone therapy and health outcomes during the intervention and extended poststopping phases of the Women's Health Initiative randomized trials. JAMA 2013;310: 1353–68.

13. Rossouw JE, Prentice RL, Manson JE, et al. Postmenopausal hormone therapy and risk of cardiovascular disease by age and years since menopause. JAMA 2007;297:1465–77.

14. Manson JE, Allison MA, Rossouw JE, et al. Estrogen therapy and coronary artery calcium. N Engl J Med 2007;356:2591–602.

15. Chlebowski RT, Anderson GL, Gass M, et al. Estrogen plus progestin and breast cancer incidence and mortality in postmenopausal women. JAMA 2010;304: 1684–92.

16. Anderson GL, Chlebowski RT, Rossouw JE, et al. Prior hormone therapy and breast cancer risk in the Women's Health Initiative randomized trial of estrogen plus progestin. Maturitas 2006;55:103–15.

17. Prentice RL, Manson JE, Langer RD, et al. Benefits and risks of postmenopausal hormone therapy when it is initiated soon after menopause. Am J Epidemiol 2009; 170:12–23.

18. Anderson GL, Chlebowski RT, Aragaki AK, et al. Conjugated equine oestrogen and breast cancer incidence and mortality in postmenopausal women with hysterectomy: extended follow-up of the Women's Health Initiative randomised placebo-controlled trial. Lancet Oncol 2012;13:476–86.

19. Stuenkel CA, Gass ML, Manson JE, et al. A decade after the Women's Health Initiative—the experts do agree. J Clin Endocrinol Metab 2012;97:2617–8.

20. de Villiers TJ, Gass MLS, Haines CJ, et al. Global consensus statement on menopausal hormone therapy. Maturitas 2013;74:391–2.

21. Stuenkel CA, Davis SR, Gompel A, et al. Treatment of symptoms of the menopause: an Endocrine Society Clinical Practice Guideline. J Clin Endocrinol Metab, in press.

22. ACOG Practice Bulletin No. 141: management of menopausal symptoms. Obstet Gynecol 2014;123:202–16.

23. Reid R, Abramson BL, Blake J, et al. Managing menopause. J Obstet Gynaecol Can 2014;36:830–3.

24. North American Menopause Society. The 2012 hormone therapy position statement of: the North American Menopause Society. Menopause 2012;19:257–71.

25. Goodman NF, Cobin RH, Ginzburg SB, et al. American Association of Clinical Endocrinologists Medical Guidelines for Clinical Practice for the diagnosis and treatment of menopause. Endocr Pract 2011;17(Suppl 6):1–25.

26. Management of symptomatic vulvovaginal atrophy: 2013 position statement of The North American Menopause Society. Menopause 2013;20:888–902.

27. Sturdee DW, Panay N, on behalf of the International Menopause Society Writing Group. Recommendations for the management of postmenopausal vaginal atrophy. Climacteric 2010;13:509–22.

28. Moyer VA, On behalf of the U.S. Preventive Services Task Force. Menopausal hormone therapy for the primary prevention of chronic conditions: U.S. Preventive Services Task Force Recommendation Statement. Ann Intern Med 2013;158: 47–54.

29. Lobo RA, Davis SR, de Villiers TJ, et al. Prevention of diseases after menopause. Climacteric 2014;17:1–17.
30. Deeks A, Zoungas S, Teede H. Risk perception in women: a focus on menopause. Menopause 2008;15:304–9.
31. Kenemans P, van Unnik GA, Mijatovic V, et al. Perspectives in hormone replacement therapy. Maturitas 2001;38(Suppl 1):S41–8.
32. McBane SE, Borgelt LM, Barnes KN, et al. Use of compounded bioidentical hormone therapy in menopausal women: an opinion statement of the Women's Health Practice and Research Network of the American College of Clinical Pharmacy. Pharmacotherapy 2014;34:410–23.
33. Committee on Gynecologic Practice and the American Society for Reproductive Medicine Practice Committee. Committee opinion No. 532: compounded bioidentical menopausal hormone therapy. Obstet Gynecol 2012;120(2 Pt 1):411–5.
34. Goff DC, Lloyd-Jones DM, Bennett G, et al. 2013 ACC/AHA Guideline on the assessment of cardiovascular risk: a report of the American College of Cardiology/American Heart Association Task Force on Practice Guidelines. Circulation 2014;129:S49–57.
35. Manson JE, Ames JM, Shapiro M, et al. Algorithm and mobile app for menopausal symptom management and hormonal/non-hormonal therapy decision making: a clinical decision-support tool from The North American Menopause Society. Menopause 2015;22:247–53.
36. Bushnell C, McCullough LD, Awad IA, et al. Guidelines for the prevention of stroke in women. A statement for healthcare professionals from the American Heart Association/American Stroke Association. Stroke 2014;45:1545–88.
37. Amir E, Freedman OC, Seruga B, et al. Assessing women at high risk of breast cancer: a review of risk assessment models. J Natl Cancer Inst 2010;102:680–91.
38. Moyer VA, On behalf of the U.S. Preventive Services Task Force. Medications for risk reduction of primary breast cancer in women: U.S. Preventive Services Task Force Recommendation Statement. Ann Intern Med 2013;159:698–708.
39. Ursin G, Ma H, Wu AH, et al. Mammographic density and breast cancer in three ethnic groups. Cancer Epidemiol Biomarkers Prev 2003;12:332–8.
40. Kerlikowske K, Cook AJ, Buist DS, et al. Breast cancer risk by breast density, menopause, and postmenopausal hormone therapy use. J Clin Oncol 2010;28:3830–7.
41. Hou N, Hong S, Wang W, et al. Hormone replacement therapy and breast cancer: heterogeneous risks by race, weight, and breast density. J Natl Cancer Inst 2013;105:1365–72.
42. Visvanathan K, Hurley P, Banting E, et al. Use of pharmacologic interventions for breast cancer risk reduction: American Society of Clinical Oncology Clinical Practice Guideline. J Clin Oncol 2013;31:2942–62.
43. Utian WH, Shoupe D, Bachmann G, et al. Relief of vasomotor symptoms and vaginal atrophy with lower doses of conjugated equine estrogens and medroxyprogesterone acetate. Fertil Steril 2001;75:1065–79.
44. Hedrick RE, Ackerman RT, Koltun WD, et al. Transdermal estradiol gel 0.1% for the treatment of vasomotor symptoms in postmenopausal women. Menopause 2009;16:132–40.
45. Grodstein F, Manson JE, Stampfer MJ, et al. Postmenopausal hormone therapy and stroke: role of time since menopause and age at initiation of hormone therapy. Arch Intern Med 2008;168:861–6.
46. Shufelt CL, Merz CN, Prentice RL, et al. Hormone therapy dose, formulation, route of delivery, and risk of cardiovascular events in women: findings from the Women's Health Initiative Observational Study. Menopause 2014;21:260–6.

47. Lokkegaard E, Andreasen AH, Jacobsen RK, et al. Hormone therapy and risk of myocardial infarction: a national register study. Eur Heart J 2008;29: 2660–8.

48. Ettinger B, Ensrud KE, Wallace R, et al. Effects of ultralow-dose transdermal estradiol on bone mineral density: a randomized clinical trial. Obstet Gynecol 2004;104:443–51.

49. Schaefers M, Muysers C, Alexandersen P, et al. Effect of microdose transdermal 17beta-estradiol compared with raloxifene in the prevention of bone loss in healthy postmenopausal women: a 2-year, randomized, double-blind trial. Menopause 2009;16:559–65.

50. Bachmann GA, Schaefers M, Uddin A, et al. Lowest effective transdermal 17beta-estradiol dose for relief of hot flushes in postmenopausal women: a randomized controlled trial. Obstet Gynecol 2007;110:771–9.

51. Huang A, Yaffe K, Vittinghoff E, et al. The effect of ultralow-dose transdermal estradiol on sexual function in postmenopausal women. Am J Obstet Gynecol 2008;198:265.e1–7.

52. Bachmann GA, Schaefers M, Uddin A, et al. Microdose transdermal estrogen therapy for relief of vulvovaginal symptoms in postmenopausal women. Menopause 2009;16:877–82.

53. Johnson SR, Ettinger B, Macer JL, et al. Uterine and vaginal effects of unopposed ultralow-dose transdermal estradiol. Obstet Gynecol 2005;105:779–87.

54. Gupta P, Ozel B, Stanczyk F, et al. The effect of transdermal and vaginal estrogen therapy on markers of postmenopausal estrogen status. Menopause 2008;15: 94–7.

55. Grady D, Vittinghoff E, Lin F, et al. Effect of ultra-low-dose transdermal estradiol on breast density in postmenopausal women. Menopause 2007;14:391–6.

56. Renoux C, Dell'aniello S, Garbe E, et al. Transdermal and oral hormone replacement therapy and the risk of stroke: a nested case-control study. BMJ 2010;340: c2519.

57. Scarabin PY. Hormones and venous thromboembolism among postmenopausal women. Climacteric 2014;17(Suppl 2):34–7.

58. American College of Obstetricians and Gynecologists. ACOG committee opinion no. 556: postmenopausal estrogen therapy: route of administration and risk of venous thromboembolism. Obstet Gynecol 2013;121:887–90.

59. Fournier JP, Duijnhoven RG, Renoux C, et al. Concurrent use of statins and hormone therapy and risk of venous thromboembolism in postmenopausal women: a population-based case-control study. Menopause 2014;21:1023–6.

60. Fournier A, Dossus L, Mesrine S, et al. Risks of endometrial cancer associated with different hormone replacement therapies in the E3N cohort, 1992–2008. Am J Epidemiol 2014;180:508–17.

61. Fournier A, Mesrine S, Dossus L, et al. Risk of breast cancer after stopping menopausal hormone therapy in the E3N cohort. Breast Cancer Res Treat 2014;145: 535–43.

62. Wildemeersch D, Pylyser K, DeWever N, et al. Endometrial safety after 5 years of continuous combined transdermal estrogen and intrauterine levonorgestrel delivery for postmenopausal hormone substitution. Maturitas 2007;57:205–9.

63. Orbo A, Vereide A, Arnes M, et al. Levonorgestrel-impregnated intrauterine device as treatment for endometrial hyperplasia: a national multicentre randomised trial. BJOG 2014;121:477–86.

64. Morelli M, Di Cello A, Venturella R, et al. Efficacy of the levonorgestrel intrauterine system (LNG-IUS) in the prevention of the atypical endometrial hyperplasia and

endometrial cancer: retrospective data from selected obese menopausal symptomatic women. Gynecol Endocrinol 2013;29:156–9.

65. Soini T, Hurskainen R, Grenman S, et al. Cancer risk in women using the levonorgestrel-releasing intrauterine system in Finland. Obstet Gynecol 2014; 124:292–9.

66. Mirkin S, Pickar JH. Management of osteoporosis and menopausal symptoms: focus on bazedoxifene/conjugated estrogen combination. Int J Womens Health 2013;5:465–75.

67. Mirkin S, Komm BS. Tissue-selective estrogen complexes for postmenopausal women. Maturitas 2013;76:213–20.

68. Pinkerton JV, Harvey JA, Lindsay R, et al. Effects of bazedoxifene/conjugated estrogens on the endometrium and bone: a randomized trial. J Clin Endocrinol Metab 2014;99:E189–98.

69. Portman DJ, Gass JL. Vulvovaginal Atrophy Terminology Consensus Conference Panel. Genitourinary syndrome of menopause: new terminology for vulvovaginal atrophy from the International Society for the Study of Women's Sexual Health and the North American Menopause Society. Menopause 2014;21:1063–8.

70. Manson JE, Goldstein SR, Kagan R, et al. Why the product labeling for low-dose vaginal estrogen should be changed. Menopause 2014;21:911–6.

71. Santen R. Vaginal administration of estradiol: effects of dose, preparation and timing on plasma estradiol levels. Climacteric 2015;18(2):121–34.

72. Archer DF, Carr BR, Pinkerton JV, et al. Effects of ospemifene on the female reproductive and urinary tracts: translation from preclinical models into clinical evidence. Menopause 2014. [Epub ahead of print].

73. Archer DF, Dorin M, Lewis V, et al. Effects of lower doses of conjugated equine estrogens and medroxyprogesterone acetate on endometrial bleeding. Fertil Steril 2001;75:1080–7.

74. Ockene JK, Barad DH, Cochrane BB, et al. Symptom experience after discontinuing use of estrogen plus progestin. JAMA 2005;294:183–93.

75. Arafah BM. Increased need for thyroxine in women with hypothyroidism during estrogen therapy. N Engl J Med 2001;344:1743–9.

The Effect of Menopausal Hormone Therapies on Breast Cancer: Avoiding the Risk

Valerie A. Flores, MD[a], Hugh S. Taylor, MD[b],*

KEYWORDS

- Estrogens • Progestogen • Hormone therapy • Breast cancer • Menopause

KEY POINTS

- Menopause is often accompanied by significant symptoms that affect quality of life; concerns over breast cancer risk is the principle reason women may choose to avoid treatment.
- Data from prospective randomized trials confirm an increased risk of breast cancer associated with long term use of combined estrogen and progestin (P) hormone therapy.
- In contrast with the effects of combined estrogen and P, the risk of breast cancer was decreased after use of estrogen in the WHI estrogen alone trial.
- Progestogens, not E, seem to convey the risk of breast cancer; however, estrogen cannot be used alone in a woman with a uterus, given the known risks of long-term exposure.
- The recent addition of bazedoxifene combined with conjugated estrogen provides a progestin-free regimen that can be used in a woman with a uterus.

INTRODUCTION

Menopausal hormone therapy (MHT) is an effective treatment for menopausal symptoms, and based on observational studies demonstrating numerous beneficial effects, was popularized as a first-line approach to menopause management. MHT was found to be very effective in treating vasomotor symptoms and preventing osteoporosis.[1] It was also thought to reduce the risk of coronary heart disease.[1] These findings provided support for broadening the use of MHT in an effort to help prevent age-related deficits associated with loss of sex steroid hormones. Thus, MHT was heralded for use in the prevention of disease in postmenopausal women.[2] Although

The authors have nothing to disclose.
^a Women and Infants Hospital, Warren Alpert Medical School of Brown University, 222 Richmond Street, Providence, RI 02903, USA; ^b Department of Obstetrics, Gynecology and Reproductive Sciences, Yale University School of Medicine, 333 Cedar Street, New Haven, CT 06520, USA
* Corresponding author.
E-mail address: hugh.taylor@yale.edu

breast cancer has always been a risk associated with MHT, the effects of treatment on other life-threatening diseases, namely cardiovascular disease, were thought to outweigh the risk of breast cancer. However, randomized controlled trials (RCTs) demonstrated that MHT did not afford the positive benefits that had previously been predicted from observational studies.[1] On the contrary, in some instances, it was found to increase the risks for breast cancer, heart disease, and pulmonary embolism.[1] The Women's Health Initiative (WHI) Trial, in its landmark study findings in 2002, reversed many of the perceptions of positive health benefits of MHT that were seen in observational studies.[1,2] Briefly, the WHI hormone trials were RCTs of postmenopausal women aged 50 to 79 (average age, 63) designed to determine whether or not MHT (estrogen only, and estrogen plus progestin combination) prevented cardiovascular disease. A global index was designed to assess the risks and benefits of MHT with respect to coronary heart disease, breast cancer, stroke, pulmonary embolism, endometrial cancer, colorectal cancer, hip fracture, and death by other causes. The WHI trials looked at combination of conjugated equine estrogen (CEE) and medroxyprogesterone acetate (MPA; together referred to as EPT) use in postmenopausal women with an intact uterus, and conjugated estrogen therapy (ET) use in those with prior hysterectomy. In the WHI EPT arm, women were randomized to receive 0.625 mg/d of CEE plus 2.5 mg MPA or placebo, whereas CEE alone was compared with placebo in the ET trial.[1]

Although the WHI trials failed to demonstrate reduction in risk or coronary heart disease with use of MHT, with regard risk to the breast cancer, these trials yielded paradoxic and intriguing data. Long-term use of EPT was associated with an increased risk of breast cancer (hazard ratio [HR], 1.25; 95% CI, 1.07–1.46; $P = .004$)[3]; the risk, however, was reversed in women who had had a hysterectomy and were randomized to estrogen alone (HR, 0.82; 95% CI, 0.65–1.04).[4]

In this review, we specifically focus on the risk of breast cancer associated with MHT. Without the potential to extend life through reduction of cardiovascular disease, a risk/benefit analysis on the use of MHT is rendered substantially less favorable. The risk of breast cancer has become the greatest concern to women considering the use of MHT to avoid hot flashes. Breast cancer is the second leading cause of cancer death in women and the most commonly diagnosed cancer. The risk of a woman in the United States developing breast cancer over her lifetime is approximately 1 in 8. Most women have experienced breast cancer in their lives, either personally or through an afflicted relative or friend. It is thus important to address this prevalent concern and put patient perceived risks in perspective.

MENOPAUSAL HORMONE THERAPY IN CLINICAL TRIALS

Although there are many factors that influence a woman's risk of breast cancer, the role of MHT deserves special consideration. Although the absolute risk of breast cancer associated with use of MHT is quite small, a lack of appreciation of the distinction between absolute and relative risks has influenced both the public and prescribers.

In observational studies, inconsistent effects of estrogen alone or estrogen combined with a progestogen (P) were seen in postmenopausal women. In the largest observational study to date—the Million Women Study—it was found that estrogen plus P treatment increased postmenopausal women's risk of breast cancer; treatment with estrogen alone, as commonly undertaken in women who have had hysterectomies, increased this risk slightly, but far less than seen with combination therapy.[5] Current users of MHT were more likely than never users to develop breast cancer (adjusted relative risk [RR], 1.66; 95% CI, 1.58–1.75; $P<.0001$) and to die from it

(RR, 1.22; 95% CI, 1.00–1.48; P = .05). Past users of MHT were, however, not at an increased risk of disease.[5] The incidence of breast cancer was significantly increased with estrogen (RR, 1.30; 95% CI, 1.21–1.40; P<.0001) as well as with combination of estrogen plus P (RR, 2.00; 95% CI, 1.88–2.12; P<.0001).[5] In this study, the results did not vary significantly by the type of progestogen used or the route of administration. Time since menopause seemed to influence MHT-related breast cancer risk. Women starting MHT (whether estrogen alone or in combination with P) less than 5 years since menopause had a small increased risk of breast cancer (RR, 1.43 [95% CI, 1.36–1.49] in the estrogen alone group and 2.04 [95% CI, 1.97–2.12] in the EPT group) compared with women initiating MHT more than 5 years since menopause (RR, 1.05 [95% CI, 0.89–1.23] in the estrogen alone group and RR, 1.53 [95% CI, 1.38–1.69]). The risk of breast cancer declined to levels seen in never-users of MHT after cessation of treatment (RR, 1.00; 95% CI, 0.97–1.03).[6]

Similar to the Million Women Study, The Nurses' Health Study was a large, observational study conducted in the United States that linked long-term MHT use with breast cancer.[7] The risk of breast cancer was increased significantly among users of estrogen alone (RR, 1.32; 95% CI, 1.14–1.54) or of combination MHT (estrogen plus P; RR, 1.41; 95% CI, 1.15–1.74), compared with postmenopausal women who had never used MHT.[7]

The E3N French cohort, another observational study, found that risk of breast cancer was greatest among women using an estrogen in combination with synthetic progestogens, but not with use of natural progesterone.[8] Unlike the WHI ET arm, but similar to the Million Woman Study, the E3N French cohort study found an increased risk of breast cancer in estrogen alone users (the majority being estradiol (E2) rather than conjugated estrogen), although this risk was still lower compared with the substantially elevated risk seen with estrogen plus progestagen (ie, not including progesterone) treatment (RR, 1.29 [95% CI, 1.02–1.65] and RR, 1.69 [95% CI, 1.50- 1.91], respectively).[8]

Similarly, in the California Teachers Study, a prospective observational study, use of combination MHT with estrogen + P was associated with a greater increase in breast cancer risk (RR, 1.65; 95% CI, 1.48–1.84) when compared with estrogen use alone (RR, 1.17; 95% CI, 1.04–1.31), and when compared with those classified as never-hormone users (RR, 1). The type of estrogen and progestogen used among women were not specified.[9]

The Heart and Estrogen/Progestin Replacement Study (HERS) was a randomized, controlled study that assessed CEE plus MPA's effects on cardiovascular disease prevention.[10] In their follow-up observational study, HERS II, the effects of EPT on non-cardiovascular disease outcomes were also assessed. This follow-up study found no significantly increased risk of breast cancer, although the study was underpowered to evaluate this endpoint.[11]

Although observational studies assist in understanding relationships, a definitive conclusion as to cause and effect cannot be drawn from these studies. Thus, RCTs like the WHI Trials offer the best available insight into the role MHT plays in breast cancer risk.

Discrepancies in breast cancer outcomes, especially with ET use, between the WHI and observational trials may be owing to selection bias, confounding, or the type of hormones used. The use of CEE, a mixture of multiple estrogens—some with selective estrogen modulator (SERM)-like properties, in the WHI may have had distinct advantages to the breast. Last, because use of the combination of estrogen and P results in a greater risk of breast cancer than estrogen alone, further research has been aimed toward understanding the role that progestogens play in this risk. Data from RCTs are deemed more reliable compared with those accrued from observational studies given a potential for bias introduced by measurable and nonmeasurable confounders inherent to any observational study design. Results of the large WHI hormone trials thus offer high-quality evidence of the effect of MHT on breast cancer risk.

MAMMARY GLAND BIOLOGY AND BREAST CANCER

During normal mammary gland development, both E2 and progesterone are responsible for enhancing cellular division and promoting lobular–alveolar breast development.[12] The mammary epithelium expresses both estrogen and progesterone receptors, and progesterone is needed for proper breast development and differentiation.[13] Similarly in the adult, during the luteal phase of the menstrual cycle and during pregnancy, progesterone facilitates breast cell proliferation, migration, and invasion.[14] In normal breast cells, proliferation occurs via paracrine interactions—because dividing epithelial cells do not contain estrogen and progesterone receptors—relying on growth factors secreted by adjacent stromal cells, which do contain sex hormone receptors.[14] In the progression from normal breast development to carcinoma, it is postulated that there is a transition from paracrine to autocrine signaling, because neoplastic cells express estrogen and progesterone receptors.[14]

Previous studies have demonstrated that estrogen plus progestogen results in increased breast proliferation compared with what is seen with estrogen treatment alone.[15] This suggests that the progestogen component itself may contribute to the carcinogenic effect of sex steroids.[16] Progestogens exert their intracellular effect by modulating the transcription of various target genes. As such, it is hypothesized that progestogens alter the normal signaling pathways facilitating normal proliferation; however, with increased proliferation and DNA replication comes an increased potential for new mutations and subsequent malignant transformation.[16] The exact pathway by which progestogens affect breast cancer cell proliferation/progression to breast cancer has not been characterized fully; however, studies on human breast cancer cells, as well as animal models, have contributed to a better understanding of the effects of progestogen in the mammary glands.

BREAST CANCER CELLS: STUDIES IN VITRO

Because both the WHI hormone trials, as well as most observational studies, have clearly demonstrated an increased risk of breast cancer with combined EPT, understanding the mechanism by which this may occur is critical. Studies using breast cancer cell culture systems have demonstrated that the effects of progestogens in vitro are influenced by progestogen type, dose, and duration of exposure, as well as cell culture conditions. Research using human breast cells has demonstrated that progestogens differentially affect breast cell proliferative activity.[17] A study by Courtin and colleagues[18] analyzed the effects of E2 alone, E2 plus progesterone (P4), and E2 plus MPA on cellular proliferation and apoptosis in breast cancer cells, as well as normal human breast cells. Treatment with E2 alone in all cell types resulted in increased cell proliferation. In normal human breast cells, the addition of P4 blocked the proliferative effect of E2, and also resulted in an increased number of apoptotic cells. When normal cells were treated with E2 plus MPA however, there was little effect on cellular proliferation, and the number of apoptotic cells was decreased. In MCF-7 and T47-D breast cancer cell lines, MPA did not induce cellular proliferation and neither MPA nor P4 affected apoptosis in these cells.[18] Microarray studies revealed induction of different sets of genes in hormonally treated cells, compared with control cells. E2 plus MPA modified genes in a distinctly different pattern from E2 plus P4.

Sweeney and colleagues[19] found that MPA combined with E2 stimulated proliferation in long-term estrogen-deprived MCF-7 (MCF-7:5C) cells, whereas E2 alone resulted in cell death.

The progesterone receptor exists as 2 isoforms (PR-A and PR-B) and is present in the female reproductive tract, mammary glands, brain, and in some immune cells.[20] In addition, some progestogens can bind to other steroid receptors, including the glucocorticoid receptor (GR), as well as the androgen receptor (AR).[20] Progestogens exert their effect via interactions of steroid receptors with growth factors, oncogenes, and estrogen metabolizing enzymes.[21] Changes in the ratio of PR-A to PR-B are thought to be involved in the development of breast cancer.[20] The aberrant effects of progestogens in breast cancer pathogenesis may also be mediated by binding to steroid receptors other than PR, such as GR and/or AR. Sweeney and colleagues[19] identified a potential role for GR in breast cancer pathogenesis by studying MPAs effect on breast cancer cells as compared with that of dexamethasone and norethindrone acetate. Like dexamethasone, MPA blocked E2-induced apoptosis, allowing for continued proliferation of these cells. In addition, like dexamethasone, MPA blocked E2-induced genes related to apoptosis. Although this is not the first study to demonstrate MPA's function as a glucocorticoid,[21,22] it differs from others in implying that the increased proliferation of human breast cancer cells is mediated through MPA binding to the GR.

A role for the AR as a mediator of progestogens' carcinogenic effect was assessed in a study using an ex vivo culture system.[23] Breast explant tissue from postmenopausal women was cultured and exposed to MPA at concentrations similar to those seen in women taking an MPA-containing formulation of EPT. Although the normal physiologic role of AR signaling results in inhibition of breast cell proliferation,[24] this study found that in postmenopausal women MPA blocked the normal signaling effect of AR, preventing AR from inhibiting epithelial cell growth.[23]

Further support for the role of progestogens in breast cancer comes from studies analyzing the effects of progestogen on estrogen-metabolizing enzymes in breast cancer cells. Using T47-D and MCF-7 cells, Xu and colleagues[25] demonstrated that E2 plus MPA increased the expression of estrogen-activating enzymes—namely, aromatase, 17 β-hydroxysteroid dehydrogenase type 1, and sulfatase—but did not increase expression of the estrogen inactivating enzymes, 17 β-hydroxysteroid dehydrogenase type 2 and sulfotransferase. The increase in cellular expression of estrogen-activating enzymes with E2 plus MPA was greater than that seen when cells were treated with E2 alone. Interestingly, the increase in estrogen-activating enzymes was not associated with an increase in cell proliferation, although there was an increase in estrogen levels. It is known, however, that locally increased estrogen levels are seen in the breast cancer cell environment, and this high-estrogen environment facilitates cancer cell growth.[25] Thus, it is postulated that MPA may exert its carcinogenic effect via induction of a local hyperestrogenic state, rather than directly through cell proliferation.

PROGESTOGEN REGIMENS

The regimen of progestogen administration has also been suggested to influence breast cancer risk.[26] Analysis of the effects of combined continuous, versus a combined sequential regimen of E2 plus MPA in vitro demonstrated that estrogen-activating enzymes were stimulated by the continuous regimen, but not the sequential regimen.[25] Lyytinen and colleagues[27] found that sequential progestin use resulted in a trend toward a smaller increase in relative risk of breast cancer compared with continuous progestin use. Within the EPT arm of the WHI, more women in the treatment group reported breast pain. Although the association between breast pain and breast cancer is uncertain, more women who were ultimately diagnosed with breast cancer reported breast pain during EPT use,[28] and breast discomfort seems to be a marker of breast gland stimulation. An ancillary study of the Kronos Early Estrogen Prevention Study (KEEPs)—an RCT designed to assess route of estrogen administration on cardiovascular effects (with cyclic progesterone administered daily for 12 days)—found that breast pain did not differ between MHT and placebo groups. Whereas MPA was given continuously in the EPT WHI trial, progesterone was given cyclically in KEEPs, suggesting differential effects of progesterone regimen on breast cancer risk. However, one must exercise caution in extrapolating information solely from this ancillary study, because sample sizes were small; future studies will facilitate the understanding of the role progestogen type, and the timing of progestogen administration, play in influencing breast cancer risk.

BREAST CANCER IN ANIMAL MODELS

Studies in animal models have contributed further to our understanding of role of progestogens in breast cancer. The characteristic response of breast cells to progesterone is ductal side branching and alveolar budding.[14] Studies in ovariectomized mice have demonstrated that estrogen plus progestogen therapy results in significantly increased breast cell proliferation when compared with estrogen treatment alone.[29–31] It is well-known that mammary gland proliferation increases during the luteal phase, when progesterone levels are higher than the estrogen levels. In progesterone receptor knockout (PRKO) mice, estrogen plus progestogen treatment did not result in the lobular–alveolar changes characteristic of EPT, suggesting that PR signaling plays an important role in breast gland tumorigenesis.[32–35]

A randomized trial in adult, ovariectomized, female macaques was used to study the effects of progestogens on risk markers for breast cancer.[36] This primate model is ideal for studying hormonal effects on breast tissue, because they have greater than a 90% average genetic coding sequence identity to humans.[37,38] In addition, the steroid receptor response to sex hormone administration, and the development of neoplastic breast tissue in this model, is similar to what occurs in humans.[36] The postmenopausal animals received 1 of 4 treatment regimens, with doses reflecting commonly prescribed doses in MHT for postmenopausal women—placebo, E2 daily, E2 plus P4 daily, or E2 plus MPA daily. After 2 months of treatment, macaques given E2 plus MPA demonstrated a significant increase in proliferation of breast lobular and ductal cells compared with placebo; this proliferative activity was not seen with E2 plus P4 treatment.[36] There was also increased expression of proliferation markers Ki67 and cyclin B1 in the E2 plus MPA–treated monkeys, but not in the E2 plus P4 treatment group. In a follow-up study using this same animal model, Wood and colleagues[15] also demonstrated differences in gene expression profiles for a given progestogen treatment. Breast biopsies were collected after 2 months of treatment, and analyzed for differences in gene expression. Breast tissue exposed to E2 plus MPA demonstrated increased expression of genes in the ErbB proliferative pathway—epidermal growth factor (EGF) and transforming growth factor-α. Genes of the Jak/Stat signal transduction pathway, including c-MYC gene expression were also differentially expressed, with a 2.5-fold change in the E2 plus MPA treatment when compared with control ($P<.01$). cMYC induces signals for cell proliferation, and is known to be involved in tumorigenesis.[15] There were no effects on genes related to apoptosis (transforming growth factor-β pathway), or genes related to estrogen receptor activity (Trefoil 1, stanniocalcin, cyclin D) seen in any group of treated animals. Thus, rather than directly enhancing the mediated response of ER to increase breast cell proliferation, MPA may instead act via modulation of growth factor pathways. E2 plus MPA enhanced the effect of E2 on ErbB pathway–related genes, providing further support for the role of MPA in promoting breast cell proliferation through growth factor signaling mechanisms.[15]

The EGF receptor is present in normal epithelial cells, and is overexpressed in more than one-half of breast cancers.[39] It is postulated that EGF receptor contributes to tumorigenesis not only by increasing cellular proliferation, but also by increasing angiogenesis and promoting cell survival. In vitro studies on breast cancer cells have also demonstrated that PR may result in EGF receptor activation, suggesting that progestogens exert their carcinogenic effect via PR-mediated regulation of downstream growth factor pathways.[40,41]

Using a human–mouse model system, Liang and colleagues[42] analyzed the effects of progestogens on xenograft tumors. BT-474 breast cancer cells, which expressed PR and mutant p53, grown on a Matrigel substrate were used to create the tumors. These cells were then injected into nude mice, which had been pretreated with E2 before cancer cell transfer. The study found that in the presence of E2 alone, xenograft tumors underwent growth initially, followed by tumor regression. However, with administration of either progesterone or MPA, tumor regrowth ensued. The mechanism by which this occurs was felt to be related to expression of vascular endothelial growth factor (VEGF), mediated by PR. Support for the role of PR was further confirmed by addition of the PR antagonist mifepristone, which inhibited the proliferative capacity of tumor cells. VEGF has been implicated previously in tumor growth.[30,43] VEGF is proangiogenic, and promotes endothelial cell survival and proliferation.[44,45] An increased expression of VEGF in tumors after administration of progestogens suggests a progestogen-dependent regulatory mechanism. In MCF-7 cells that do not express mutant p53, there is no induction of VEGF expression and no associated growth of tumors in response to progestogens, which supports the hypothesis that acquisition of mutations predispose to breast cancer, with progestogens potentially acting on cells with existing mutations.[46] Interestingly, and in support of the ET arm of the WHI, although estrogen was needed initially to facilitate tumor growth, it did not enhance tumor growth over time but instead resulted in tumor regression, again suggesting that it is the progestogen component itself that is responsible for inducing breast tumorigenesis in vivo.[46]

Although these studies provide insight into the mechanisms involved in breast cancer acquisition, there are several differences exist in mammary development in murine models compared with humans; thus, results from such studies must be interpreted with caution. As mentioned, given the marked similarities between Macaque and human gene coding sequences, this primate serves as a more reliable model for studying the effects of MHT on breast cancer acquisition and risk.

BREAST CANCER AND THE WOMEN'S HEALTH INITIATIVE: POSTINTERVENTION CLINICAL DATA

After the initial results of the WHI Hormone Trials, the significantly increased risk of invasive breast cancer with EPT use was affirmed on long-term follow-up after the intervention was stopped.[47] Both intervention and postintervention follow-up in the EPT arm of the WHI demonstrated an increased risk of breast cancer and breast cancer mortality.[3] The intervention phase of the EPT ended in 2002, after a median of 5.6 years, owing to increased breast cancer risk and an unfavorable risk–benefit ratio.[1]

Extended follow-up continued through 2010, with a median postintervention follow-up of 8.2 years. The significantly increased risk of breast cancer incidence seen in the intervention phase remained significantly increased during the postintervention phase (HR, 1.27, 95% CI, 0.91–1.78).[1] In a sensitivity analysis adjusting for adherence, a significant difference in the HR slopes for the 2 study phases was found. There was a trend toward mitigation of breast cancer risk in EPT users in the postintervention phase (HR, 1.26; 95% CI, 0.73–2.20) compared with a hazard ratio of 1.62 (95% CI, 1.10–2.39) in the intervention phase.[48] In a sensitivity analysis adjusting for continued EPT use during the postintervention phase; however, ongoing EPT use had a higher association with breast cancer than was seen with EPT use in the intervention phase of the clinical trial (P<.001). Breast cancer mortality was greater in the EPT group compared with the placebo group (P = .049).[3] The breast tumors diagnosed in the postintervention phase were also larger than those seen in the placebo group (P = .03); however, there was no difference in receptors status based on EPT use.[3,48]

Chlebowski and colleagues[49] analyzed the effect of EPT on the ability of mammography and breast biopsy to detect breast cancer in the WHI EPT. There were significantly more abnormal mammograms in the EPT group compared with the placebo group. Interestingly, the number of breast cancers diagnosed by biopsy in the hormone group was less than that in the placebo group, despite the fact that breast cancers were not only increased in the EPT group, but also more cancers were diagnosed at a higher stage and were more likely to be lymph node positive. Women who began EPT within 5 years of menopause were at greater risk of breast cancer compared with women who were greater than 5 years since menopause; however, the risk did not attain significance and did not substantiate the gap hypothesis, which states there is a time frame at which administration of HRT would be most protective/beneficial, whereas administration past this optimum time frame may result in more harmful effects.[50] Subgroup analyses demonstrated no significant relationship in EPT and breast cancer incidence with respect to age, body mass index, or the Gail breast cancer risk assessment tool score.[49] Postmenopausal women aged 50 to 59 years in the hormone group were also found to have a shorter time to first biopsy and, overall, more biopsies after 5 years of EPT compared with placebo. After discontinuation of study medications, abnormal mammograms persisted for women in the EPT group for 1 year; however, postintervention data demonstrated that thereafter there were no differences.[3]

The intervention and postintervention WHI data highlight several important points. First, the increased risk in breast cancer is significant, and although it decreases over time, the risk persists even after discontinuation of hormone therapy.[51] In addition, although the absolute risk of death after breast cancer diagnosis in the EPT users was 2 per 10,000 women, caution and extensive counseling for women is important when considering long-term EPT use for relief of menopausal symptoms.[51]

An unanswered question regarding breast cancer and EPT is this: if cessation of EPT results in fewer breast cancer cases, where do the cancers go? More than 5 years are needed for a new breast cancer to be clinically detected. The time frame of the WHI is too brief to account for a new breast cancer arising de novo, and subsequently resolving within 1 year of MHT termination. A more plausible explanation is that EPT acts on a preexisting, subclinical breast cancer, spurring the initial growth of precancerous cells, which then slow or regresses after cessation of hormone therapy.[26,48] This explanation is further supported by the WHI data, demonstrating that there were no more in situ lesions in the EPT users compared with the placebo group, nor were there more new in situ lesions found upon discontinuation of EPT.[49] New cancers were not forming in response to EPT therapy.

The breast cancer data from the ET arm of the WHI trials are distinct from the EPT arm. Not only was use of estrogen alone not associated with an increased risk in breast cancer, but in contrast with the EPT data, ET data even suggested an element of risk reduction with use of estrogen alone (RR, 0.80; 95% CI, 0.62–1.04).[52] Age-specific comparisons also demonstrated fewer invasive breast cancers in the ET group compared with placebo in all age groups.[52] The intervention phase of the ET trial ended in 2004, after a median of 7.2 years of follow-up. The postintervention phase began shortly after the intervention phase was stopped, and continued through 2010. The decreased risk of breast cancer in the CEE group reached statistical significance in the postintervention phase.[53] In the postintervention phase of the WHI, women with prior hysterectomy were followed for 11.8 years. Users of CEE for a median of 5.9 years had a significantly decreased risk of developing breast cancer (HR, 0.77; 95% CI, 0.62–0.95).[53] Tumor receptor status, size, and nodal status were not different between ET users and placebo. Unlike the EPT postintervention phase, there was a significantly lesser mortality risk from breast cancer in the ET group compared with placebo (HR, 0.37; 95% CI, 0.13–0.91).[53] Despite both trials having an increased number of mammograms in participants randomized to receive hormone therapy, those in the ET group did not have a significant increase in mammographic abnormalities compared with placebo (5.4% vs 5.1%; $P = .53$) and the diagnostic utility of mammograms was not compromised significantly.[54] The specificity and negative predictive value of mammograms between the ET group and placebo group were comparable, except during the first 2 years of estrogen use, where the diagnostic performance of mammography was inferior to that seen in the placebo group. Estrogen use for 2 years did increase breast density compared with placebo to some degree, but did not affect interpretation of mammograms.[54] As such, there was no delay in breast cancer diagnosis in the CEE group. Although more biopsies were needed in the ET group to find tumors, when compared with the placebo group, a diagnosis of breast cancer was made in 8.9% and 15.8% of biopsies in the ET and placebo groups, respectively ($P = .04$).[54]

The use of ET for more than 5 years was safe, decreased breast cancer, and was associated with lower breast cancer mortality; these findings are in stark contrast with EPT use, which had an associated increased risk of breast cancer, delay in diagnosis, and increased breast cancer mortality.[3,53] As previously discussed, the progestin component itself is highly implicated, because cessation of EPT was associated with a decline in breast cancer, and the breast cancer rates for the placebo groups in both arms of the WHI were the same.[47,53]

The choice of CEE in the ET arm of the WHI may explain the favorable effects seen on the breast. CEE contains a mixture of multiple estrogens, and each estrogen type not only preferentially binds the 2 estrogen receptors, but may also exert differential actions depending on the target tissue.[55,56] Whereas E2 is the well-characterized estrogen, less is known about the many estrogenic components of CEE.[56] Unlike E2, these other estrogens differ in their B-ring saturation and in their chemical moieties at the 17 position.[55] In a study assessing the activity of an estrogenic compound with similarities to several estrogens in CEE (NCI 122–17 β-methyl-17α-dihydroequilenin), it was found that NCI 122, as well as 2 other equine estrogens, were estrogen agonists that binds both ER-α and -β, but are less potent estrogens than E2.[55] Despite their lower potency, NCI 122 and equine estrogens are able to exert transcriptional changes distinct from E2, which are postulated to account for the positive effects seen in several tissue types.[57–60] Bhavnani and colleagues[61] analyzed the effects of 11 equine estrogens (in CEE preparations) on the transcriptional activity of ER-α and -β, and found that many of the equine estrogens preferentially bind ER-β. ER-β activation can inhibit ER-α activity on cell proliferation.[62,63] This inhibition induced by equine estrogens may in part explain the decreased risk of breast cancer observed in the WHI ET study. Further support for beneficial SERM-like properties of CEE comes from work by Song and colleagues,[64] where the effects of CEE and E2 on breast cancer cells were compared. CEE and E2 were noted to have distinct effects on gene expression. Research by Berrodin and colleagues[65] also demonstrated that several estrogenic compounds in CEE act as partial estrogen agonists; thus, like SERMs, the differences in binding and downstream cell signaling may afford CEE with specific tissue manifestations that are unlike the purely stimulatory effects of E2.[64] Additional research identifying which equine estrogens exert more SERM-like properties is needed, because they cannot only be preferentially used in MHT, but perhaps may even be of benefit in the treatment of breast cancer.

TISSUE SELECTIVE ESTROGEN RECEPTOR COMPLEX AND BREAST CANCER

Whereas MHT is the most effective pharmacologic treatment for vasomotor symptoms, the risks that MHT imposes on cancers, including breast and endometrial cancer risk, cannot be ignored. Efficacious treatment options for addressing menopausal symptoms that do not inherently increase cancer risk are needed, and research and development efforts to identify such alternative options are ongoing. Recently, a SERM and CEE have been paired to form a tissue selective estrogen complex (TSEC). TSECs pair a SERM with an estrogen, ideally blending the effects of the SERM and estrogen in a way that is more favorable than treating with 1 form of therapy alone.[66–68] The first TSEC to be approved by the US Food and Drug Administration (FDA) pairs bazedoxifene (BZA), a SERM, with CEE. In the phase 3 Selective Estrogen Menopause and Response to Therapy (SMART) trials, enrolling postmenopausal women at risk for osteoporosis with a uterus, BZA/CEE improved hot flashes and prevented bone loss.[66,69] There were no associated adverse effects on the breast, uterus, or ovary. Importantly, given the anti-estrogen effects of BZA on the uterus, combined treatment with BZA and CEE does not require the addition of a progestin, thus likely reducing the probability of breast cancer risk that has been associated with EPT treatment.[68–70] Furthermore BZA neither stimulates breast cells nor increases mammographic breast density.[68,71,72] Data from the SMART trials were reassuring, with the incidence of breast cancer being comparable in the BZA/CEE and placebo groups, although these trials were underpowered to evaluate fully this end point.[72] Additional insight comes from an in vitro study assessing the effect of BZA/CEE on MCF-7 breast cancer cells.[64] BZA was found to block the effects of CEE on breast cancer cell proliferation, and blocked antiapoptotic effects of CEE. Furthermore, like tamoxifen and raloxifene, BZA used alone did not induce estrogen agonist effects on breast cancer cells.[64] Furthermore, in tamoxifen-resistant breast tumor xenografts, BZA was able to inhibit cancer cell growth.[73] BZA seems to have an effect of breast tissue that is similar or superior to other commonly used SERMs.

For menopausal women with a uterus, a TSEC offers theoretic advantage over traditional combined MHT because the risk of breast cancer is theoretically absent.

ALTERNATIVES TO TRADITIONAL MENOPAUSAL HORMONE THERAPY AND BREAST CANCER RISK

As their name implies, SERMs are compounds that are capable of exerting both agonist and antagonist effects on estrogen receptors, depending on their target tissue.[67,74] When bound to estrogen receptors in the breast, SERMs act as estrogen antagonists, inhibiting the stimulatory action of estrogen on breast tissue.[74] Tamoxifen and raloxifene were initially classified as anti-estrogens, given their effects on breast tissue; however, they were subsequently renamed SERMs once they were found to exert estrogenlike effects in bone and the endometrium.[75,76] Tamoxifen is used as an adjuvant treatment for breast cancer. It also reduces invasive breast cancer risk in women with ductal carcinoma in situ, and women at high risk of breast cancer.[77] Raloxifene also reduces breast cancer incidence and ductal carcinoma in situ.[78,79] Raloxifene is approved for treating and preventing osteoporosis as well as preventing breast cancer in postmenopausal women.[80] Tamoxifen and raloxifene, unlike estrogen, do not improve vasomotor symptoms, but instead can even cause worsening of vasomotor symptoms.[81–83] Although early SERMs were not developed for the purpose of treating menopausal symptoms, newer SERMs, such as ospemifene, have been developed with the intent of treating specific menopausal symptoms. Although oral ospemifene is fairly effective for the treatment of the genitourinary syndrome of menopause, it can exacerbate hot flushes.[68,84,85] There are currently no clinical data on the effects of ospemifene on breast cancer risk.

SUMMARY

Treatment with the combination of estrogen and P results in a greater risk of breast cancer than placebo. In contrast, not only does treatment with estrogen alone not increase the risk of breast cancer, but estrogen alone use by women who have had a hysterectomy may even result in a decreased risk of breast cancer. The 2 prevailing theories to explain the increased risk with combination MHT focus on estrogen and progesterone acting in concert to increase breast cancer risk, versus progesterone alone having carcinogenic properties. Given the rapid development of clinically apparent tumors and the lack of new in situ lesions seen with MHT use, it is logical to surmise the carcinogenic effect of progesterone to a mechanism that involves hormone actions on pre-existing, small lesions.[86,87] Variations in the various progestogens differing in their affinity for PR, GR, and AR, variability of progestogen component of different MHT regimens, and variability in the duration of progestogen use across MHT regimens may all modulate EPT's deleterious effects on breast tissue. Continued research using breast cancer cell culture systems and animal models will hopefully allow for an improved understanding of the interplay between estrogen and progestogens that predispose to adverse effects on breast tissue. The FDA-approved TSEC (BZA/conjugated estrogen) holds promise as a treatment option that will eliminate the increased risk of breast cancer by avoiding administration of a progestogen along with estrogen in symptomatic menopausal women with intact uteri. Caution over this hypothesized benefit is warranted until it is substantiated by data on the incidence of breast cancer in TSEC users.

REFERENCES

1. Manson JE, Chlebowski RT, Stefanick ML, et al. Menopausal hormone therapy and health outcomes during the intervention and extended poststopping phases of the Women's Health Initiative randomized trials. JAMA 2013;310(13):1353–68.
2. Grady D, Rubin SM, Petitti DB, et al. Hormone therapy to prevent disease and prolong life in postmenopausal women. Ann Intern Med 1992;117(12):1016–37.
3. Chlebowski RT, Anderson GL, Gass M, et al. Estrogen plus progestin and breast cancer incidence and mortality in postmenopausal women. JAMA 2010;304(15):1684–92.
4. Stefanick ML, Anderson GL, Margolis KL, et al. Effects of conjugated equine estrogens on breast cancer and mammography screening in postmenopausal women with hysterectomy. JAMA 2006;295(14):1647–57.

5. Beral V. Breast cancer and hormone-replacement therapy in the Million Women Study. Lancet 2003;362(9382):419–27.
6. Beral V, Reeves G, Bull D, et al. Breast cancer risk in relation to the interval between menopause and starting hormone therapy. J Natl Cancer Inst 2011; 103(4):296–305.
7. Colditz GA, Hankinson SE, Hunter DJ, et al. The use of estrogens and progestins and the risk of breast cancer in postmenopausal women. N Engl J Med 1995; 332(24):1589–93.
8. Fournier A, Berrino F, Clavel-Chapelon F. Unequal risks for breast cancer associated with different hormone replacement therapies: results from the E3N cohort study. Breast Cancer Res Treat 2008;107(1):103–11.
9. Saxena T, Lee E, Henderson KD, et al. Menopausal hormone therapy and subsequent risk of specific invasive breast cancer subtypes in the California Teachers Study. Cancer Epidemiol Biomarkers Prev 2010;19(9):2366–78.
10. Hulley S, Grady D, Bush T, et al. Randomized trial of estrogen plus progestin for secondary prevention of coronary heart disease in postmenopausal women. Heart and Estrogen/progestin Replacement Study (HERS) Research Group. JAMA 1998;280(7):605–13.
11. Hulley S, Furberg C, Barrett-Connor E, et al. Noncardiovascular disease outcomes during 6.8 years of hormone therapy: Heart and Estrogen/progestin Replacement Study follow-up (HERS II). JAMA 2002;288(1):58–66.
12. Kuhl H, Schneider HP. Progesterone–promoter or inhibitor of breast cancer. Climacteric 2013;16(Suppl 1):54–68.
13. Diaz J, Aranda E, Henriquez S, et al. Progesterone promotes focal adhesion formation and migration in breast cancer cells through induction of protease-activated receptor-1. J Endocrinol 2012;214(2):165–75.
14. Conneely OM, Jericevic BM, Lydon JP. Progesterone receptors in mammary gland development and tumorigenesis. J Mammary Gland Biol Neoplasia 2003;8(2):205–14.
15. Wood CE, Register TC, Cline JM. Transcriptional profiles of progestogen effects in the postmenopausal breast. Breast Cancer Res Treat 2009;114(2):233–42.
16. Hapgood JP, Africander D, Louw R, et al. Potency of progestogens used in hormonal therapy: toward understanding differential actions. J Steroid Biochem Mol Biol 2014;142:39–47.
17. Stanczyk FZ, Hapgood JP, Winer S, et al. Progestogens used in postmenopausal hormone therapy: differences in their pharmacological properties, intracellular actions, and clinical effects. Endocr Rev 2013;34(2):171–208.
18. Courtin A, Communal L, Vilasco M, et al. Glucocorticoid receptor activity discriminates between progesterone and medroxyprogesterone acetate effects in breast cells. Breast Cancer Res Treat 2012;131(1):49–63.
19. Sweeney EE, Fan P, Jordan VC. Molecular modulation of estrogen-induced apoptosis by synthetic progestins in hormone replacement therapy: an insight into the women's health initiative study. Cancer Res 2014;74(23):7060–8.
20. Conneely OM, Mulac-Jericevic B, DeMayo F, et al. Reproductive functions of progesterone receptors. Recent Prog Horm Res 2002;57:339–55.
21. Wan Y, Nordeen SK. Overlapping but distinct gene regulation profiles by glucocorticoids and progestins in human breast cancer cells. Mol Endocrinol 2002; 16(6):1204–14.
22. Africander D, Verhoog N, Hapgood JP. Molecular mechanisms of steroid receptor-mediated actions by synthetic progestins used in HRT and contraception. Steroids 2011;76(7):636–52.

23. Ochnik AM, Moore NL, Jankovic-Karasoulos T, et al. Antiandrogenic actions of medroxyprogesterone acetate on epithelial cells within normal human breast tissues cultured ex vivo. Menopause 2014;21(1):79–88.
24. Birrell SN, Bentel JM, Hickey TE, et al. Androgens induce divergent proliferative responses in human breast cancer cell lines. J Steroid Biochem Mol Biol 1995; 52(5):459–67.
25. Xu B, Kitawaki J, Koshiba H, et al. Differential effects of progestogens, by type and regimen, on estrogen-metabolizing enzymes in human breast cancer cells. Maturitas 2007;56(2):142–52.
26. Taylor HS, Manson JE. Update in hormone therapy use in menopause. J Clin Endocrinol Metab 2011;96(2):255–64.
27. Lyytinen H, Pukkala E, Ylikorkala O. Breast cancer risk in postmenopausal women using estradiol-progestogen therapy. Obstet Gynecol 2009;113(1):65–73.
28. Files JA, Miller VM, Cha SS, et al. Effects of different hormone therapies on breast pain in recently postmenopausal women: findings from the Mayo Clinic KEEPS breast pain ancillary study. J Womens Health (Larchmt) 2014;23(10): 801–5.
29. Raafat AM, Hofseth LJ, Haslam SZ. Proliferative effects of combination estrogen and progesterone replacement therapy on the normal postmenopausal mammary gland in a murine model. Am J Obstet Gynecol 2001;184(3):340–9.
30. Wang S, Counterman LJ, Haslam SZ. Progesterone action in normal mouse mammary gland. Endocrinology 1990;127(5):2183–9.
31. Said TK, Conneely OM, Medina D, et al. Progesterone, in addition to estrogen, induces cyclin D1 expression in the murine mammary epithelial cell, in vivo. Endocrinology 1997;138(9):3933–9.
32. Allan GF, Leng X, Tsai SY, et al. Hormone and antihormone induce distinct conformational changes which are central to steroid receptor activation. J Biol Chem 1992;267(27):19513–20.
33. Meyer ME, Quirin-Stricker C, Lerouge T, et al. A limiting factor mediates the differential activation of promoters by the human progesterone receptor isoforms. J Biol Chem 1992;267(15):10882–7.
34. Lydon JP, Ge G, Kittrell FS, et al. Murine mammary gland carcinogenesis is critically dependent on progesterone receptor function. Cancer Res 1999;59(17): 4276–84.
35. Kastner P, Krust A, Turcotte B, et al. Two distinct estrogen-regulated promoters generate transcripts encoding the two functionally different human progesterone receptor forms A and B. EMBO J 1990;9(5):1603–14.
36. Wood CE, Register TC, Lees CJ, et al. Effects of estradiol with micronized progesterone or medroxyprogesterone acetate on risk markers for breast cancer in postmenopausal monkeys. Breast Cancer Res Treat 2007;101(2):125–34.
37. Magness CL, Fellin PC, Thomas MJ, et al. Analysis of the Macaca mulatta transcriptome and the sequence divergence between Macaca and human. Genome Biol 2005;6(7):R60.
38. Gibbs RA, Rogers J, Katze MG, et al. Evolutionary and biomedical insights from the rhesus macaque genome. Science 2007;316(5822):222–34.
39. Carpenter G. The EGF receptor: a nexus for trafficking and signaling. Bioessays 2000;22(8):697–707.
40. Faivre EJ, Lange CA. Progesterone receptors upregulate Wnt-1 to induce epidermal growth factor receptor transactivation and c-Src-dependent sustained activation of Erk1/2 mitogen-activated protein kinase in breast cancer cells. Mol Cell Biol 2007;27(2):466–80.

41. Daniel AR, Qiu M, Faivre EJ, et al. Linkage of progestin and epidermal growth factor signaling: phosphorylation of progesterone receptors mediates transcriptional hypersensitivity and increased ligand-independent breast cancer cell growth. Steroids 2007;72(2):188–201.

42. Liang Y, Besch-Williford C, Brekken RA, et al. Progestin-dependent progression of human breast tumor xenografts: a novel model for evaluating antitumor therapeutics. Cancer Res 2007;67(20):9929–36.

43. Folkman J. Angiogenesis in cancer, vascular, rheumatoid and other disease. Nat Med 1995;1(1):27–31.

44. Liang Y, Hyder SM. Proliferation of endothelial and tumor epithelial cells by progestin-induced vascular endothelial growth factor from human breast cancer cells: paracrine and autocrine effects. Endocrinology 2005;146(8):3632–41.

45. Shibuya M, Claesson-Welsh L. Signal transduction by VEGF receptors in regulation of angiogenesis and lymphangiogenesis. Exp Cell Res 2006;312(5):549–60.

46. Liang Y, Wu J, Stancel GM, et al. p53-dependent inhibition of progestin-induced VEGF expression in human breast cancer cells. J Steroid Biochem Mol Biol 2005; 93(2–5):173–82.

47. Heiss G, Wallace R, Anderson GL, et al. Health risks and benefits 3 years after stopping randomized treatment with estrogen and progestin. JAMA 2008; 299(9):1036–45.

48. Chlebowski RT, Kuller LH, Prentice RL, et al. Breast cancer after use of estrogen plus progestin in postmenopausal women. N Engl J Med 2009;360(6):573–87.

49. Chlebowski RT, Anderson G, Pettinger M, et al. Estrogen plus progestin and breast cancer detection by means of mammography and breast biopsy. Arch Intern Med 2008;168(4):370–7 [quiz: 345].

50. Harman SM, Vittinghoff E, Brinton EA, et al. Timing and duration of menopausal hormone treatment may affect cardiovascular outcomes. Am J Med 2011;124: 199–205.

51. Chlebowski RT, Manson JE, Anderson GL, et al. Estrogen plus progestin and breast cancer incidence and mortality in the Women's Health Initiative Observational Study. J Natl Cancer Inst 2013;105(8):526–35.

52. LaCroix AZ, Chlebowski RT, Manson JE, et al. Health outcomes after stopping conjugated equine estrogens among postmenopausal women with prior hysterectomy: a randomized controlled trial. JAMA 2011;305(13):1305–14.

53. Anderson GL, Chlebowski RT, Aragaki AK, et al. Conjugated equine oestrogen and breast cancer incidence and mortality in postmenopausal women with hysterectomy: extended follow-up of the Women's Health Initiative randomised placebo-controlled trial. Lancet Oncol 2012;13(5):476–86.

54. Chlebowski RT, Anderson G, Manson JE, et al. Estrogen alone in postmenopausal women and breast cancer detection by means of mammography and breast biopsy. J Clin Oncol 2010;28(16):2690–7.

55. Hsieh RW, Rajan SS, Sharma SK, et al. Molecular characterization of a B-ring unsaturated estrogen: implications for conjugated equine estrogen components of premarin. Steroids 2008;73(1):59–68.

56. Heldring N, Pike A, Andersson S, et al. Estrogen receptors: how do they signal and what are their targets. Physiol Rev 2007;87(3):905–31.

57. Bhavnani BR, Cecutti A, Gerulath A, et al. Comparison of the antioxidant effects of equine estrogens, red wine components, vitamin E, and probucol on low-density lipoprotein oxidation in postmenopausal women. Menopause 2001;8(6):408–19.

58. Subbiah MT, Kessel B, Agrawal M, et al. Antioxidant potential of specific estrogens on lipid peroxidation. J Clin Endocrinol Metab 1993;77(4):1095–7.

59. Bhavnani BR, Berco M, Binkley J. Equine estrogens differentially prevent neuronal cell death induced by glutamate. J Soc Gynecol Investig 2003;10(5): 302–8.

60. Zhang Y, Lu X, Bhavnani BR. Equine estrogens differentially inhibit DNA fragmentation induced by glutamate in neuronal cells by modulation of regulatory proteins involved in programmed cell death. BMC Neurosci 2003;4:32.

61. Bhavnani BR, Tam SP, Lu X. Structure activity relationships and differential interactions and functional activity of various equine estrogens mediated via estrogen receptors (ERs) ERalpha and ERbeta. Endocrinology 2008;149(10):4857–70.

62. Lazennec G, Bresson D, Lucas A, et al. ER beta inhibits proliferation and invasion of breast cancer cells. Endocrinology 2001;142(9):4120–30.

63. Strom A, Hartman J, Foster JS, et al. Estrogen receptor beta inhibits 17beta-estradiol-stimulated proliferation of the breast cancer cell line T47D. Proc Natl Acad Sci U S A 2004;101(6):1566–71.

64. Song Y, Santen RJ, Wang JP, et al. Inhibitory effects of a bazedoxifene/conjugated equine estrogen combination on human breast cancer cells in vitro. Endocrinology 2013;154(2):656–65.

65. Berrodin TJ, Chang KC, Komm BS, et al. Differential biochemical and cellular actions of Premarin estrogens: distinct pharmacology of bazedoxifene-conjugated estrogens combination. Mol Endocrinol 2009;23(1):74–85.

66. Lobo RA, Pinkerton JV, Gass ML, et al. Evaluation of bazedoxifene/conjugated estrogens for the treatment of menopausal symptoms and effects on metabolic parameters and overall safety profile. Fertil Steril 2009;92(3):1025–38.

67. Taylor HS. Tissue selective estrogen complexes (TSECs) and the future of menopausal therapy. Reprod Sci 2013;20:118.

68. Santen RJ, Kagan R, Altomare CJ, et al. Current and evolving approaches to individualizing estrogen receptor-based therapy for menopausal women. J Clin Endocrinol Metab 2014;99(3):733–47.

69. Taylor HS, Ohleth K. Using bazedoxifene plus conjugated estrogens for treating postmenopausal women: a comprehensive review. Menopause 2012;19(4): 479–85.

70. Harvey JA, Pinkerton JV, Baracat EC, et al. Breast density changes in a randomized controlled trial evaluating bazedoxifene/conjugated estrogens. Menopause 2013;20(2):138–45.

71. Pinkerton JV, Harvey JA, Pan K, et al. Breast effects of bazedoxifene-conjugated estrogens: a randomized controlled trial. Obstet Gynecol 2013;121(5):959–68.

72. Pinkerton JV, Thomas S. Use of SERMs for treatment in postmenopausal women. J Steroid Biochem Mol Biol 2014;142:142–54.

73. Wardell SE, Nelson ER, Chao CA, et al. Bazedoxifene exhibits antiestrogenic activity in animal models of tamoxifen-resistant breast cancer: implications for treatment of advanced disease. Clin Cancer Res 2013;19(9):2420–31.

74. Riggs BL, Hartmann LC. Selective estrogen-receptor modulators – mechanisms of action and application to clinical practice. N Engl J Med 2003;348(7):618–29.

75. Love RR, Mazess RB, Barden HS, et al. Effects of tamoxifen on bone mineral density in postmenopausal women with breast cancer. N Engl J Med 1992;326(13): 852–6.

76. Kedar RP, Bourne TH, Powles TJ, et al. Effects of tamoxifen on uterus and ovaries of postmenopausal women in a randomised breast cancer prevention trial. Lancet 1994;343(8909):1318–21.

77. McDonnell DP. The Molecular Pharmacology of SERMs. Trends Endocrinol Metab 1999;10(8):301–11.

78. Cauley JA, Norton L, Lippman ME, et al. Continued breast cancer risk reduction in postmenopausal women treated with raloxifene: 4-year results from the MORE trial. Multiple outcomes of raloxifene evaluation. Breast Cancer Res Treat 2001; 65(2):125–34.

79. Vogel VG, Costantino JP, Wickerham DL, et al. Update of the National Surgical Adjuvant Breast and Bowel Project Study of Tamoxifen and Raloxifene (STAR) P-2 Trial: Preventing breast cancer. Cancer Prev Res (Phila) 2010;3(6):696–706.

80. Siris ES, Harris ST, Eastell R, et al. Skeletal effects of raloxifene after 8 years: results from the continuing outcomes relevant to Evista (CORE) study. J Bone Miner Res 2005;20(9):1514–24.

81. Stovall DW, Utian WH, Gass ML, et al. The effects of combined raloxifene and oral estrogen on vasomotor symptoms and endometrial safety. Menopause 2007;14(3 Pt 1):510–7.

82. Glusman JE, Huster WJ, Paul S. Raloxifene effects on vasomotor and other climacteric symptoms in postmenopausal women. Prim Care Update Ob Gyn 1998;5(4):166.

83. Davies GC, Huster WJ, Lu Y, et al. Adverse events reported by postmenopausal women in controlled trials with raloxifene. Obstet Gynecol 1999;93(4):558–65.

84. Portman DJ, Bachmann GA, Simon JA. Ospemifene, a novel selective estrogen receptor modulator for treating dyspareunia associated with postmenopausal vulvar and vaginal atrophy. Menopause 2013;20(6):623–30.

85. Kelly CM, Juurlink DN, Gomes T, et al. Selective serotonin reuptake inhibitors and breast cancer mortality in women receiving tamoxifen: a population based cohort study. BMJ 2010;340:c693.

86. Narod SA. Hormone replacement therapy and the risk of breast cancer. Nat Rev Clin Oncol 2011;8(11):669–76.

87. Horwitz KB, Sartorius CA. Progestins in hormone replacement therapies reactivate cancer stem cells in women with preexisting breast cancers: a hypothesis. J Clin Endocrinol Metab 2008;93(9):3295–8.

Menopause and Cancers

Mark H. Einstein, MD[a,b], Nanci F. Levine, MD[a],
Nicole S. Nevadunsky, MD[a,b],*

KEYWORDS

- Menopause • Cancer • Hormone replacement • Cancer screening
- Cancer prevention • Lifestyle modification

KEY POINTS

- Cancer is a disease of aging, and therefore is more prevalent after menopause.
- Preventive screening as informed by genetic and lifestyle risk, and lifestyle modification, may mitigate the risk of cancer and cancer mortality.
- Hormone replacement, though not contraindicated, is rarely prescribed to survivors of gynecologic malignancies despite potential benefits to quality of life.

INTRODUCTION

There are important changes in cancer risk after menopause occurs and, conversely, cancer treatment has implications for early menopause. Moreover, menopausal symptoms that are a result of cancer treatments are an important survivorship issue in cancer care. The goal of this article is to review the preventive strategies, utilization of health resources, and management of menopausal symptoms after cancer treatment. In general, cancer is a disease of aging. Seventy-seven percent of all cancers occur in people who are 55 years or older.[1] Although hormonal and metabolic changes that occur at the time of menopause may affect cancer risk, the predominant attributable risk for the development of cancer after menopause relates to the aging processes.[2,3] In developed regions of the world the cause of death for 20% to 25% of women is cancer, compared with 35% to 40% of deaths attributable to cardiopulmonary diseases.[4] One in 3 women will be diagnosed with a cancer during her lifetime,

The authors have nothing to disclose.
[a] Division of Gynecologic Oncology, Department of Obstetrics & Gynecology and Women's Health, Montefiore Medical Center, 1300 Morris Park Avenue, Bronx, NY 10461, USA;
[b] Albert Einstein Cancer Center, Albert Einstein College of Medicine, Bronx, 1300 Morris Park Avenue, NY 10461, USA
* Corresponding author. Department of Obstetrics, Gynecology and Women's Health, Montefiore Medical Center, Albert Einstein College of Medicine, 3332 Rochambeau Avenue, Bronx, NY 10467.
E-mail address: nnevadun@montefiore.org

Endocrinol Metab Clin N Am 44 (2015) 603–617
http://dx.doi.org/10.1016/j.ecl.2015.05.012   **endo.theclinics.com**

and current cancer survivorship of both women and men in the United States is estimated at 13.7 million people and is rapidly growing.[1] Cancer risk can be mitigated by lifestyle maintenance and modification in addition to preventive screening.[4] Genetic mutations and previous cancers may affect screening modalities and frequencies.[5] Women who have had cancer treatments, namely cytotoxic chemotherapy or radiation therapy, may undergo premature menopause.[6] Special considerations are needed for treatment and supportive care of menopausal symptoms in cancer survivors.[7–10]

INCIDENCE

In 2014 an estimated 810,320 women were diagnosed with a new cancer in the United States, and 275,710 women died of cancer.[1] For all disease sites, 265,140 women aged 45 and older compared with 10,570 women younger than 45 years died of cancer in the United States in 2014. The risk of developing invasive cancers increases exponentially after menopause, from 1 in 17 at age 50 to 59 to 1 in 10 at age 60 to 69, compared with 1 in 4 for women aged 70 years and older.[1] The most common sites of cancer diagnosis in the United States in 2014 were breast (29%), lung and bronchus (13%), colon and rectum (8%), uterine corpus (6%), thyroid (6%), non-Hodgkin lymphoma (4%), melanoma of the skin (4%), kidney and renal pelvis (3%), pancreas (3%), and leukemia (3%).[1] Estimated death distribution was lung (26%), breast (15%), colon and rectum (9%), pancreas (7%), ovary (5%), leukemia (4%), uterine corpus (3%), non-Hodgkin lymphoma (3%), liver and bile duct (3%), and brain and nervous system (2%). In 2014, lung cancer surpassed breast cancer as the leading cause of cancer death for women in economically developed regions of the world.[3] Breast cancer remains the leading cause of death among women in less developed countries.[4] The importance of this finding is a reflection on the intimate relationship between modifiable lifestyle risks, namely smoking, and cancer death. Incidence rates of cancers for women are twice as high in the developed regions; however, mortality rates are only 8% to 15% higher than those in low- and middle-income countries. The disparity in incidence and mortality rates likely reflects the detection and treatment of risk factors.[4]

COMMON CANCERS

Gynecologic malignancies are not the most common cancers found in perimenopausal and menopausal women. The most common, breast cancer, is discussed elsewhere in this issue. The diagnosis, screening, preventive measures, treatment, and implications for menopause and from menopause for lung/bronchus, colon, and rectum and other cancers are reviewed here. Although they are not the most common types, cancers of the female reproductive organs are discussed because of the intimate relationship between the hormonal milieu and diagnosis, treatment, and survival of these cancers.

Endometrial Cancer

Endometrial cancer is the most common cancer of the female reproductive tract.[1] The mean age of diagnosis in the United States is 61 years.[1] In developed regions of the world, endometrial cancer has an incidence of 12.9 per 100,000 women and a mortality rate of 2.4 per 100,000.[11] The most common histopathologic type of endometrial cancer is type I, or endometrioid adenocarcinoma; most of these endometrial cancers are highly curable, with 5-year survival rates for surgical extirpation alone being at the 96th percentile.[1] The explanation for the favorable prognosis of most endometrial cancers is that approximately 90% are diagnosed as stage I disease, before spread beyond the uterus. The harbinger of early diagnosis is abnormal vaginal bleeding or spotting. Type II, or nonendometrioid endometrial cancers, have poorer prognosis and are more commonly diagnosed in the nonwhite and Hispanic ethnic minorities.[12]

Risk factors for endometrial cancers are primarily related to long-term exposure to excess estrogen without progestin opposition.[13] Chronic estrogen exposure may be the result of exogenous hormone use, early menarche, late menopause, or obesity. Other risk factors include tamoxifen therapy, obesity, nulliparity, unopposed estrogen therapy, chronic anovulation, estrogen-secreting tumors (such as granulosa cell tumors), Lynch syndrome, Cowden syndrome, type II diabetes, hypertension, and a personal history of breast cancer.[13] These estrogens may be the result of exogenous hormone use, early menarche, late menopause, or obesity. Obesity is linked to estrogen by the aromatization of hormones in peripheral adipose tissue.[13] There is a linear relationship between younger age at development of endometrial cancer and obesity.[14] An association has been made between insulin resistance and some types of endometrial cancer, and data support improved survival for women with type II endometrial cancers who use metformin and statin therapy.[15,16] A minority of endometrial cancers (10% or less) are linked to genetic mutations and chromosomal abnormalities such as Lynch syndrome, which results from aberrations in the hMLH1, hMSH2, hMSH6, and PMS2 genes.[17,18] Use of oral contraceptive pills and progesterone-secreting intrauterine devices has been proved to be protective against the development of endometrial cancer.[19,20] Women who take hormone replacement therapy, and have their uterus, must take estrogen and progesterone to prevent endometrial hyperplasia and carcinoma.[21] Factors found to be protective for endometrial cancer include increasing parity, older age at last birth, smoking, and exercise.[22–25]

Approximately 75% to 95% of women with endometrial carcinoma present with abnormal uterine bleeding before diagnosis.[26] For most women who do not have a genetic predisposition, there is no effective cancer screening test. Women must have an evaluation if they present with vaginal bleeding, spotting, or staining after the cessation of menstruation for 1 year or more. Of these postmenopausal women, 5% to 15% will have endometrial hyperplasia and 3% to 20% will have endometrial carcinoma.[27] Pipelle evaluation should be undertaken in women aged 45 to menopause with abnormal uterine bleeding as defined by cycles less than 21 days, heavy volume (>80 mL), or intermenstrual bleeding.[28] Recommendations for women younger than 45 years include endometrial evaluation for those with persistent abnormal uterine bleeding, those with history or profile of unopposed estrogen exposure, such as obesity or anovulation, those failing medical management of bleeding, and in those for whom Lynch syndrome is diagnosed or suspected.[28] Women with Lynch syndrome should be screened every 1 to 2 years beginning at age 20 to 35 with endometrial biopsy and a record of menstrual calendar.[28]

Surgical staging for endometrial cancer includes total extrafascial hysterectomy, bilateral salpingo-oophorectomy, and pelvic and para-aortic lymph node dissection.[29] High-risk cancers, as defined by stage, grade, histology, myometrial invasion, lymphovascular space invasion, and patient age, may be treated after surgery with vaginal brachytherapy with or without whole pelvic irradiation.[30,31] Patients who are unwilling or medically unable to undergo surgery may be treated primarily with radiation therapy. High-risk patients may also benefit from chemotherapy and radiation.[32,33] For women who desire to maintain fertility, or who are not able to undergo surgery or radiation therapy for medical reasons, progesterone therapy may be attempted.[34]

As the prognosis for most endometrial cancers is favorable, issues regarding long-term survivorship and quality of life are very important. Despite high-quality evidence for surveillance after treatment, consensus-based guidelines from the United States National Comprehensive Cancer Network include pelvic examination every 3 to 6 months for 2 years and then every 6 months or yearly thereafter.[35] For menopausal survivors with low-grade and early-stage endometrial cancers, with intractable menopausal symptoms of hot flushing and vaginal dryness, local vaginal estrogen and low-dose hormone replacement therapy has not been associated with cancer recurrence or decreased survival.[36] Despite data from 8 randomized and 1 prospective study supporting that there is no harm from menopausal hormone replacement therapy for survivors of endometrial cancer, rates of patient adherence to estrogen therapy in this population are unknown.[37,38] However, it has been reported that only 15% to 48% of medical prescribers will give estrogen to survivors of endometrial and ovarian cancer.[39,40] Because of the associated relationship between obesity and the development of endometrial cancer, there have been clinical trials of diet and lifestyle modification for survivors. Results of the SUCCEED trial, which included a 6-month program of cognitive behavioral therapy and counseling to improve diet and exercise, demonstrated improvement in quality of life in the physical domain in the intervention group, as measured by the Functional Assessment of Cancer Therapy.[41]

Ovarian Cancer

Ovarian cancer is the most deadly gynecologic malignancy, and is the second most common gynecologic cancer in the United States.[42] It is the seventh most common and eighth most deadly cancer worldwide.[43] Ninety-five percent are of epithelial histologic subtypes, as opposed to germ cell or stromal tumors.[44] The average age for diagnosis of these cancers is 63 and the average of death is 71 years.[1] Most of these cancers are diagnosed after menopause (85%–90%). Even with advanced disease (stage 3) up to 80% of women will enter remission after primary therapy, although 25% of women with early-stage and 80% of women with advanced-stage disease will recur within 5 years.[45] Despite the aggressive nature of ovarian cancer, 5-year survival as high as 43% and 10-year survival rates as high as 33% have been reported.[46]

Ovarian cancer was once described as the "silent killer"; however, retrospectively queried patients often report new onset and persistent symptoms of bloating, urinary urgency or frequency, difficulty with eating, early satiety, and abdominal and pelvic pain as an antecedent phenomenon.[47,48] There is approximately a threefold increased risk for venous thromboembolism (VTE) in patients with ovarian cancer, and diagnosis often follows an initial VTE event. Indeed, screening for occult malignancy is suggested at the time of a VTE diagnosis.[49] A common presentation of ovarian cancer is the presence of a pelvic mass, found secondary to evaluation of pelvic pain or abnormality on physical examination, or incidentally during evaluation for a different medical concern.

Asymptomatic women at average risk for ovarian cancer should not undergo screening. Numerous trials, including prospective evaluation using multiple tumor markers for screening that generally include CA-125, have shown no evidence of mortality reduction, and increased harm resulting from unnecessary evaluation of numerous false-positive results.[50] The strongest risk factor for ovarian cancer is genetic predisposition, although these familial ovarian cancer syndromes only account for 5% to 10% of cases of ovarian cancer.[51] Hereditary cancer syndromes include Lynch II syndrome (hereditary nonpolyposis colorectal cancer [HNPCC]), which predisposes to cancers of the colon, breast, endometrium, and ovary, and breast-ovarian cancer syndrome (BRCA1 and BRCA2). The lifetime risk of ovarian cancer for women with Lynch syndrome is 3% to 14%, compared with 1.8% in the general population.[52] For women with BRCA1 and BRCA2 mutations, the lifetime risk for developing ovarian cancer is 35% to 45% and 15% to 25%, respectively.[53] Despite a lack of evidence showing benefit from randomized trials, the American College of Obstetricians and Gynecologists and the National Comprehensive Cancer Network (NCCN) recommend routine screening of women with BRCA mutations at age 30 to 35 years or 5 to 15 years before the earliest diagnosed family member with serum CA-125, and transvaginal ultrasonography every 6 to 12 months.[5] Risk-reducing surgery with bilateral salpingo-oophorectomy is recommended for women after age 35 up to 40 or when childbearing is complete.[5] Factors found to be protective for development of ovarian cancer included pregnancy, use of oral contraceptive pills, breastfeeding, tubal ligation, or hysterectomy. Factors associated with increased risk of ovarian cancer include infertility, endometriosis, and perimenopausal or postmenopausal hormone therapy. Despite reports to the contrary, there has been no prospectively identified association between fertility treatment and development of ovarian cancer.[6]

Ovarian cancer is a histopathologically diagnosed disease.[30] Tissue evaluation is usually confirmed at the time of surgical removal of pelvic mass and staging if frozen section indicates malignancy. However, some patients may not be able to tolerate surgery, and radiographic-assisted biopsy is necessary to confirm diagnosis.[54,55] Surgical resection of all grossly visible disease, if possible, and chemotherapy constitute the standard management approach to diagnosis of ovarian cancer. Following treatment, up to 25% and 80% of women with early-stage and late-stage disease, respectively, will recur.[45]

Despite the poor prognosis of many women diagnosed with ovarian cancer, it is estimated that in 2014 there were approximately 200,000 survivors in the United States alone.[56] The 4 main domains of concern for survivors can be classified as physical, emotional, spiritual, and social.[57] Fatigue, cognitive dysfunction, gastrointestinal complaints, loss of fertility, and sexual dysfunction are common problems reported in up to 50% of the survivors.[58,59] Anxiety, depression, and guilt are not uncommon, and up to 23% of patients decline to below the 25th percentile of social functioning.[60] Many women with ovarian cancer will become menopausal as a result of surgical and medical treatments.[8] Data do not show increased mortality or recurrence risk with menopausal hormonal therapy for survivors of ovarian cancer.[9,61] However, increased risk for ovarian cancer has been reported with long duration of the use of unopposed estrogen and estrogen plus progestin in menopausal women.[62] The benefits of lifestyle modification for survivors of ovarian cancer is not well defined; however, increased physical activity has been associated with lower depression and higher quality-of-life scores for women undergoing treatment with chemotherapy.[63] Increased physical activity and diet is currently being studied prospectively by the National Cancer Institute–sponsored NRG Oncology group.

Cervical Cancer

Cervical cancer is the fourth most common cancer in the world and the fourth most common cause of death for women worldwide.[3] More than 70% of cases occur in resource-poor countries and in countries that do not have organized screening programs for cervical cancer. It remains the second most common cancer and second most common cause of cancer death in women in low- and middle-income countries.[3] In the United States cervical cancer is the third most common gynecologic cancer and cause of death from gynecologic cancer.[42] The mean age for development of cervical cancer is 50 years.[1] Screening has resulted in a continuous decrease in the number of cases in regions were programs have been implemented.[3]

The most important risk factor for the development of cervical cancer is the human papillomavirus (HPV), which is found in 99.7% of cervical cancers.[64] Experts predict a decrease in new cases of cervical cancer related to HPV vaccination. In Australia, which has achieved a vaccination rate of greater than 70%, a 38% decreased incidence in high-grade dysplasia has already been observed.[65] Most of the risk factors related to cervical cancer are associated with risk of acquiring HPV, including early onset of sexual activity, multiple sexual partners, high-risk sexual partners (partner with known HPV infection), history of sexually transmitted infections (chlamydia, genital herpes), history of vaginal or vulvar squamous intraepithelial neoplasia or cancer, and immunosuppression (human immunodeficiency virus infection). Worldwide and in the United States, low socioeconomic status is associated with an increased risk for and increased mortality from cervical cancer.[66] There is also a higher incidence and mortality in the United States for Nonwhite in comparison with white women with cervical cancer.[67] Although there are no clearly defined genes associated with cervical cancer, studies of familial clustering have demonstrated that heritable risk factors contribute more to the development of cervical cancer then shared environmental risk factors.[68] Focus of these genetic risk factors has been on genetic alterations that inhibit clearance of the HPV virus.[68]

Although most early cervical cancers are asymptomatic, the most common presentation includes heavy or irregular vaginal bleeding and postcoital bleeding.[69] Critical to the diagnosis and prevention of cervical cancer is screening. Invasive cervical cancer is evaluated by clinical staging, and treatment can be surgery with or without adjuvant radiation therapy, radiation therapy, or concomitant chemoradiotherapy. Early stage is defined as a lesion less than 4 cm in size, and can be treated by radical surgery or concomitant chemoradiotherapy.[70] Side effects related to radical surgery, pelvic lymphadenectomy, and chemoradiotherapy include lower extremity lymphedema, which is reported as one of the most concerning symptoms for survivors of cervical cancer.[71–73] In women seeking fertility preservation, an attempt is often made to remove ovaries from the field of radiation to maintain ovarian function, the procedure being termed oophoropexy. Survivors should be followed every 3 months for the first 3 years, every 6 months from years 3 to 5, and yearly thereafter. Surveillance should include annual cytology; routine imaging is not necessary. Surveillance is recommended although not well studied, although the Society of Gynceologic Oncology recommendations include examination every 3 months for the first 24 months, then annually thereafter, in addition to an annual Papanicolaou smear.[35]

Long-term sequelae related to radical hysterectomy include sympathetic and parasympathetic denervation and resulting urinary urgency, frequency, incontinence, incomplete evacuation, and constipation. Women may also suffer from sexual dysfunction as a result of radical hysterectomy with upper vaginectomy, radiation therapy, or both.[74] Up to 60% of women treated with radiation therapy after radical surgery report that bowel symptoms are the most concerning.[73] Twenty-five percent of women with radical hysterectomy reported sexual dysfunction in one study, including decreased lubrication and vaginal length.[75] Comparing women with and without irradiation, irradiation had a stronger negative effect on menopausal symptoms and sexual activity, including hot flushes, vaginal dryness, difficulty in achieving sexual arousal, and sexual satisfaction.[74] Hormone therapy is not contraindicated in women with cervical cancer and should be considered for the treatment of menopausal symptoms.[75,76]

Vulvar and Vaginal Cancers

Vulvar cancer is the fourth most common gynecologic malignancy, with almost 5000 cases in the United States annually with 1000 attributable deaths.[42] The average age at diagnosis of vulvar cancer is 65 years.[1] Risk factors include cigarette smoking, vulvar dystrophy, intraepithelial neoplasia of the vulva or cervix, immune deficiency, HPV infection, northern European ancestry, and history of cervical cancer.[77,78] Signs and symptoms of vulvar cancer include a plaque, ulcer, or mass on the perineum, pruritus, bleeding, discharge, dysuria, and enlarged groin nodes.[79] Treatments include surgery, radiation, lymph node dissection, and chemotherapy as directed by clinical and surgicopathologic findings as per the International Federation of Gynecology and Obstetrics staging system.[80] These cancers may be particularly debilitating for patients because of the long-term sequelae of both cancers and their treatments on the external genitalia.[81]

Vaginal cancers occur much more infrequently, with a frequency of 1 in 100,000 women.[42] Postmenopausal women who present with vaginal bleeding, the primary clinical symptom associated with vaginal cancer, should be evaluated with cytology and colposcopy.[82] Treatment consists of surgery, chemotherapy, or radiation. It is estimated that 10% to 15% of women treated for vaginal cancer will develop complications including rectovaginal or vesicovaginal fistulas, radiation cystitis, and radiation proctitis.[82] Women who are sexually active should be counseled to continue to engage in intercourse after treatment, and if they are not sexually active they may require topical estrogen and vaginal dilator therapy.[82] As vaginal and vulvar cancers are not considered hormonally responsive cancers, estrogen replacement therapy is not contraindicated.[81] In rare instances the histologic subtype of vulvar cancer may be melanoma.[83] Although there are no data on vulvar melanoma specifically, retrospective cohort analysis of postmenopausal women with vulvar cancer showed a survival advantage associated with hormone use (hazard ratio [HR] 0.17, 95% confidence interval [CI] 0.05–0.62).[84]

Lung Cancer

Lung cancers are the second most common type of cancers and the leading cause of cancer deaths for women in developed regions of the world.[3] In comparison with breast cancer, it is estimated that twice as many women in the United States will die in 2015 from lung cancer than breast cancer (72,710 vs 40,290).[42] The average age at lung cancer diagnosis is 80 years. Eighty percent of cases of lung cancer in women are attributable to smoking.[85] Other risk factors include air pollution (nonventilated charcoal or wood burning stoves), radiation therapy, endocrine factors, and family history of lung cancer.[86–88] In the Women's Health Initiative there was a trend toward increased incidence of non–small cell lung cancer in women taking estrogen-progestin therapy verses placebo, and an increased number of deaths from lung cancer (0.11% vs 0.06%; HR 1.71, 95% CI 1.16–2.52).[89] Secondary to these data, it is suggested that women on hormone replacement therapy who develop lung cancer should discontinue hormone use.[89] Discontinuation of smoking is the most effective intervention. Guidelines for screening as developed by the NCCN support low-dose computed tomography scans for identified high-risk groups and no screening for low-to-moderate risk and low-risk individuals.[90]

Colon Cancer

The lifetime risk for colorectal cancer in the United States is approximately 5%, with 90% of cases occurring after the age of 50 years.[3] The incidence of colon cancer is 25% higher in men than in women. The death rate in the United States has been declining since the 1980s, and at present data from the Surveillance, Epidemiology, and End Results reporting program suggest a median 5-year survival of 61% for all colorectal cancers at 5 years.[91] Familial colorectal cancer syndromes including familial adenomatous polyposis and HNPCC contribute to approximately 5% of cases of colorectal cancer.[92–94] Up to 3% of patients with a personal history of colorectal cancer or adenomatous polyps are at risk for development of colon cancer in the first 5 postoperative years.[95] There is a 2-fold increased cancer risk for patients with one first-degree relative with colorectal cancer, and even greater risk if there are 2 relatives younger than 50 years.[92] The American Cancer Society recommends early colonoscopic surveillance at age 40 or 10 years earlier than the youngest family member who developed adenomatous polyps.[96] Additional nonmodifiable risk factors that lower the recommended age of screening include ulcerative colitis, Crohn disease, abdominal irradiation, nonwhite race, acromegaly, and renal transplantation.[97] Risk factors that do not lower the age of recommended screening include diabetes and insulin resistance, cholecystectomy, alcohol, and obesity.[97]

Several lifestyle factors have been associated with decreased colorectal cancer, including physical activity, dietary modification, aspirin or nonsteroidal anti-inflammatory drug (NSAID) use, and hormone replacement therapy in postmenopausal women.[98] However, none of these factors change screening recommendations. Up to a 27% decreased risk of colorectal cancer has been shown in a meta-analysis of 21 studies of lifestyle modifications (relative risk 0.73, 95% CI 0.66–0.81).[99,100] Decreased risk colorectal cancer with dietary lifestyle modification is less well defined, although a meta-analysis of 19 cohort studies suggests a threshold level of protection associated with more than 100 g/d of fruits and vegetables.[101] Some studies also suggest that diets with decreased red meat, cholesterol, and animal fat are protective.[101–103] The role of fiber in protecting against colorectal cancer is controversial. A 20% to 40% decreased risk of colorectal cancer has been reported with regular use of aspirin and NSAIDs.[104]

PREMATURE MENOPAUSE AND CANCER

Premature menopause is a recognized consequence of cancer diagnosis and subsequent treatment. Cytotoxic chemotherapeutic agents may damage the ovarian follicles, the oocytes, and the endocrine cells (ovarian granulosa and theca cells), which produce estrogen and progesterone.[105] The degree of infertility and premature menopause consequent to chemotherapy depends on the cytotoxic chemotherapeutic agent.[106] Alkylating agents have an incidence of ovarian failure of up to 70%.[107] Commonly used alkylating agents include cyclophosphamide, chlorambucil, and melphalan. Ovarian failure has been extensively studied in breast cancer, and persistent amenorrhea has been reported in a wide range of 30% to 70%.[108] Twenty-four percent of premenopausal women treated with FOLFOX (5-fluorouracil, leucovorin, and oxaliplatin) for stage 2 and 3 colorectal cancers experience persistent amenorrhea.[109] Cumulative nonsurgical premature menopause risk in survivors of childhood cancers is 8%. These women have been reported to experience more infertility than siblings, and are less likely to be prescribed medications for infertility.[110] Options for preservation of hormonal and reproductive ovarian function include treatment with a gonadotropin-releasing hormone agonist during chemotherapy, embryo cryopreservation, oocyte cryopreservation, and ovarian tissue cryopreservation.[105] These options should be offered to all women of reproductive age who will be offered chemotherapy and who have a high risk of premature ovarian failure. Important considerations also include prevention of menopausal bone loss through an increase in weight-bearing exercise, calcium, and vitamin D supplementation.

SEXUAL DYSFUNCTION

Sexual dysfunction is common among cancer survivors, with as many as 40% of women cancer survivors having sexual complaints.[111] The American Psychiatric Association defines sexual disorders as: (1) sexual interest/arousal, (2) orgasmic, and (3) genitopelvic pain/penetration.[112] Mechanisms of sexual dysfunction include hypoestrogenism, altered anatomy, mucosal alterations, vaginal obstruction, and psychological impact of cancer diagnosis and treatment. Bilateral oophorectomy in premenopausal women can result in physical and hormonal changes, and the impact of bilateral salpingo-oophorectomy on postmenopausal women is controversial. Chemotherapy itself is also a risk factor for sexual dysfunction in cancer survivors.[113]

FUTURE DIRECTIONS

Because of the increased life expectancy of the world's population, cancer incidence is increasing. However, cancer survival is also increasing because of improvements in early detection and treatment. Improved education to help women identify personal health changes that may be signs of cancer in addition to lifestyle modifications to mitigate cancer risk may reduce morbidity and mortality. Further research is needed to characterize the impact of cancer on menopausal symptoms including sexual dysfunction, and the influence of menopausal symptoms or treatments on cancer therapies and survivors' quality of life. Judicious utilization of hormone replacement therapy is not contraindicated for menopausal cancer survivors and may significantly improve their quality of life.

REFERENCES

1. American Cancer Society. Cancer facts and figures 2014. Atlanta (GA): American Cancer Society; 2014.
2. Gunter M, Hoover D, Yu H, et al. Insulin, insulin-like growth factor-I, and risk of breast cancer in postmenopausal women. J Natl Cancer Inst 2009;101(1): 48–60.
3. Torre L, Bray F, Siegel R, et al. Global cancer statistics. CA Cancer J Clin 2015; 65:87–108.
4. Gompel A, Baber R, Villers T, et al. Oncology in midlife and beyond. Climacteric 2013;16:522–35.
5. American College of Obstetricians and Gynecologists, ACOG Committee on Practice Bulletins—Gynecology, ACOG Committee on Genetics, Society of Gynecologic Oncologists. ACOG Practice Bulletin No. 103. Hereditary breast and ovarian cancer syndrome. Obstet Gynecol 2009;113:957.
6. Bristow R, Karlan B. Ovulation induction, infertility and ovarian cancer risk. Fertil Steril 1996;66:499.
7. Siris E, Leventhal B, Vaitukaitis J. Effects of childhood leukemia and chemotherapy n puberty and reproductive function in girls. N Engl J Med 1976;294: 1143.
8. Mascarenhas C, Lambe M, Bellocco R, et al. Use of hormone replacement therapy before and after ovarian cancer diagnosis and ovarian cancer survival. Int J Cancer 2006;119:2907.
9. Eeles R, Ran S, Wiltshaw E, et al. Hormone replacement therapy and survival after surgery for ovarian cancer. BMJ 1991;302:259.

10. Ursic-Vrscaj M, Bebar S, Zakelj M. Hormone replacement therapy after invasive ovarian serous cystadenocarcinoma treatment: the effect on survival. Menopause 2001;8:70.

11. Jemal A, Bray F, Cnetr M, et al. Global cancer statistics. CA Cancer J Clin 2011; 61:69.

12. Smotkin D, Nevadunsky N, Harris K, et al. Histopathologic differences account for racial disparity in uterine cancer survival. Gynecol Oncol 2012;127(3):616–9.

13. Brinton L, Berman M, Mortel R, et al. Reproductive menstrual and medical risk factors for endometrial cancer: results form a case-control study. Am J Obstet Gynecol 1992;167:1317.

14. Nevadunsky N, Van Arsdale A, Strickler H, et al. Obesity and age at diagnosis of endometrial cancer. Obstet Gynecol 2014;124(2):300–6.

15. Nevadunsky N, Van Arsdale A, Strickler H, et al. Metformin use and endometrial cancer survival. Gynecol Oncol 2014;132(1):236–40.

16. Soliman P, Wu D, Tortolero-Luna G, et al. Association between adiponectin, insulin resistance, and endometrial cancer. Cancer 2006;106:2376.

17. Sandels L, Shulman L, Elias S, et al. Endometrial adenocarcinoma: genetic analysis suggesting heritable site-specific uterine cancer. Gynecol Oncol 1992;47:16720.

18. Win A, Reece J, Ryan S. Family history and risk of endometrial cancer: a systematic review and meta-analysis. Obstet Gynecol 2015;125:89.

19. Vesey M, Painter R. Oral contraceptive use and cancer. Findings in a large cohort study, 1968-2004. Br J Cancer 2006;95:385.

20. Soini T, Hurskainen R, Grenman S, et al. Cancer risk in women using the levonorgestrel-releasing intrauterine system in Finland. Obstet Gynecol 2014; 124:292.

21. Anderson G, Judd H, Kaunitz A, et al. Effects of estrogen plus progestin on gynecologic cancers and associated diagnostic procedures: the Women's Health Initiative randomized trial. JAMA 2003;290:1739.

22. McPherson C, Sellers T, Potter J, et al. Reproductive factors and risk of endometrial cancer. The Iowa Women's Health Study. Am J Epidemiol 1996;143:1195.

23. Zhou B, Yang L, Sun Q, et al. Cigarette smoking and risk of endometrial cancer: a meta-analysis. Am J Med 2008;121:501.

24. Setiawan V, Pike M, Karageorgi S, et al. Age at last birth in relation to risk of endometrial cancer: pooled analysis in the epidemiology of endometrial cancer consortium. Am J Epidemiol 2012;176:269.

25. Moore S, Gierach G, Schatzkin A, et al. Physical activity, sedentary behaviors, and the prevention of endometrial cancer. Br J Cancer 2010;103:933.

26. Seerbacher V, Schmid M, Polterauer S, et al. The presence of postmenopausal bleeding as a prognostic parameter in patients with endometrial cancer: a retrospective multi-center study. BMC Cancer 2009;9:460.

27. Espindola D, Kennedy K, Fischer E. Management of abnormal uterine bleeding and the pathology of endometrial hyperplasia. Obstet Gynecol Clin North Am 2007;34:717.

28. American College of Obstetricians and Gynecologists, ACOG Committee on Practice Bulletins—Gynecology, ACOG Committee on Genetics, Society of Gynecologic Oncologists. ACOG Practice Bulletin No. 147. Lynch Syndrome. Obstet Gynecol 2014;124(5):1042–54.

29. Pecorelli S. Revised FIGO staging for carcinoma of the vulva, cervix and endometrium. Int J Gynaecol Obstet 2000;70:209.

30. Creutzberg C, van Putten W, Koper P, et al. Surgery and postoperative radiotherapy versus surgery alone for patient s with stage -1 endometrial carcinoma: mulicentre randomized trial. PORTEC Study Group. Post Operative Radiation Therapy in Endometrial Carcinoma. Lancet 2000;335:1404.
31. Keys H, Roberts J, Brunetto V, et al. A phase III trial of surgery with or without adjunctive external pelvic radiation therapy in intermediate risk endometrial adenocarcinoma: A Gynecologic Oncology Group study. Gynecol Oncol 2004;921:744.
32. Einstein M, Klobocista M, Hou JY, et al. Phase II trial of adjuvant pelvic radiation "sandwiched" between ifosfamide or ifosfamide plus cisplatin in women with uterine carcinosarcoma. Gynecol Oncol 2012;124(1):126–30.
33. Einstein M, Frimer M, Kuo D, et al. Phase II trial of adjuvant pelvic radiation "sandwiched" between combination paclitaxel and carboplatin in women with uterine papillary serous carcinoma. Gynecol Oncol 2012;124(1):21–5.
34. Gunderson C, Fander A, Carson K, et al. Oncologic and reproductive outcomes with progestin therapy in women with endometrial hyperplasia and grade 1 adenocarcinoma: a systematic review. Gynecol Oncol 2012;125:477.
35. Salani R, Backes F, Fung M, et al. Posttreatment surveillance and diagnosis of recurrence in women with gynecologic malignancies: Society of Gynecologic Oncologists recommendations. Am J Obstet Gynecol 2011;204:466.
36. Shim S, Lee S, Kim S. Effects of hormone replacement therapy on the rate of recurrence n endometrial cancer survivors: a meta-analysis. Eur J Cancer 2014;50:1628–37.
37. Guidozzi F, Daponte A. Estrogen replacement therapy for ovarian carcinoma survivors: a randomized controlled trial. Cancer 1999;86:1013–8.
38. Ibeanu O, Modesitt S, Ducie J, et al. Hormone replacement therapy in gynecologic cancer survivors: why not? Gynecol Oncol 2011;12(2):447–54.
39. Hancke K, Foeldi M, Zahradnik H, et al. Estrogen replacement therapy after endometrial cancer: a survey of physicians' prescribing practice. Climacteric 2010;13:271–7.
40. Vavillis D, Tsolakidis D, Goulis D, et al. Hormonal replacement therapy in ovarian cancer survivors: a survey among obstetricians-gynaecologists. Eur J Gynaecol Oncol 2011;32:81–93.
41. McCarrol M, Armbruster S, Frasure H, et al. Self-efficacy, quality of life and weight loss in overweight/obese endometrial cancer survivors (SUCCEED); a randomized controlled trial. Gynecol Oncol 2014;132(2):397–402.
42. Siegel R, Naishadham D, Jemal A. Cancer statistics, 2014. CA Cancer J Clin 2012;64:9.
43. Yancik R, Ries L. Population aging and cancer: a cross-national concern. Cancer J 2005;11:437.
44. Lacey J, Sherman M. Ovarian neoplasia. In: Robboy S, Mutter G, Prat J, et al, editors. Robboy's pathology of the female reproductive tract. 2nd edition. Oxford (United Kingdom): Churchill Livingstone Elsevier; 2009. p. 601.
45. Armstrong D, Bundy B, Wenzel L, et al. Intraperitoneal cisplatin and paclitaxel in ovarian cancer. N Engl J Med 2006;354:34.
46. Ovarian Cancer National Alliance. Statistics. Available at: http://www.ovariancancer.org/about-ovarian-cancer/statistics. Accessed May 15, 2015.
47. Goff B, Mandel L, Melancon C, et al. Frequency of symptoms of ovarian cancer in women presenting to primary care clinics. JAMA 2004;291:2705.
48. Goff B, Mandel L, Drescher C, et al. Development of an ovarian cancer symptom index: possibilities for earlier detection. Cancer 2007;109:221.

49. White R, Chew H, Zhou H. Incidence of venous thromboembolism in the year before the diagnosis of cancer in 528,693 adults. Arch Intern Med 2005;165:1782.
50. Buys S, Partridge E, Greene M, et al. Ovarian cancer screening in the Prostate, Lung, Colorectal and Ovarian (PLCO) cancer screening trial: findings from the initial screen of a randomized trial. Am J Obstet Gynecol 2005; 193:1630.
51. Stratton J, Gayther S, Russel P, et al. Contribution of BRCA 1 mutations to ovarian cancer. N Engl J Med 1997;336:1125.
52. Barrow E, Robinson L, Alduaij W, et al. Cumulative lifetime incidence of extracolonic cancers in Lynch syndrome: a report of 121 families with proven mutations. Clin Genet 2009;75:141.
53. Rubin S, Backwood M, Bandera C, et al. BRCA 1, BRCA2 and hereditary non-polyposis colorectal cancer gene mutations in an unselected ovarian cancer population: relationship to family history and implications for genetic testing. Am J Obstet Gynecol 1998;178:670.
54. Hewitt M, Anderson K, Hall G, et al. Women with peritoneal carcinomatosis of unknown origin: efficacy of image-guided biopsy to determine site specific diagnosis. BJOG 2007;114:46.
55. Mehdi G, Maheshwari V, Afzal S, et al. Image-guided fine-needle aspiration cytology of ovarian tumors: an assessment of diagnostic efficacy. J Cytol 2010;27:91.
56. DeSantis C, Lin C, Mariotto A, et al. Cancer treatment and survivorship statistics, 2014. CA Cancer J Clin 2014;64:252.
57. Cella D. Measuring quality of life in palliative care. Semin Oncol 1995;22:73.
58. Mirabeau-Beale K, Kornblith A, Penson R, et al. Comparison of the quality of life of early and advanced stage ovarian cancer survivors. Gynecol Oncol 2009; 114:353.
59. Teng F, Kalloger S, Brotto L, et al. Determinants of quality of life in ovarian cancer survivors: a pilot study. J Obstet Gynaecol Can 2014;36:708.
60. Wenzel L, Huang H, Monk B, et al. Quality of life comparisons in a randomized trial of interval secondary cytoreduction in advanced ovarian carcinoma: a Gynecologic Oncology Group Study. J Clin Oncol 2005;23:5605.
61. Biglia N, Gadducci A, Ponzone R, et al. Hormone replacement therapy in cancer survivors. Maturitas 2004;48:222.
62. Lacey J, Brinton L, Leitzman M, et al. Menopausal hormone therapy and ovarian cancer risk in the National Institute of Health-AARP Diet and Health Study Cohort. J Natl Cancer Inst 2006;98(19):1397–405.
63. Beesley V, Price M, Butlow P, et al. Physical activity in women with ovarian cancer and its association with decreased distress and improved quality of life. Psychooncology 2011;20:1161.
64. Walboomers J, Jacobs M, Manos M, et al. Human papilloma virus is a necessary cause of invasive cervical cancer worldwide. J Pathol 1999;189(1):12–9.
65. Brotherton J, Fridman M, May C, et al. Early effect of the HPV vaccination programme on cervical abnormalities in Victoria, Australia: an ecological study. Lancet 2011;377:2085.
66. Singhm G, Milller B, Hankey B, et al. Area socioeconomic variation in U.S. Cancer incidence, 1975-1999. Bethesda (MD): National Cancer Institute; 2003.
67. Saraiya M, Ahmed F, Krishnan S, et al. Cervical cancer incidence in prevaccine era in the United States. 1998-2002. Obstet Gynecol 2007;109:360.
68. Hemminki K, Chen. Familial risks for cervical tumors in full and half siblings: etiologic apportioning. Cancer Epidemiol Biomarkers Prev 2006;15:1413.

69. Disai P, Creasman W. Invasive cervical cancer. In: Monk B, Tewari K, editors. Clinical gynecologic oncology. 7th edition. Philadelphia: Mosby Elsevier; 2007. p. 55.
70. Landoni F, Maneo A, Colombo A, et al. Randomized study of radical surgery versus radiotherapy for stage 1b-IIa cervical cancer. Lancet 1997;350:535.
71. Vistad I, Fossa S, Dahl A. A critical review of patient-related quality of life studies of long-term survivors of cervical cancer. Gynecol Oncol 2006;102:563.
72. Ferrandina G, Mantegna G, Petrillo M, et al. Quality of life and emotional distress in early stage and locally advanced cervical cancer patients: a prospective, longitudinal study. Gynecol Oncol 2012;124:389.
73. Bergmark K, Evall Lundquist E, Dickman P, et al. Patient rating of distressful symptoms after treatment for early cervical cancer. Acta Obstet Gynecol Scand 2002;81:443.
74. Frumovitz M, Sun C, Schoer L, et al. Quality of life and sexual functioning in cervical cancer survivors. J Clin Oncol 2005;23:7428–36.
75. Sturdee D, Panay N, International Menopause Society Writing Group. Recommendations for the management of postmenopausal vaginal atrophy. Climacteric 2010;13:509–22.
76. Ploch E. Hormonal replacement therapy in patients after cervical cancer treatment. Gynecol Oncol 1987;26:169–77.
77. Rubin S, Young J, Mikuta J. Squamous carcinoma of the vagina: treatment complications and long-term follow-up. Gynecol Oncol 1985;20:346.
78. Madsen B, Jensen H, van den Brule A, et al. Risk factors for invasive squamous cell carcinoma of the vulva and vagina—population-based case-control study in Denmark. Int J Cancer 2008;122:2827.
79. Zacur H, Genadry R, Woodruff J. The patient-at-risk for development of vulvar cancer. Gynecol Oncol 1980;9:199.
80. Burger M, Hollema H, Emanuels A, et al. The importance of the groin node status for the survival of T1 and T2 vulvar carcinoma patients. Gynecol Oncol 1995; 57:327.
81. Anderson B, Hacker N. Psychosexual adjustment after vulvar surgery. Obstet Gynecol 1983;62:457.
82. Kirkbride P, Fyles A, Rawlings G, et al. Carcinoma of the vagina—experience at the Princess Margaret Hospital (1974-1989). Gynecol Oncol 1995;56:435.
83. DeMatos P, Tyler D, Seigler H. Mucosal melanoma of the female genitalia: a clinicopathological study of forty-three cases at Duke University Medical Center. Surgery 1998;124:38.
84. MackKie R, Bray C. Hormone replacement therapy after surgery for stage 1 or 2 cutaneous melanoma. Br J Cancer 2004;90:770–2.
85. Wingo PA, Ries LA, Giovino GA, et al. Annual report to the nation on the status of cancer 1973-1996. With a special section on lung cancer and tobacco smoking. J Natl Cancer Inst 1999;91:675.
86. Preston D, Ron E, Tokuoka S, et al. Solid cancer incidence in atomic bomb survivors: 1958-1998. Radiat Res 2007;168:1.
87. Heiss G, Wallace R, Anderson G, et al. Health risks and benefits 3 years after stopping randomized treatment with estrogen and progestin. JAMA 2008;299:1036.
88. Horwitz R, Smaldone L, Viscoli C. An ecogenetic hypothesis for lung cancer in women. Arch Intern Med 1988;148:2609.
89. Chlewbowski R, Schwartz A, Waklee H, et al. Oestrogen plus progestin and lung cancer in postmenopausal women (Women's Health Initiative Trial): a post-hoc analysis of a randomized controlled trial. Lancet 2009;372:1243.

90. Winder R, Fontham E, Barrera E, et al. American Cancer Society lung cancer screening guidelines. CA Cancer J Clin 2013;63:107.

91. Ries L, Kosary C, Hankey B, et al. SEER cancer statistics review 1973-1995. Bethesda (MD): National Cancer Institute; 1998.

92. Burt RW, Disanio JA, Cannon-Albright L. Genetics of colon cancer: impact of inheritance on colon cancer risk. Annu Rev Med 1995;46:371.

93. Lynch H, Smyrk T, Watson P, et al. Genetics, natural history, tumor spectrum and pathology of hereditary nonpolyposis colorectal cancer: an updated review. Gastroenterology 1993;1104:1535.

94. Ponz de Leon M, Sassatelli R, Benatti P, et al. Identification of hereditary nonpolyposis colorectal cancer in the general population. The 6-year experience of a population-based registry. Cancer 1993;71:3493.

95. Atkin W, Morson B, Cuzick J. Long-term risk of colorectal cancer after excision of rectosigmoid adenomas. N Engl J Med 1992;326:658.

96. Rex D, Johnson D, Anderson J, et al. American College of Gastroenterology guidelines for colorectal cancer screening 2009. Am J Gastroenterol 2009; 104:739.

97. Levin B, Lieberman D, McFarland B, et al. Screening and surveillance for the early detection of colorectal cancer and adenomatous polyps. 2008: a joint guideline from the American Cancer Society, the US Multi-Society Task force on Colorectal Cancer and the American College of Radiology. CA Cancer J Clin 2008;58:130.

98. Janne P, Mayer R. Chemoprevention of colorectal cancer. N Engl J Med 2000; 342:1960.

99. Boyle T, Keegel T, Bull F, et al. Physical activity and risks of proximal and distal colon cancers: a systematic review and meta-analysis. J Natl Cancer Inst 2012; 104:1548.

100. Lee J, Chan A. Fruit, vegetables and folate: cultivating the evidence for cancer prevention. Gastroenterology 2011;141:16.

101. Jarvinen R, Knekt P, Hakulinen T, et al. Dietary fat, cholesterol and colorectal cancer in a prospective study. Br J Cancer 2001;85:357.

102. Butler L, Sinha R, Millikan R, et al. Heterocyclic amines, meat intake, and association with colon cancer in a population-based study. Am J Epidemiol 2003; 157:434.

103. Giovannuci E. Modifiable risk factors for colon cancer. Gastroenterol Clin North Am 2002;31:925.

104. Rothwell P, Fowkes F, Belch J, et al. Effect of daily aspirin on long-a term risk of death due to cancer: analysis of individual patient data from randomized trials. Lancet 2011;377:31.

105. Marhom E, Cohen I. Fertility preservation options for women with malignancies. Obstet Gynecol Surv 2007;62:58–72.

106. Fornier M, Modi S, Pangaea K, et al. Incidence of chemotherapy-induced, long term amenorrhea inpatient with breast carcinoma age 40 years and younger after adjuvant anthracycline and taxane. Cancer 2005;104:1575–9.

107. Koyama H, Wada T, Nishizawa Y, et al. Cyclophosphamide-induced ovarian failure and its therapeutic significance in patients with breast cancer. Cancer 1977; 39:1403.

108. Amnderson R, Cameron D. Pretreatment serum anti-mullerian hormone predicts long-term ovarian function and bone mass after chemotherapy for early breast cancer. J Clin Endocrinol Metab 2011;96:1336.

109. Cercek A, Siegel C, Capanu M, et al. Incidence of chemotherapy-induced amenorrhea in premenopausal women treated with adjuvant FOLFOX for colorectal cancer. Clin Colorectal Cancer 2013;12(3):164–7.
110. Stillman R, Schinfeld J, Schiff I, et al. Ovarian failure in long-term survivors of childhood malignancy. Am J Obstet Gynecol 1981;139:2.
111. American Psychiatric Association. Diagnostics and statistical manual of mental disorders. 5th edition. Arlington (VA): American Psychiatric Association; 2013.
112. Shifren J, Monsz B, Russo P, et al. Sexual problems and distress in United States women: prevalence and correlates. Obstet Gynecol 2008;112:970.
113. Ganz P, Desmond K, Belin T, et al. Predictors of sexual health in women after a breast cancer diagnosis. J Clin Oncol 1999;17:2371.

Complementary and Alternative Approaches to Menopause

Maida Taylor, MD, MPH

KEYWORDS

- Black cohosh • Botanic medicine • S-equol • Pine bark • Hops • Flaxseed
- Daidzein • Genistein

KEY POINTS

- Few botanic therapies suggested for menopause have robust evidence for efficacy and safety.
- Pycnogenol, pollen extract, ERr731 (rhubarb extract), S-equol, and genistein may offer some symptom mitigation.
- Soy foods offer limited symptom relief.
- Red clover, evening primrose oil, *Panax ginseng*, *Dioscorea*, and vitamin E are ineffective.
- At best, botanicals decrease vasomotor symptoms 15% to 30% better than placebo.

INTRODUCTION: WHY IS COMPLEMENTARY AND ALTERNATIVE MEDICINE SO POPULAR?

Since the publication of the Women's Health Initiative (WHI),[1] women bothered by symptoms of menopause have been desperate to find nonhormonal therapies. While professionals continue to debate the merits or deficiencies of the WHI, and as the pendulum of professional opinion keeps oscillating, women continue to be frightened by hormones and confused by alternatives. For the past decade, women have been inundated with seemingly conflicting information from multiple sources, both scientific and commercial.

What is the window of opportunity? Is estrogen good when used alone but bad when used with a progestin? Are hormones helpful if taken early in the menopausal transition but dangerous later on? What if you start, then stop, and then restart? There is no universal consensus among health care professionals regarding these

The author has nothing to disclose.
Department of Obstetrics, Gynecology, and Reproductive Sciences, University of California San Francisco, San Francisco, CA, USA
E-mail address: maida.beth@gmail.com

Endocrinol Metab Clin N Am 44 (2015) 619–648
http://dx.doi.org/10.1016/j.ecl.2015.05.008
0889-8529/15/$ – see front matter © 2015 Elsevier Inc. All rights reserved.

conundrums. Continuing uncertainty and ambiguity about hormone therapy fuels anxieties about midlife and future morbidity. As a result, many women have lost faith in conventional pharmaceutical offerings. They perceive that the medical establishment has colluded with big pharma to turn aging and menopause into diseases rather than natural processes. History does indeed document such a partnership. In 1966, Robert Wilson, MD,[2] published *Feminine Forever*, with major financial backing from the leading manufacturer of estrogens at that time. He promulgated the notion that menopause marked the end of a meaningful, healthy existence for women. He stated that he could not understand why his colleagues "simply refuse to recognize menopause for what it is—a serious, painful and often crippling disease."[2] This characterization of menopause, as an endocrine deficiency disease, not merely deficiency, was pervasive until the 1970s and is antithetical to the way many women nowadays want to approach midlife and menopausal symptoms.

Women now hold to personal beliefs and values that are more holistic and want treatments that support wellness, maintain mental and physical function, and improve quality of life. Although a complex set of variables influence each individual's personal experience of menopause and menopausal symptoms, an even more complex set of variables influence the decision to use hormone therapy. Complementary and alternative medicine (CAM) approaches to menopause seem to harmonize far better with the cultural of wellness. Women who want to take more personal responsibility for their health and well-being also want more autonomy. There is a paradigm operating that leads many women to feel like failures if, having eaten properly and exercised regularly, they have continued symptoms, rising cholesterol, or progressive bone loss. Accepting a drug treatment is viewed as a passive acquiescence, a sign that one did not work hard enough to maintain one's own health.

In the following sections, the author reviews commonly suggested CAM options for menopause and offers rational guidance based on a rubric proposed by the Natural Medicines Comprehensive Data Base—products that are safe and effective, safe but ineffective, unsafe but effective, and both unsafe and ineffective. Data are cited from peer reviewed publications, randomized trials, and well-done meta-analyses. If no quality studies are available, existing data are mentioned; but recommendation regarding use is withheld.

DEFINING COMPLEMENTARY AND ALTERNATIVE MEDICINE

Alternative medicine encompasses several systematic medical practices based on models of health and disease that differ from the medical physiology that underpins Western medicine (**Box 1**). Traditional Chinese medicine (TCM) defines health as the balance of the essential life force called qi (pronounced *chee*); acupuncture, as one of the therapeutics used in TCM, is said to support wellness and to treat disease by regulating the flow of qi along meridians that course through the body. Mind-body systems of medicine see health as a balance of conscious and unconscious influences of mind on bodily functions. Manipulative and body-based systems like chiropractic, osteopathy, and massage seek to rebalance or realign the body through manipulation. Meditation, hypnosis, music, and prayer fall under the aegis of mind-body practice. Mind-body also includes energy-modulating modalities, like therapeutic touch, qi gong, and magnets, which supposedly reorder bioelectric fields in or around the body.

The most commonly used CAM practices are biologic-based therapies, including botanic medicines, dietary supplements, vitamins, minerals, and orthomolecular medicine.

Box 1 **CAM headings in MEDLINE**
Acupuncture
Anthroposophy
Biofeedback
Chiropractic
Color therapy
Diet fads
Eclecticism
Electric stimulation
Homeopathy
Kinesiology
Massage
Medicine, traditional
Mental healing
Moxibustion
Music therapy
Naturopathy
Organotherapy
Radiesthesia
Rejuvenation
Relaxation techniques
Therapeutic touch

COMPLEMENTARY AND ALTERNATIVE MEDICINE AND MENOPAUSE

The Study of Women's Health Across the Nation (SWAN), a longitudinal study of menopause in the United States, found that use of CAM for menopausal symptoms increased dramatically in the decade after publication of the WHI. Use rates escalated from 48.5% to 51.0%, 52.7%, and 80.0% in 2002, 2005, 2007, and 2008, respectively.[3–6] In a comprehensive review on the use of CAM for menopause, Peng and colleagues[7] analyzed 49 studies of CAM use in menopause and found that these levels of use were consistent across studies from around the world. Geller and Studee[8] also reported a 70% rate of use in the United States but, perhaps more importantly, noted that 70% of women using CAM do not inform their health care providers about the supplements they are taking. Gentry found similar rates of nonreporting by women in the United Kingdom.[9]

The motivations and reasons for using CAM are consistent across surveys. Most commonly, women use CAM to treat symptoms of hot flashes and night sweats, disturbed sleep, anxiety and mood disorders, vaginal dryness, fatigue, and bodily aches and pains.[8] A recent survey in the United Kingdom of 6383 ever users of hormone therapy, of whom 79.3% had discontinued HT, found that almost 90% had tried at least one or more types of complementary and alternative medicine for vasomotor symptoms relief. Seventy percent used herbal remedies, with the two most often reported being evening primrose oil (48%) and black cohosh (30%). Of behavioral methods, exercise was cited by 68.2% of respondents.[10]

It should be noted here that the terms *herbal* and *botanic* are often used interchangeably. The term *herbal* applies to substances derived from the herbaceous portions of plants, specifically the leaves and stems. *Botanic* is the broader term and denotes products made from any plant part: leaves, stems, seeds, fruits, flowers, and roots.

BOTANICALS COMMONLY RECOMMENDED FOR MENOPAUSE

The Natural Medicines Comprehensive Database has divided botanicals used for menopause into 2 groups: those purported to be hormonally active, either as estrogens or selective estrogen receptor modulators (SERMs), and those altering symptoms by modulating the function of central neuroreceptors, perhaps mimicking the effects of neuroactive molecules like venlafaxine and other selective serotonin reuptake inhibitors (**Box 2**).

THE PHYTOESTROGENS: SOY, SOY DERIVATIVES, AND RED CLOVER EXTRACT

Three types of polyphenolic compounds are said to be estrogenic: the isoflavones, lignans, and coumestans. In animal husbandry, these phytochemicals produce disturbances in the estrus cycle: sheep grazed on red clover and cattle fed whole soy are at risk for cycle disruption and sterility.[10] One might wonder why plants make substances that act as mammalian endocrine messengers. Within an ecosystem, by interfering with the animal's reproductive life cycle, these phytosterols made by forage plants act as natural birth control, restraining the growth of the grazing population and protecting the plants themselves from overpredation. When used as animal fodder, clover and soy products are alcohol washed to remove these bioactive compounds. However, the washing solution is rich in isoflavones and, when evaporated, leaves a residue of isoflavone isolates. This waste slurry used to be discarded; but the residues are now processed, packaged, and sold as dietary supplements, supposedly offering the benefits of soy to people who do not want to eat soy foods.

In the soybean, isoflavones are bound to a sugar moiety and are classed as glycosides, the principal ones found in soy being genistin, daidzin, and glycitin. Fermentation and digestion cleaves the sugar moiety off and produce the aglyconic forms, which are more potent: genistein, daidzein, and glycitein.

Soy

Soy, or soya (scientific name: *Glycine max* L), specifically fermented soy products like tempeh, miso, and tamari, is a major source of protein in Asian diets. Tofu is a more recent invention and is the most common form of soy used in Western dishes, whereas tempeh is the mainstay in the Japanese diet.[11]

Soy is not part of Asian traditional medicine or food recommendations for menopausal women. The incorporation of soy into the natural medicine lexicon as a menopause remedy stems from the characterization of the polyphenolic isoflavones found in soy as so-called phytoestrogens. Although soy isoflavones do bind to estrogen receptor (ER) alpha and ER beta, they do not produce the same conformational changes that true estrogens produce. Thus, isoflavones function as selective ER modulators, evoking both agonist and antagonist activity. These actions are generally weak.

A second misapprehension about soy and its potential as a panacea for menopause comes from the mistaken impression that Asian women do not suffer the symptoms of

---

Box 2
Botanicals recommended for menopause: supposed mechanism of action

Hormone mediators/modulators

- Alfalfa (*Medicago sativa*)
- Black cohosh (*Actaea racemosa*)
- Chaste berry (*Vitex agnus-castus*)
- Aniseed, dill, fennel, fenugreek (all members of the dill family)
- Dong quai (*Angelica sinensis*)
- Evening primrose oil (*Oenothera biennis*)
- Flaxseed (*Linum usitatissimum*)
- Gotu kola (*Centella asiatica*)
- Green tea (Camellia sinensis)
- Hops (*Humulus lupulus*)
- Kudzu (*Pueraria lobata*)
- Licorice (*Glycyrrhiza glabra*) (also mineralocorticoid activity)
- Maca (*lepidium peruvianum*)
- Milk thistle (*Silybum marianum*)
- Red clover (*Trifolium pratense*)
- Rhubarb (*Rheum rhaponticum*)
- Sarsaparilla (*Smilax regelii*)
- Sage (*Salvia officinalis*)
- Soy (*Glycine max*) and its derivatives daidzein, genistein, S-equol, and other isoflavones
- Wild yam (*Dioscorea villosa*)

Central/neurotransmitter mediators

- Ginkgo (*Ginkgo biloba*)
- Kava kava (*Piper methysticum*)
- *Panax ginseng* (also said to be estrogenic)
- St. John's wort (*Hypericum perforatum*)
- Valerian (*Valeriana officinalis*)

---

menopause, that they sail through menopause effortlessly, and the reason is their soy-based diet. Although hot flashes are less common in Asian women, in SWAN and other studies, more than 90% of Japanese American women related having menopausal symptoms, the most common complaint being shoulder and neck pain.[12,13] And although Japanese American women report fewer hot flashes and fewer night sweats than European American women, within the Japanese American group, higher soy consumption was not associated with a reduction in vasomotor symptoms.[14]

Nonetheless, soy foods are said to ease hot flashes, preserve bone mineral density, and improve the lipid profile. In addition, specific isoflavone isolates like genistein and an isoflavone metabolite of daidzein, S-equol, are also being marketed to treat hot flashes and other symptoms. Isoflavone isolates extracted from red clover is discussed separately.

The available studies using soy foods as therapies within randomized trials are difficult to assess in the aggregate. Most experts who have attempted to perform meta-analyses have stated that the studies suffer from methodological problems, design flaws, and small samples. Studies have used different kinds of soy, with differing amounts of isoflavones. Different symptom ratings scales have been used, and often times nonvalidated measures and scales have been used.

The North American Menopause Society (NAMS) has published recommendations[15] regarding isoflavones and menopausal symptoms. There is a high degree of consistency in their recommendations and those of the other professional reviews that have been published subsequently. Soy isoflavones are seen as modestly effective, at best; genistein is thought to hold some added promise as a therapeutic modality. NAMS also mentions S-equol as an entity that might offer some therapeutic advantages.

Key conclusions of the NAMS paper were

- Soy-based isoflavones are modestly effective in relieving menopausal symptoms.
- Supplements providing higher proportions of genistein or increased S-equol may provide more benefits.
- Soy food consumption is associated with a lower risk of breast and endometrial cancer in observational studies.
- The efficacy of isoflavones on bone has not been proven, and the clinical picture of whether soy has cardiovascular benefits is still evolving.

A meta-analysis by Bolaños and colleagues[16] reviewed the use of soy dietary supplements, soy extract, or isoflavone concentrate (genistein or daidzein) for hot flashes. Overall, a measurement (applied daily, weekly, or monthly and designated as the standardized mean difference in hot flashes) was calculated to be -0.39 (95% confidence interval [CI], -0.53 to -0.25) for soy. For soy concentrate, extract, and dietary supplement, the deltas were -0.45 (95% CI, -0.64 to -0.25), -0.51 (95% CI, -0.79 to -0.22), and -0.20 (95% CI, -0.46 to -0.06), respectively. These changes, although statistically significant, may well be clinically insignificant.

The Cochrane Collaborative[17] reviewed soy and soy-derived products for menopause. The reviewers identified a total of 43 randomized controlled trials (RCTs) with 4364 subjects, including all studies using dietary soy, soy extracts, and other types of phytoestrogens. The variations in the study treatments and designs were so wide ranging that a meta-analysis could not be performed. In the resulting descriptive review, the investigators stated that, although some trials demonstrated reductions in the frequency and severity of hot flushes and night sweats, many were small and subject to possible bias. Placebo responses ranged from 1% to 59% reduction in symptoms. The trials did provide some reassurance, however, because the review found that, in the aggregate, there was no evidence of estrogenlike effects on the endometrium or vagina or other major adverse events with up to 2 years of use. The doses recommended within studies ranged from 35.0 to 134.4 mg, with overall 40% to 50% reductions in symptoms, which were 15% greater than the reductions seen within placebo-treated subjects.

The investigators surmised that there is no conclusive evidence to show "that phytoestrogen supplements effectively reduce the frequency or severity of hot flushes and night sweats in perimenopausal or postmenopausal women, although benefits derived from concentrates of genistein should be further investigated."[17]

Taku and colleagues,[18] extracting information from a larger data set, made similar determinations: a 20.6% reduction in frequency and a 26.2% reduction in severity for soy beyond that seen with placebo. The average dose was equivalent to 54 mg of aglycone forms of isoflavones. This review also mentions that genistein in higher doses might be a viable therapy.

Drawing on a similar pool of research material, Chen and colleagues[19] found 15 RCTs that met criteria for use in a meta-analysis. The mean daily hot flush frequency was statistically lower in the isoflavone study groups (reduction mean = 0.89, CI 0.2–1.52, $P<.005$). Side effects were no more common than those with placebo. Studies that used the Kupperman Index (KI) as an outcome measure evidenced no significant treatment effect. The investigators concluded that phytoestrogens seem to be effective and safe, though the hot flash reductions noted, although statistically significant, may not be clinically meaningful.

SOY-DERIVED ISOFLAVONE ISOLATES

People raised on a traditional American diet often find it difficult to incorporate soy foods into their routine. Even dedicated vegans may find certain traditional Asian soy foods, especially fermented products like seitan and natto, quite unpalatable. Many people, when trying to increase their soy intake, develop gastrointestinal symptoms, with flatulence, cramps, and bloating.[20] In fact, gastrointestinal complaints are the main reason clinical research subjects drop out of soy clinical trials.

Exploiting the American penchant for pill taking, isoflavone isolates are promoted in lieu of soy foods and are advertised as offering the same benefits as soy, but in pill or powder form.

S-Equol

Equol is a more potent metabolite of daidzein and is produced by the action of intestinal bacteria. Most individuals in Western societies lack the essential intestinal flora to produce equol, with only 28.2% of persons in Europe, 27.6% in the United States, and 31.3% in Australia being equol producers, significantly lower than the reported 50% to 60% frequency of equol producers in Japan, Korea, or China and Western adult vegetarians.[21]

Newton and colleagues[22] examined equol versus nonequol producers and vasomotor symptoms. They found that although there were no differences in VMS bother or severity in nonproducers by dietary daidzein level, dietary intake did affect symptoms in equol producers. Comparing those in the lowest quartile of dietary daidzein intake (mean, 4.9 mg/d) to those in the highest quartile (mean, 28.5 mg/d), the high-intake women were 76% less likely to have VMS, though the trend was not significant $(P = .06)$.

Using biofermentation with a strain of lactobacillus, a Japanese pharmaceutical company manufactures S-equol from soy germ (Natural S-Equol). The rationale for administering S-equol is to circumvent the lack of appropriate intestinal flora in non–equol-producing persons. Three studies have been done to date using S-equol for menopausal symptoms. All the studies have been done in Japan using a tool called the Japanese Menopausal Symptom Score, which is heavily weighted with quality-of-life scales. S-equol at a dosage of 10 mg once per day proved less than effective, whereas S-equol 10 mg 3 times a day was associated with significant improvements in measures of mood and anxiety. No changes in follicle-stimulating hormone (FSH), luteinizing hormone (LH), estradiol, or progesterone were evident.[23,24] Utian and colleagues[25] recently reviewed the aggregate evidence for S-equol. The investigators concluded that, at this time, both efficacy and safety claims for S-equol require further study.

Genistein

Genistein, an aglycone isoflavone, is being studied as single agent for menopausal symptoms. The genistein being marketed in the United States (sold as i-cool) is a non–soy-derived product. The Cochrane Collaborative review identified 4 trials and noted that extracts with high amounts (>30 mg/d) of genistein consistently reduced the frequency of hot flushes.[18]

An often-cited genistein trial was done to examine its effects on bone and cardiovascular risks.[26] The overall study randomized 389 participants, and then a subset of subjects (125 genistein/122 placebo) was segregated from the larger study after randomization. After 12 months, in this subset, researchers noted a 56.4% reduction in the mean number of hot flushes per day. Women in the placebo group evidenced no reduction in symptoms over 1 year, though one would expect some natural decrement over time. No additional reductions were seen after 2 full years of study. In the parent trial,[27] after 6 months of treatment, the genistein group evidenced improvements in cardiovascular and bone markers, including fasting glucose, insulin, insulin resistance, osteoprotegerin, fibrinogen, and sex hormone-binding globulin (SHBG).

Other studies of genistein have yielded variable degrees of symptom relief, ranging from 30% to 50%. Evans and colleagues[28] reported a 12-week randomized double-blind placebo-controlled study in which 84 postmenopausal women received placebo or a single 30-mg dose of synthetic genistein. Within both intent to treat and per protocol completers, subjects on genistein demonstrated a trend toward a greater percent reduction in the mean number of hot flushes from baseline to week 4 (28% vs 17%, $P = .150$) and week 8 (45% vs 26% $P = .067$); but this difference was not statistically significant until week 12 (38% vs 19%, $P = .026$). Subjects who were retained for the full 12 weeks of the study evidenced a greater percent reduction in the mean number of hot flushes from baseline at weeks 4, 8, and 12 compared with placebo (33% vs 19%, $P = .098$; 47% versus 29%, $P = .064$; and 51% vs 30%, $P = .049$, respectively).

Daidzein

Daidzein is another aglycone isoflavone, also abundant in soy, which is being considered as a single therapy for menopausal symptoms. Khaodhiar and colleagues[29] reported on a 12-week RCT using 2 different doses of daidzein, 40 mg and 60 mg. At 8 weeks, vasomotor symptom frequency declined by 43% in the 40-mg and 41% in the 60-mg daidzein group, versus only 32% in the placebo arm. By 12 weeks the rate of reduction was 52% for 40 mg, 51% for 60 mg, and 39% for placebo subjects. These differences, however, are not statistically significant. The investigators pooled the data from both doses and observed a 43% reduction in vasomotor symptoms at 8 weeks ($P = .1$) and 52% at 12 weeks ($P = .048$). Menopausal quality-of-life measures improved in all study groups but were not statistically significant. Although these findings are marginal at best, the investigators nonetheless concluded that daidzein might be a viable alternative therapy.

RECOMMENDATIONS FOR SOY, SOY FOODS, SOY EXTRACTS, AND SOY METABOLITES

Soy is one of the major sources of protein in many types of diets. Large, population-based studies of Asian, vegetarian, and vegan diets have demonstrated incontrovertible health benefits of diets rich in soy. The Adventist Health Study 2[30] found significant reductions in cardiovascular mortality, noncardiovascular noncancer mortality, renal mortality, and endocrine mortality in vegans and vegetarians. Eating whole soy foods with intact soy protein and isoflavones is also associated with lower rates of breast and endometrial cancer. Vegetarian and vegan diets also hold great ethical and environmental appeal for many people and; incidentally, eating soy may help hot flashes.

Women should be advised to keep their dietary soy intake within the range of intake observed in Asian diets, 90 g of soy per day. Different types of soy provide differing amounts of isoflavones; but generally speaking, 6 to 11 g of soy protein will provide 25 to 50 mg of total soy isoflavones, one-half of which are the active aglyconic forms. Note that tofu in the 3-layer box, such as the long shelf-life brand, Silken, contains isoflavones. Soy packed in water in the white tubs typically found in grocery dairy cases is alcohol washed and isoflavone poor (**Table 1**).

Two isoflavone isolates, S-equol and genistein, may offer some symptom relief. Data are less compelling for daidzein. Genistein is marketed as i-cool, which contains 30 mg of a proprietary, non–soy-derived genistein called geniVida. S-equol (Natural S-Equol) will be marketed in the United States by NatureMade, a vitamin manufacturer with a reputation for reliable products that are independently tested and verified for purity and consistency. The product is made from soy. Pricing information is not available at this time. Both products are probably safe.

Red Clover–Based Isoflavone Supplements

Red clover (scientific name: *Trifolium pratense*) contains the most isoflavones of any plant. The principal isoflavones in red clover are daidzein, genistein, formanectin, and biochanin, along with coumestans, coumarinlike substances, and salicylates. Red clover is not a human foodstuff. In botanic medicine, it has been recommended to treat asthma, pertussis, bronchitis, cancer, bladder infections, liver disease, and skin disorders.

Embedded within the Cochrane Collaborative review of isoflavones[22] is a meta-analysis of 4 studies that used a proprietary brand of red clover extract, Promensil. Across all trials, the mean daily reduction in hot flashes was −0.6 (95% CI −1.8 to 0.6) per day. Safety assessments were reassuring, with no increase in endometrial thickness or breast density. There was a single report of increased vaginal maturation index with red clover, suggesting some estrogenlike activity. Hence, caution should be exercised in recommending red clover extracts to women with a history of estrogen-dependent neoplasms. In another study by Geller and Studee,[31] red clover, black cohosh, and conjugated estrogens plus medroxyprogesterone acetate (CEE/MPA) were compared head-to-head. Only the CEE/MPA produced a statistically significant reduction in symptoms.

THE SAFETY OF SOY

Most studies in the literature have failed to demonstrate estrogenic activity from naturally occurring soy. Clinical trials that have measured estrogen and estrogen-dependent markers found no change in serum hormone levels, vaginal maturation index, FSH, SHBG, and markers of bone turnover. Soy ingested in amounts found in Asian diets is generally regarded as safe. There is no evidence that women in Japan, who eat 20 to 50 times more soy than women in Western societies, experience higher rates of estrogen-dependent tumors or have higher rates of recurrence if they are diagnosed with estrogen-dependent cancers.

In a study of breast tissue excised from women with known breast cancer, who were given 200 mg of isoflavones per day for 2 to 6 weeks before surgery, the investigators found a nonsignificant trend toward cancer growth inhibition in the isoflavone-treated subjects, with higher apoptosis/mitosis ratios versus untreated controls.[32] In another study, breast cancer survivors on a soy-rich diet had a 23% reduction in risk of recurrence compared with women on a standard diet.[33]

Table 1
Isoflavones in food (derived from US Department of Agriculture data)

Food Product	Total Isoflavones	Daidzein	Genistein
Soy flour, full fat	177.89	71.19	96.83
Soy flour, textured	148.61	59.62	78.90
Soy flour, defatted	131.19	57.47	71.21
Soybeans	128.34	46.46	73.76
Soy protein concentrate, aqueous washed	102.07	43.04	55.59
Soy protein isolate	97.43	33.59	59.62
Natto	58.93	21.85	29.04
Soybean chips	54.16	26.71	27.45
Tempeh	43.52	17.59	24.85
Miso	42.55	16.13	24.56
Soybean sprouts	40.71	19.12	21.60
Tofu, soft	29.24	8.59	20.65
Tofu, silken	27.91	11.13	15.58
Tofu, firm	22.70	8.00	12.75
Soy hot dog	15.00	3.40	8.20
Soy protein concentrate, alcohol extracted	12.47	6.83	5.33
Soy milk	9.65	4.45	6.06
Vegetarian burger	9.30	2.95	5.28
Soy cheese, mozzarella	7.70	1.10	3.60
Soy cheese, cheddar	7.15	1.80	2.25
Soy drink	7.01	2.41	4.60
Split peas	2.42	2.42	0.00
Shoyu	1.64	0.93	0.82
Pigeon peas	0.56	0.02	0.54
Clover sprouts	0.35	0.00	0.35
Peanuts	0.26	0.03	0.24
Navy beans	0.21	0.01	0.20
Mung beans	0.19	0.01	0.18
Chickpeas	0.10	0.04	0.06
Green tea	0.05	0.01	0.04
Broad beans	0.03	0.02	0.00
Cowpeas	0.03	0.01	0.02
Lima beans	0.03	0.02	0.01
Lentils	0.01	0.00	0.00

Isoflavones are in milligrams per 100 g.

Eating soy in amounts higher than traditional Asian diets is inadvisable, and the safety assumptions about soy foods cannot be extrapolated to high doses of soy extracts or isoflavone isolates[34] or to synthetic isoflavones. Two cautionary reports follow.

A recent publication reported on 376 healthy postmenopausal women, all with intact uteri. They were randomized to 5 years of treatment with either soy tablets (150 mg of isoflavones per day) or placebo. Endometrial biopsies were obtained at baseline, 30 months, and 5 years after the beginning of the treatment. Two hundred ninety-eight women completed the 5-year of study. Seventy percent of soy-treated women had atrophic or nonassessable biopsies versus 81% receiving placebo. Although there were no cases of endometrial carcinoma, endometrial hyperplasia was significantly more prevalent among women in the soy group (3.37% vs 0%). These findings raise concerns about the long-term safety of isoflavone supplementation.[35]

Ipriflavone (IP) is a synthetic isoflavone synthesized from the soy isoflavone daidzein. Although it is not a naturally occurring compound, it is regarded as a food derivative and sold as a supplement without prescription. IP is often combined with vitamin D, calcium, boron, and other vitamins and minerals as a bone tonic.

IP was heavily promoted in the European Union (EU), with a seemingly profound body of support coming from 18 randomized clinical trials, approximately half of which demonstrated greater bone density or reduced bone loss among IP-treated women compared with those receiving calcium alone. Three studies suggested that IP reduced vertebral fractures.

A large, independent trial, the Ipriflavone Multicenter European Fracture Study, was then designed, which enrolled 474 postmenopausal women aged 45 to 75 years with low bone mass. They were assigned to IP at the same dosage that is sold on the Internet (200 mg 3 times daily) or to placebo. Both groups received 500 mg of calcium daily. The study failed to demonstrate any bone protection for IP. Bone mineral density and bone markers were no different in treatment versus placebo groups. However, 31 women (13.2%) in the IP group were found to have subclinical lymphocytopenia; in 29 of these women, the lymphocytopenia emerged during IP treatment. Most women recovered 2 years after discontinuing the study medication.[36]

IP continues to be marketed and is easily available over the counter as Ostovone in the United States. On one of the Web sites where IP is sold, there is no mention of the risk of lymphocytopenia.[37] Because it is considered a dietary supplement, it is not subject to the same level of regulation and disclosure of risks as are drugs approved by the Food and Drug Administration (FDA). Additional issues around safety of botanicals are discussed later in the section "Sold does not mean safe."

OTHER BOTANICALS USED FOR MENOPAUSE (LISTED ALPHABETICALLY)
Black Cohosh

Black cohosh, scientific name *Actaea racemosa* L (previously *Cimicifugae racemosae*), goes by a variety of common names: black snakeroot, rattlesnake root, squawroot, rich weed, rattle root, rattle snakeroot, rattle top, and rattle weed. A Native American plant, exported to Europe during colonial times, it lacks an extensive history of use in traditional folk medicine as a menopause remedy. Yet, it has become the most commonly recommended botanic for menopausal symptoms. The most popular black cohosh extract marketed in the United States and Europe is Remifemin. It is also the product used in most of the clinical trials reported in peer-reviewed journals.

The active ingredients in black cohosh extract have not been defined, and the mechanism of action has not been clearly elucidated. Extracts are usually standardized to the triterpene glycosides content in the preparation. Remifemin is standardized to the triterpene glycoside 27-deoxyactein.

Early efforts tried to promote black cohosh as a phyto-therapeutic with estrogenlike effects. In vitro and in vivo testing demonstrated possible estrogenlike activity in initial studies.[38] When publications began surfacing positing a possible link between estrogen and breast cancer, black cohosh was revitalized as a nonestrogen, as a possible selective ER modulator.[39] More recently, the proposed mechanisms of action include modulation of serotonergic pathways and antioxidant or antiinflammatory effects.

More than 19 clinical trials of black cohosh appear in the literature, but most suffer from significant methodological deficits. Newton and colleagues[40] conducted a well-designed, 12-month study and found no effect studied used 40 mg/d black cohosh (Remifemin) versus placebo in a 9-week crossover design: 1 week run in, placebo or product for 4 weeks, and then subjects were crossed over for an additional 4 weeks of study. Women who received black cohosh reported a 20% reduction in their hot flash scores, whereas women on placebo evidenced a 27% decrease.[41] In the Geller and Studee[30] study cited earlier, black cohosh reduced VMS by 34%, red clover by 57%, and placebo by 63%. The hormone therapy arm, CEE/MPA yielded a highly significant 94% reduction in VMS.

Although early preclinical assessments of the effects of black cohosh in in vitro and animal models are conflicting, human studies have confirmed that black cohosh has no effect on circulating LH, FSH, prolactin, or estradiol. A 52-week study reassuringly demonstrated that black cohosh does not increase endometrial thickness on ultrasound.[42] In studies of up to 6 months' duration, there have been no reports of vaginal bleeding.

A series of case reports of hepatotoxicity possibly associated with black cohosh surfaced in the medical literature. This prompted regulatory authorities to investigate whether, indeed, black cohosh was implicated. The analysis was complicated by the fact that often the product used could not be conclusively identified, the identified subject had taken multiple supplements with multiple components, the subject had also take prescription drugs that might potentiate hepatotoxic effects or the subject may have had preexisting liver disease. The US Pharmacopeia Botanic Expert Committee examined the reported cases of hepatotoxicity and identified 30 nonduplicate reports. All cases were rated as "possible causality," although thought to be "probable" or "certain causality."[43]

The committee issued a directive that black cohosh products should carry a statement of caution regarding the use in persons with compromised liver function: "Discontinue use and consult a healthcare practitioner if you have a liver disorder or develop symptoms of liver trouble, such as abdominal pain, dark urine, or jaundice." Although these precautions remain in place, the National Institutes of Health has stated that there is no plausible mechanism that might explain a link between black cohosh and hepatotoxicity.

Recommendations

When taken in the aggregate, the data do not support the use of black cohosh for vasomotor symptoms; but given the lack of effective alternatives to estrogen, many practitioners continue to recommend it.

Newer studies suggest that black cohosh may improve mood, sleep, and other complaints, consistent with a new proposed mechanism of action for black cohosh, which is now postulated to act via serotonergic pathways. These claims seem to be an attempt to revive black cohosh after sales plummeted in reaction to the reports of hepatotoxicity. A product containing black cohosh combined with valerian, lemon balm, and hops is being promoted for sleep disturbance (Remifemin Goodnight) and another combining black cohosh with St. John's Wort is recommended for mood (Remifemin Plus).

Crinum

Crinum is a large genus within the family Amaryllidaceae, which also includes the decorative amaryllis plant. There are some 130 tropical species, and the plant is widely used in folk medicine in South Asia. Extracts are supposed to exert antitumor, immune-modulating, analgesic, and antimicrobial effects.[44] The branded product Crila is being promoted to treat vasomotor symptoms, and to promote uterine and prostate health. No studies can be found in the available medical research literature. No recommendations regarding efficacy or safety can be made.

Dioscorea villosa (Wild Yam)

Also known as Mexican yam, shan yao, white yam, wild yam root, yam, yellow yam, and yuma, several varieties of yam plants are sources of diosgenin, which is used in the manufacture of synthetic steroids. The varieties most often used include *Dioscorea barbasco, D mexicana*, and *D villosa*. Diosgenin, in a chemical process known as marker degradation, is converted in vitro to progesterone in a 5-step process (**Fig. 1**). There is no biopathway for this conversion in vivo. Despite this fact, researchers in Japan fed women *Dioscorea alata* or sweet potato 2 times a day for 30 days replacing rice as the staple in their diet and found significant increases in serum concentrations of estrone (26%), SHBG (9.5%), and a near-significant increase in estradiol (27%) in the yam group.[45] The mechanism of action for these changes may reside in metabolic changes other than steroidal conversion, such as changes in enterohepatic circulation.

Folk medicine practitioners assert that yams have dehydroepiandrosterone-like activity and act as precursors for the endogenous production of sex hormones like estrogen and progesterone. Again there is no mammalian biopathway for this bioconversion. Ingesting yams (or diosgenin) has no effect on endogenous steroid production. One trial of yam cream yielded nonsignificant improvements in symptoms.[46]

Recommendation

Yam creams are ineffective. Most yam creams do not contain any yam extract. The yams and sweet potatoes at the local supermarket are not related to the *Dioscorea*

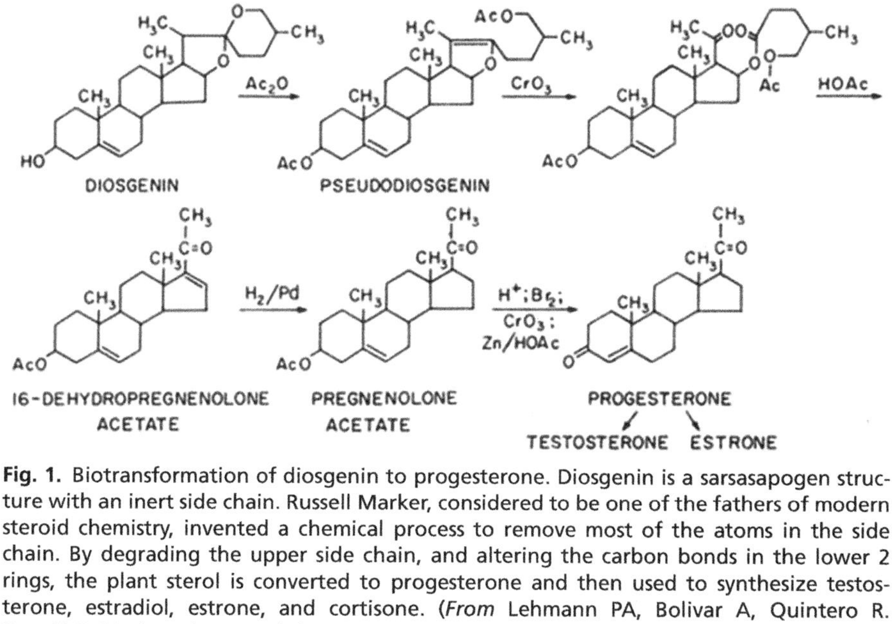

Fig. 1. Biotransformation of diosgenin to progesterone. Diosgenin is a sarsasapogen structure with an inert side chain. Russell Marker, considered to be one of the fathers of modern steroid chemistry, invented a chemical process to remove most of the atoms in the side chain. By degrading the upper side chain, and altering the carbon bonds in the lower 2 rings, the plant sterol is converted to progesterone and then used to synthesize testosterone, estradiol, estrone, and cortisone. (*From* Lehmann PA, Bolivar A, Quintero R. Russell E. Marker pioneer of the Mexican steroid industry. J Chem Educ 1973;50(3):195–9, with permission. Copyright © 1973 American Chemical Society.)

species used in commercial steroid production. Yam creams are often adulterated with undisclosed naturally occurring or synthetic sex steroids, including estrogens, progesterone, and medroxyprogesterone acetate. Given the high rate of adulteration, and the risk of inadvertent hormone exposure, women should be advised to not to buy these products.

Dong Quai

Dong quai, also know as *Angelica sinensis*, Dang Gui, and Tang Kuei, is the root of the plant Angelica, botanical name *Angelica polymorpha* Maxim, var *sinensis* Oliv. It has been used as the female balancing agent in TCM and is a panacea for a wide array of gynecologic ailments, including hot flashes, dysmenorrhea, oligomenorrhea, premenstrual syndrome (PMS), amenorrhea, and menopausal syndrome.

In the lexicon of TCM, dong quai is "a warm herb that both circulates and nourishes blood, strengthening someone who is underweight, frail, anemic and chilly."[47] Dong quai is reputed to be estrogenic owing to reports of uterine bleeding with use and uterotropic effects in ovariectomized rats.[48] Human clinical studies, however, have found no evidence of estrogenic activity.

There is only one study investigating the efficacy of dong quai for menopausal symptoms. Hirata and colleagues[49] enrolled 71 women in a randomized clinical trial, with subjects receiving either 4.5 g dong quai per day or placebo. After 24 weeks, there were no differences in the number of vasomotor flushes or in KI of menopausal symptoms. There also were no differences in FSH, LH, estradiol, vaginal maturation index, and endometrial thickness, again documenting a lack of estrogenic activity at the dose of dong quai administered. Critics of the study have stated that the dose of dong quai used is much lower than the dose used in TCM formulations and that dong quai is never used alone but rather must be given in concert with other botanicals to promote the synergies needed for therapeutic effect.

Dong quai was sold as a single agent, Rejuvex, which also contained bovine ovarian, uterine, mammary, and pituitary tissues. This product was discontinued by the manufacturer owing to the 2004 FDA ban on dietary supplements containing brain or spinal cord material from cows more than 30 months of age and the potential risk of prion-related bovine spongiform encephalopathy. Nonetheless, this banned product can still be ordered online at theherbalhealthstore.com.

Recommendation

Dong quai is ineffective and potentially unsafe as commercially prepared. It also has anticoagulant effects, is photosensitizing, and is possibly carcinogenic. Women should be advised against using it.

Evening Primrose

Evening Primrose, also known as evening star and often delineated by the acronym *EPO* (evening primrose oil) is known by the scientific name *Oenothera biennis* L, family Onagraceae. The evening primrose, a flowering plant, is rich in linolenic acid, an omega-3 essential fatty acid, and gamma linolenic acid (GLA). GLA, along with other omega-3 fatty acids, helps to regulate inflammatory processes via T-lymphocyte activity. GLA also inhibits angiogenesis. EPO is recommended for a wide array of inflammatory and autoimmune disorders, including allergies, eczema, arthritis, diabetic neuropathy, mastalgia/mastodynia, and inflammatory or irritable bowel disease.

EPO is commonly recommended for PMS, not menopause. All 5 randomized trials of EPO in the treatment of PMS were negative. There is no scientific rationale for the use of EPO for menopause-related hot flashes. There is one published study of EPO in menopause, with 56 women randomized to EPO 500 mg per day or placebo for 6 months. Only 18 women on EPO and 17 on placebo completed the trial. A significant decrease was seen in the placebo group for daytime and nighttime flushes and in nighttime flushes only for the EPO group. Overall, flushes declined by 1.0 per day with EPO and by 2.6 per day with placebo.[50]

Recommendation

Although ineffective for menopausal symptoms, EPO is safe and is a good source of omega-3 essential fatty acids in dietary supplements.

Flaxseed

Flaxseed or linseed (*Linum usitatissimum*) is a rich source of lignans, which are poly-phenolic sterols that, when acted on by gut microbiota, produce enterodiol and enter-olactone, both of which are weak estrogenic sterols. Flaxseed is grown to produce linseed oil as well as for animal fodder. One of the best sources of lignans, flaxseed offers 10 times the lignan content found in sesame seeds. Lignans reside in cell walls and are not bioavailable without extensive crushing, like the action of ruminants (graz-ing animals) chewing cud. For humans to gain the benefits of flax-derived lignans, the best food sources are flaxseed flour and flaxseed meal. Flaxseed oil, although a good source of polyunsaturated fatty acids such as alpha-linolenic acid, provides no lignans, though many women mistakenly take flax oil thinking it provides all of the ther-apeutic benefits of milled flaxseed.

There are 3 trials of flaxseed to treat hot flashes. Lewis and colleagues[51] gave women 25 g of flaxseed with 50 mg of lignans daily (N = 28), or 25 g of soy with 42 mg of isoflavones (N = 31), or a wheat placebo (N = 28) baked into muffins. Using hot flash diaries and the menopause-specific quality-of-life index, neither flax nor soy provided symptom relief greater than placebo.

Colli and colleagues[52] randomized 90 women to 3 study groups: group I received 1 g per day of flaxseed extract containing at least 100 mg of secoisolariciresinol diglu-coside (SDG); group II received 90 g per day of flaxseed meal containing at least 270 mg of SDG; and group III received 1 g per day of collagen (placebo group). There were significant reductions in VMS in both flax groups, but the KI remained unchanged despite a trend toward improvement. The most reassuring aspect of this trial is that neither the flaxseed extract nor the flaxseed meal imposed any sort of estrogenic effects on vaginal maturation index or endometrial thickness, and there were no changes in levels of FSH and estradiol.

Pruthi and colleagues[53] did a randomized trial, enrolling 188 women to eat a flax-seed nutritional bar with 410 mg of lignans or a placebo bar for 6 weeks. The mean hot flash severity score decreased 4.9 in the flaxseed group and 3.5 in the placebo group (*P* = .29).

Recommendations

Flaxseed meal, flour, and oil are safe as food. To date, the accumulated evidence for flaxseed as a menopausal remedy is weak. Therefore, flaxseed should be regarded as safe and possibly ineffective.

Ginseng (Panax ginseng)

There are 2 distinct types of ginseng in common use, American ginseng (white or yellow) and Asiatic ginseng (Korean or Chinese red ginseng). In herbal medicine, American ginseng is said to be cooling, whereas Asiatic ginseng is warming and en-hances the ability of the body to tolerate and acclimate to environmental challenges, physical and emotional stress, and illness. Korean/Chinese ginseng is said to be a stimulant, aphrodisiac, and digestive aid. Asian ginseng is supposedly anabolic and used to enhance sexual function. It is used as a health tonic for the frail elderly.

A third substance promoted as an adaptogenic ginseng, Siberian ginseng (scientific name: *Acanthopanax senticosus* or *Eleutherococcus senticosus*), is not a true ginseng. It is a member of a closely related family of plants, Araliaceae, which also includes sarsaparilla. *Eleutherococcus* was intensively studied and used by Soviet military and Olympic trainers to enhance athletic performance and endurance.[54]

Panax ginseng, a specific product named G115, was studied specifically for the treatment of menopausal complaints in 384 postmenopausal women. After 16 weeks, women taking G115 showed slightly better overall symptom relief; but changes were not statistically significant ($P<.1$) and only accrued from improvements in depression, well-being, and health scores and not hot flashes. Ginseng had no effect on hot flashes; there were no changes in FSH, estradiol, endometrial thickness, maturity index, and vaginal pH.

Ginseng is often mixed into energy drinks along with other stimulants; these energy beverages have been reported to cause agitation, diarrhea, headache, nervousness, and insomnia. Anaphylaxis has also been reported as having drug-herb interactions. When advising the use of ginseng, consult a drug interaction database against patients' current medications.

Recommendations

Although *Panax ginseng* is widely reputed to be estrogenic, the one trial in the accessible literature found no evidence of estrogenic activity and no significant change in menopausal symptoms. Other forms of ginseng have not been studied specifically for menopausal symptoms. Ginseng is generally well tolerated by most people; when used at recommended doses, serious side effects are rare.

Hops

Hops (*Humulus lupulus*) are female flowers (seed cones or strobiles); although they can be used to brew a weak beer, hops are most often used to add a bitter, tart flavor to beers made from other grains. The plant makes a flavonoid, 8-prenylnaringenin, which is said to have greater estrogenic activity than soy isoflavones. There are 2 trials using hops to treat symptoms of menopause.

The first, by Heyerick and colleagues,[55] was a randomized, double-blind, placebo-controlled study over 12 weeks with 67 menopausal women, given 2 standardized doses of hop extract (100 or 250 mcg). Hop extract at the 100-mcg dose was better than placebo at 6 weeks ($P = .023$) but not at 12 weeks ($P = .086$). The higher dose (250 mcg) offered no therapeutic efficacy over placebo.

The second study[56] enrolled only 36 women in a 16-week randomized, double-blind, placebo-controlled, crossover study, with 8 weeks on hops or placebo, then 8 weeks in the opposite treatment arm. Outcome measures included the KI, the Menopause Rating Scale (MRS), and a multifactorial visual analog scale (VAS) at baseline and after 8 and 16 weeks. There was no significant change in symptoms in those women who did active treatment followed by placebo. The researchers did additional modeling using different statistical methods and found improvements using "time-specific estimates of treatment efficacy"[56] in KI ($P = .02$) and VAS ($P = .03$) and a marginally significant reduction ($P = .06$) for MRS after 16 weeks. These results are not robust, given the small sample size and large number of variables included in the statistical analysis.

Recommendations

Hops are safe as a food additive and when used in beverages. There is scant evidence of therapeutic efficacy for treatment of menopausal symptoms.

Maca

Maca (*Lepidium meyenii* Walp, *Lepidium peruvianum* Chacon), a traditional foodstuff from South America, is a cruciferous root grown exclusively in the central Peruvian Andes at 12,000 to 14,000 feet altitude. It is recommended as a tonic and adaptogen, characterized as Peruvian ginseng, and is used to enhance strength, stamina, and athletic performance and for anemia, fertility-enhancement, and aphrodisiac properties. Maca is suggested as a remedy for female hormonal imbalances and menstrual irregularities. It is also said to have antineoplastic activity.

The mechanism of action of maca on male and female hormones remains to be elucidated. Maca contains a weak phytosterol, β-sitosterol. Both methanolic and aqueous extracts of maca exhibit estrogenic activity in vitro, but studies have found no in vivo estrogen effects. The proposed mechanism of action for maca in treating menopause, osteoporosis, and sexual function is via modulation of sex steroid receptor dynamics.

Lee and colleagues[57] did a systematic review of the literature on maca and menopause. Only 4 studies reported their methodologies adequately. Brooks and colleagues[58] did an RCT with crossover design in 14 postmenopausal women. They received 3.5 g/d of either powdered maca for 6 weeks or a matching placebo for 6 weeks over a 12-week period. The main outcome measure was the Greene Climacteric Scale (GCS). Significant improvements in the total GCS score ($P<.05$), sexual function ($P<.001$), and psychological symptoms ($P<.001$), such as anxiety ($P<.001$) and depression ($P<.001$), were reported after maca consumption compared with placebo. The other 3 studies were done by Meissner and colleagues[59]. In the first, one group (n = 62) was given a placebo for 1 month and maca for 2 months (commercial Maca-GO, 2 g/d); a second group (n = 40) was given maca for 2 months and placebo for 1 month. Overall menopausal symptoms as measured with both the GCS ($P<.001$) and KI ($P<.001$) were improved while taking maca. In a second randomized trial, 66 postmenopausal women were divided into 6 different treatment arms, with outcomes reported for only 4 groups. Improvements on the GCS ($P<.001$) and KI ($P<.001$) were seen with maca compared with placebo.[59] The third study included 20 perimenopausal women randomized to maca (n = 10) or placebo (n = 10), with maca observed to be superior to placebo ($P<.05$).[60] Although maca offered some apparent benefits, Lee and colleagues[57] suggested "that the total number of trials, the total sample size, and the average methodological quality of the primary studies were too limited to draw firm conclusions. Furthermore, the safety has not yet been proven."

Recommendations

Evidence for the efficacy of maca in treating menopausal symptoms is uncertain, given that studies are small, short in duration, and have methodological challenges. Maca is safe as a foodstuff.

Pine Bark

Pine bark from the Mediterranean pine (*Pinus pinaster*) is a good source of proanthocyanidins, the same group of compounds found in grape seeds, peanut skins, and other plant material. Proanthocyanidins are heavily promoted as antioxidants and are sold in the United States under the registered trademark name, Pycnogenol, (which is derived from the pine bark). Other pine bark extracts are marketed in a wide variety of formulations. The historical record claims that in 1535, the explorer Jacques Cartier and his crew were ice-bound in the Saint Lawrence River. The crew became ill with scurvy and was purportedly saved when Native Americans showed them how to brew a tea, now thought to have been concocted from the bark of the eastern white cedar tree and reputed to contain large amounts of vitamin C. In the mid last century a French researcher, expanding on the historical record, processed the bark of the European coastal pine tree, extracted the proanthocyanidins, patented the process, and named the compound Pycnogenol. Proanthocyanidins are heavily promoted as antioxidants.

There are 3 trials testing the efficacy of Pycnogenol in perimenopause and menopause, the first randomizing 200 women to 200 mg or placebo,[61] the second treating 38 women with 100 mg for 8 weeks comparing them to 33 controls who did not receive a placebo,[62] and lastly 170 women given 30 mg Pycnogenol or placebo twice daily for 3 months.[63] In all studies, there were trends toward improvements, with the larger trials offering more robust statistically significant improvements. The studies suffer from the fact that the scales used are not validated. The Women's Health Rating Scale used in 2 of the 3 studies does not give a numerical count of VMS.

Recommendation

Pycnogenol (proprietary) might offer some benefits in relieving symptoms. The studies to date are not of sufficient quality to document the degree of therapeutic benefit. The effective dose has yet to be determined. Pycnogenol is possibly safe, but the safety of other pine bark preparations cannot be assured.

Pollen Extract

A proprietary extract made from flower pollen, Relizen, has been recently introduced in the United States. This product has been available in the EU since 1999 and sold under the brand names Serelys, Femal, and Femalen. Its constituents are pollen cytoplasmic extract (GC Fem) and pistil extract (PI 82), and the proposed mechanism of action is said to be antioxidant and antiinflammatory. The current product contains 40 mg of GC Fem and 120 mg of PI 82. Some earlier formulations sold in the EU also contained vitamin E.

According to research papers supplied by the manufacturer, the pollen and pistil come from selected grass species (Poaceae) cultivated and harvested in accordance with the directives of the European Medicine Agency. In vitro and animal studies demonstrate a lack of binding to estrogen receptors and no estrogenic activity (Munoz E. Final report. Effect of PE-F/A on estrogenic activity. unpublished, 2012).[64]

There is only one RCT testing pollen extracts in menopausal women.[65] Sixty-four women were randomized, 54 of whom completed the trial, though only 53 are enumerated in the hot flash data. Hot flashes are reported as number per month, not a conventional analytical measure. There was a trend for hot flashes to increase over the course of the trial in the placebo group, a finding that contradicts the trends in other similar studies. Hot flashes decreased 23% in the active treatment arm ($P<.021$) at 2 months and 22.0% ($P<.027$) at 3 months. Because hot flashes seemed to increase in the placebo group, the between-group difference at 3 months was greater, 27% ($P<.026$). The MRS evidenced significant improvements in other quality-of-life parameters in the pollen extract group ($P<.031$).

Recommendations

Pollen extract is probably safe and possibly effective. The manufacturer attests that there is no pollen in the product and that it is safe for persons with pollen allergies. The one clinical trial is small and has methodological issues.

Siberian Rhubarb

Siberian rhubarb (scientific name: *Rheum rhaponticum*) is used as a food and as a medicinal plant for constipation, diarrhea, and other gastrointestinal complaints. It has laxative qualities that are similar to extracts from senna plants. Two hydrostilbenes found in rhubarb, rhapontigenin and desoxyrhapontigenin, have very weak binding affinity for ER alpha but higher affinity for ER beta. In vitro and in vivo studies support the hypothesis that the hydrostilbenes in rhubarb act as SERMs with mixed agonist/antagonist activity.[66]

A single commercial preparation of rhubarb extract has been studied for menopause. The product has been in use in Germany for more than 20 years and was introduced in the United States as Estrovera. The product contains a proprietary extract called rhaponticin or extract ERr 731.

Published studies have been done on symptomatic perimenopausal, but not menopausal, women. Heger and colleagues[67] randomized 109 women with climacteric complaints to one enteric-coated tablet of ERr 731 (n = 54) or placebo (n = 55) daily for 12 weeks. At 4 weeks, ERr 731 significantly decreased the number and severity of hot flushes ($P<.0001$). At 12 weeks, the MRS II total score, and each symptom within the scale, significantly improved in the active treatment group versus placebo ($P<.0001$). It is noteworthy that only 7 of the 55 women randomized to placebo (12.7% retention rate) and 39 of the 54 randomized to active treatment actually completed the trial. Two women in the active treatment arm developed endometrial hyperplasia. The Hamilton Anxiety Scale and other measures of health and well-being improved in women taking ERr 731. Owing to the small number of completers, the study seems to be underpowered.

Safety data on ERr 731 were gathered from a subset of women drawn from an earlier study, in which 23 subjects were followed for 48 weeks; but only 20 women completed the full 96-week observational period. Few adverse events were reported.[68]

Recommendations

Rhubarb should be regarded as possibly safe and possibly effective. There is limited evidence that applies to only one specific product, Estrovera. The manufacturer has performed long-term safety studies in beagle dogs; no abnormal hematological or metabolic trends have been seen, even at high doses.[69] The long-term human safety data, however, are slim. Additional evidence is needed for both efficacy and safety.

Multiple Botanic Remedies for Menopause

Combination botanicals are frequently recommended by herbal medicine practitioners, owing to the use of multiple botanicals in TCM. Such formulations are said to have advantages over single agents because of the complexity and variety of menopause-related symptoms. Whether this is sound or logical thinking remains to be seen, given that estrogen effectively mitigates most, if not all, menopausal symptoms.

Botanic combinations offer the hope of better symptom relief, but given the complexity of the formulation, offer more potential for adverse events and drug-herb interaction. The following list is to inform the reader of the array of products being promoted and is by no means exhaustive. A few of the products have been tested in RCTs; some have demonstrated some efficacy, but many of the trials listed suffer from the same types of methodological problems noted earlier for single-agent products.

The botanic combinations in **Table 2** have at least one published clinical trial available for review.

BOTANICALS: THE BOTTOM LINE

Few botanic therapies used during menopause have robust evidence of efficacy. Pycnogenol, pollen extract, ERr 731 (rhubarb extract), S-equol, and genistein all have limited evidence of efficacy. Black cohosh is plagued by questions about both efficacy

Table 2
Botanical Combinations

Traditional Name/ Trade Name	Constituents	Reference
Climex	Dong quai (*Angelica sinensis*) + chamomile (*Matricaria chamomilla*)	Kupfersztain et al,[70] 2003
Dang Gui Buxue Tang	1:5 Dang quai (*Angelica sinensis*) + huang qi (*Astragalus membranaceus*)	Haines et al,[71] 2008
Dr Tagliaferri's Formula	Shu Di Huang (*Radix rehnmanniae*) Shan Zhu Yu (*Fructus corni officinalis*) Shan Yao (*Radix dioscoreae oppositae*) Fu Ling (*Sclerotium poriae cocos*) Mu Dan Pi (*Cortex moutan radicis*) Ze Xie (*Rhizoma alismatis orientalis*) Zhi Mu (*Anemarrhena rhizome*) Gan Cao (*Glycyrrhiza uralensis*) Huang qi (*Radix astragali*) Bai Zhu (*Atractylodis macrocephalae rhizoma*)	Clinical trial completed, not yet in press
CuraTrial Research Group	125 mg soy extract daily (providing 50 mg isoflavones including 24 mg genistein and 21.5 mg daidzein) 1500 mg evening primrose oil extract (providing 150 mg gamma linoleic acid) 100 mg *Actaea racemosa* L extract (providing 8 mg deoxyacetein) 200 mg calcium 1.25 mg vitamin D 10 IU vitamin E	Verhoeven et al,[72] 2005
Er-Xian decoction, Er xian tang, Menofine	*Rhizoma curculiginis orchioidis* (Xian Mao) *Herba epimedii grandiflori* (Yin Yang Huo) *Radix morindae officinalis* (Yin Yang Huo) *Radix angelica sinensis* (Dang Gui) *Cortex phellodendri chinensis* (Huang Bo) *Rhizoma anemarrhenae asphodeloidis* (Zhi Mu)	Zhong et al,[73] 2013
Estro G-100	*Cynanchum wilfordii* *Phlomis umbrosa* *Angelica gigas* Kakai extracts Isoflavones, lignans and black cohosh	Sammartino et al,[74] 2006
Jiawei Qing'e Fang	*Cortex eucommiae* *Fructus psoraleae* *Semen juglandis* Rhizoma garlic	Xia et al,[75] 2012
		(continued on next page)

Table 2 *(continued)*		
Traditional Name/ Trade Name	**Constituents**	**Reference**
Menoprogen	Chinese wolfberry Safflower Sea kelp Hawthorne berry Mulberry	Liu et al,[76] 2009
Naturopathic remedy (Herbal Alternatives for Menopause)	Black cohosh, alfalfa, chaste tree, dong quai, false unicorn, licorice, oats, pomegranate, Siberian ginseng, boron	Aso et al,[23] 2012
Nutrafem	*Eucommia ulmoides* bark extract 75 mg plus vigna radiata beans 150 mg.	Garcia et al,[77] 2010
Phytoestrol	Soy extract (Glycine max) (Non-GMO) Red clover extract 30:1 (*Trifolium pratense*) Wild yam root extract 6:1 (*Dioscorea villosa*) Black cohosh extract 15:1 (*Cimicifuga racemosa*) Chaste tree berry extract 4:1 (*Vitex agnus-castus*) Dong quai extract 10:1 (*Angelica sinensis*) Passion flower 8:1 (*Passiflora incarnate*) Burdock root extract 15:1 (*Arctium lappa*)	Informational only. Note that this is not Estrovera, which has been marketed under the brand name Phytoestrol
Phyto-Female Complex	Standardized extracts of black cohosh Dong quai Milk thistle Red clover American ginseng Chaste tree berry	Rotem & Kaplan,[78] 2007
Zhi Mu 14 (with and without acupuncture)	Zhi Mu14 is based on modification of Gan Mai Da Zao Tang *Radix glycyrrhizae uralensis* (Gan Cao) *Semen tritici levis* (Xiao Mai) *Fructus jujubae* (Da Zao) *Radix curcumae* (Yu Jin) *Radix polygalae tenuifoliae* (Yuan Zhi) *Rhizoma acori tatarinowii* (Shi Chang Pu) With "Qing Hao Bie Jia Tang" *Artemisia Annua* and soft-shelled turtle shell decoction	Nedeljkovic et al,[79] 2014

Abbreviation: GMO, genetically modified organism.

and safety. Soy foods are safe and may offer some very limited treatment effects. Red clover, EPO, *Panax ginseng*, *Dioscorea*, and vitamin E are ineffective therapies for vasomotor symptoms. For most botanicals, the decrement in hot flashes is 15% to 30% greater than that seen with placebo.

Researchers in this field do not to adhere to any standardized protocol and do not use any consistent, validated outcome measures. Therefore, it is extremely difficult to make any comparison between products or to assess how these products perform relative to HT. In the few studies that have compared botanicals head to head with HT, botanicals are dismal failures.

SOLD DOES NOT MEAN SAFE: REGULATORY ISSUES AND BOTANIC MEDICINES

Botanic medicines are not subject to the regulatory statutes that apply to pharmaceutical drugs. The US Pharmacopeia (USP) sets the manufacturing standards, but the organization has no legal enforcement power. Potential defects in manufacturing include

- Lack of standardization of active ingredients (if known)
- Adulteration (active drugs, steroids, unknown substances)
- Contamination (heavy metal, pesticides)
- Variation in constituents caused by growing conditions and extraction techniques

On March 29, 2015, Consumer Lab, an independent health and nutritional testing service, under the Freedom of Information Act obtained results from the FDA of its inspections of 483 dietary supplement manufacturing facilities.[80] Over the course of 2014, 62% of the sites had received letters of noncompliance with current Good Manufacturing Practices (cGMPs). Sixty-two percent of the sites (N = 255) were in the United States and 16 were in China (of which 58% received citations). More than 75% of sites in Mexico, India, Spain, and South Korea received citations. Sites averaged 6 infractions.

The most common infractions were failure to verify the identity of a dietary supplement ingredient and failure to establish specifications for identity, purity, strength, and/or composition of the finished product.

Only a small fraction of such facilities are inspected each year because of a lack of funding and personnel at the FDA. Consumer Lab has listed offenders and nonoffenders on their Web site and plans to do updates on an annual basis.

This report dovetails with the investigation initiated by the Attorney General of the State of New York, reported on February 3, 2015 in the *New York Times*.[81] The Office of the Attorney General (AG) bought herbal products from 4 leading national retailers: GNC, Target, Walmart and Walgreens. Four out of 5 products tested using DNA bar coding (in essence a genetic fingerprint for the plant type) did not contain any of the herbs listed on the label. Many products contained nothing but fillers, like rice powder, radish powder, legume powder, asparagus, and houseplant material. The AG issued cease and desist letters to all the retailers involved. Apologists for the supplement manufacturers argued that the DNA testing was flawed and that perhaps the DNA for the active materials was destroyed in manufacturing. The AG's office responded that the DNA signature of the contaminants and adulterants were easily identifiable, and if any real herbal material was present, it should have been verifiable. GNC initially defended their products, claiming a vigorous independent testing program for their products. Nonetheless, 6 weeks later, GNC announced that they were initiating a rigorous new testing program. Although the trade associations and supplement manufacturers continue to defend their products, other states' AGs around the country, stepping around the FDA, are initiating their own fraud investigations. These states include Connecticut, the District of Columbia, Hawaii, Idaho, Indiana, Iowa, Kentucky, Massachusetts, Mississippi, New Hampshire, Pennsylvania, and Rhode Island.[82]

Two major dilemmas remain: First, is the material in the bottle really what is specified on the label. Second, if the material is true, does it work and is it safe?

Women should be directed to buy botanicals from reliable sources. The USP logo on a product indicates that it has been tested for quality, standardization, and purity.

Retailers who submit their products for testing are listed on the USP Web site.[83] Consumer Lab offers manufacturers testing and verification services. Access to their list of verified products requires a nominal subscription fee.[84] Verification processes include testing to assure that the product

- Contains the ingredients listed on the label, in the declared potency and amounts
- Does not contain harmful levels of specified contaminants
- Will break down and release into the body within a specified amount of time
- Has been made according to FDA cGMPs using sanitary and well-controlled procedures

Botanic medicines are more tightly regulated in Europe; brands from Germany, Switzerland, and the United Kingdom may offer more consistent quality.

As discussed at the start of this article, after the publication of WHI, as use of hormone therapy plummeted, the use of alternatives seems to have accelerated. A woman who distrusts the medical establishment and who suspects the pharmaceutical industry of evil intentions, will suspend all disbelief when she walks into a health food store. Menopausal women, despite the absence of quality evidence, continue to perceive CAM as highly effective for menopausal symptoms, with a low risk of side effects or adverse events.[8] Most Americans, until the recent events discussed earlier, thought that over-the-counter drugs, vitamins, botanic products, and dietary supplements are all regularly tested by the FDA. In actuality, these alternatives are marketed without documentation of efficacy or safety.

On its Web site, the FDA clearly answers whether dietary supplements are FDA approved: *Dietary supplement manufacturers and distributors are not required to obtain approval from FDA before marketing dietary supplements. Before a firm markets a dietary supplement, the firm is responsible for ensuring that:*

- *The products it manufactures or distributes are safe*
- *Any claims made about the products are not false or misleading*
- *The products comply with the Federal Food, Drug, and Cosmetic Act and FDA regulations in all other respects*[85]

BRINGING COMPLEMENTARY AND ALTERNATIVE MEDICINE INTO A TREATMENT PLAN

When a health care professional advises, recommends, or supports the use of a specific CAM product, even an over-the-counter remedy, that provider is judged to be a learned expert and, in this role, incurs responsibility and liability for poor outcomes. Moreover, if a practitioner decides to sell and distribute supplements and botanic medicines in the office, responsibility and liability are heightened.

Because botanic medicines are exempt from the statutes that govern drug safety, the health care provider who recommends botanic medicine assumes most of the burden for the risks that might be incurred. The following recommendations should help to protect both the patients and provider:

1. Document major symptoms and severity of symptoms and acknowledge drug-herb interactions before making recommendations.
2. Provide handouts with basic information about any botanic products when recommending their use. WebMD, Medline Plus, and other sites have well-researched, herb-specific patient information online.
3. Provide women with clear warnings on the potential for adverse events with botanicals, especially for those products with limited documentation of safety and/or efficacy.

Box 3
Botanicals and coagulation

Botanicals that interfere with clotting and should be discontinued before surgery

Salicylate-containing supplements

  Black cohosh

  Meadowsweet flower

  Poplar bark or buds

  Sweet birch bark

  Willow bark

  Wintergreen leaf

Supplements inhibiting platelet function

  Angelica

  Bromelain

  Cayenne fruit

  Chinese skullcap root

  Danshen

  Dong quai

  Feverfew

  Fish oil

  Garlic

  Ginger

  Ginkgo

  Ginseng

  Licorice

  Papain

  Policosanol

  Pycnogenol (in smokers)

  Red clover

  Reishi

  Relshi fruit bodies

  Resveratrol

  Saw palmetto

  Turmeric root

  Tocopherols, mixed

  Tocotrienols

  Vitamin E

4. Document the information you provide by placing printouts of materials into patients' medical record.
5. Document your informed consent discussion with patients.
6. Provide a list of quality products from reputable manufacturers or refer patients to the USP or Consumer Lab Web site for lists of verified products.
7. Schedule a follow-up appointment at a reasonable interval, usually 6 to 12 weeks, to assess compliance and satisfaction with treatment and to query about possible adverse events.
8. Monitor and report adverse events through MEDWATCH or through your local poison control network.
9. Be aware that many herbal/botanic medicines affect coagulation. Stop all supplements at least 4 to 6 weeks before any scheduled major surgical procedures. See **Box 3** for a list of supplements known to affect clotting.

REFERENCES

1. Rossouw JE, Anderson GL, Prentice RL, Writing Group for the Women's Health Initiative Investigators. Risks and benefits of estrogen plus progestin in healthy postmenopausal women: principal results From the Women's Health Initiative randomized controlled trial. JAMA 2002;288(3):321–33.
2. Wilson RA. Feminine Forever. New York: M Evans Co; 1966.
3. Bair YA, Gold EB, Greendale GA, et al. Ethnic differences in use of complementary and alternative medicine at midlife: longitudinal results from SWAN participants. Am J Public Health 2002;92:1832–5.
4. Bair YA, Gold EB, Azari RA, et al. Use of conventional and complementary healthcare during the transition to menopause: longitudinal results from the Study of Women's Health Across the Nation (SWAN). Menopause 2005;12:31–9.
5. Gold EB, Bair Y, Zhang G, et al. Cross-sectional analysis of specific complementary and alternative medicine (CAM) use by racial/ethnic group and menopausal status: the Study of Women's Health Across the Nation (SWAN). Menopause 2007;14:612–23.
6. Bair YA, Gold EB, Zhang G, et al. Use of complementary and alternative medicine during the menopause transition: longitudinal results from the Study of Women's Health Across the Nation. Menopause 2008;15:32–43.
7. Peng W, Adams J, Sibbritt DW, et al. Critical review of complementary and alternative medicine use in menopause: focus on prevalence, motivation, decision-making, and communication. Menopause 2014;21(5):536–48.
8. Geller SE, Studee L. Botanical and dietary supplements for menopausal symptoms: what works, what doesn't. J Womens Health 2005;14(7):634–49.
9. Gentry-Maharaj A, Karpinskyj C, Glazer C, et al. Use and perceived efficacy of complementary and alternative medicines after discontinuation of hormone therapy: a nested United Kingdom Collaborative Trial of Ovarian Cancer Screening cohort study. Menopause 2015;22(4):384–90.
10. Adams NR. Detection of the effects of phytoestrogens on sheep and cattle. J Anim Sci 1995;73(5):1509–15.
11. Kim J, Kang M, Lee JS, et al. Fermented and nonfermented soy food consumption and gastric cancer in Japanese and Korean populations: a meta-analysis of observational studies. Cancer Sci 2011;102(1):231–44.
12. Green R, Santoro N. Menopausal symptoms and ethnicity: the Study of Women's Health Across the Nation. Womens Health (London England) 2009;5(2):127–33.

13. Ishizuka B, Kudo Y, Tango T. Cross-sectional community survey of menopause symptoms among Japanese women. Maturitas 2008;61(3):260–7.
14. Sievert LL, Morrison L, Brown DE, et al. Vasomotor symptoms among Japanese-American and European-American women living in Hilo, Hawaii. Menopause 2007;14(2):261–9.
15. North American Menopause Society. The role of soy isoflavones in menopausal health: report of The North American MenopauseSociety/Wulf H. Utian Translational Science Symposium in Chicago, IL (October 2010). Menopause 2011; 18(7):732–53.
16. Bolaños R, Del Castillo A, Francia J. Soy isoflavones versus placebo in the treatment of climacteric vasomotor symptoms: systematic review and meta-analysis [review]. Menopause 2010;17(3):660–6.
17. Lethaby A, Marjoribanks J, Kronenberg F, et al. Phytoestrogens for menopausal vasomotor symptoms. Cochrane Database Syst Rev 2013;(12):CD001395.
18. Taku K, Melby MK, Kronenberg F, et al. Extracted or synthesized soybean isoflavones reduce menopausal hot flash frequency and severity: systematic review and meta-analysis of randomized controlled trials. Menopause 2012;19(7): 776–90.
19. Chen MN, Lin CC, Liu CF. Efficacy of phytoestrogens for menopausal symptoms: a meta-analysis and systematic review. Climacteric 2015;18(2):260–9.
20. Suarez FL, Springfield J, Furne JK, et al. Gas production in human ingesting a soybean flour derived from beans naturally low in oligosaccharides. Am J Clin Nutr 1999;69(1):135–9.
21. Setchell KDR, Clerici C. Equol: history, chemistry, and formation. The J Nutr 2010; 140(7):1355S–62S.
22. Newton KM, Reed SD, Uchiyama S, et al. A cross-sectional study of equol producer status and self-reported vasomotor symptoms. Menopause 2015;22(5): 489–95.
23. Aso T, Uchiyama S, Matsumura Y, et al. A natural S-(-)equol supplement alleviates hot flushes and other menopausal symptoms in equol nonproducing postmenopausal Japanese women. J Womens Health (larchmt) 2012;21(1):92–100.
24. Aso T. Equol improves menopausal symptoms in Japanese women. J Nutr 2010; 140(7):1386S–9S.
25. Utian WH, Jones M, Setchell KD. S-equol: a potential nonhormonal agent for menopause-related symptom relief. J Womens Health (Larchmt) 2015;24(3): 200–8.
26. D'Anna R, Cannata ML, Atteritano M, et al. Effects of the phytoestrogen genistein on hot flushes, endometrium, and vaginal epithelium in postmenopausal women: a 1-year randomized, double-blind, placebo-controlled study. Menopause 2007; 14(4):648–55.
27. Crisafulli A, Altavilla D, Marini H, et al. Effects of the phytoestrogen genistein on cardiovascular risk factors in postmenopausal women. Menopause 2005;12(2): 186–92.
28. Evans M, Elliott JG, Sharma P, et al. The effect of synthetic genistein on menopause symptom management in healthy postmenopausal women: a multi-center, randomized, placebo-controlled study. Maturitas 2011;68(2):189–96.
29. Khaodhiar L, Ricciotti HA, Li L, et al. Daidzein-rich isoflavone aglycones are potentially effective in reducing hot flashes in menopausal women. Menopause 2008;15(1):125–32.
30. Orlich MJ, Singh PN, Sabaté J, et al. Vegetarian dietary patterns and mortality in Adventist Health Study 2. JAMA Intern Med 2013;173(13):1230–8.

31. Geller S, Studee L. Soy and red clover for mid-life and aging. Climacteric 2006; 9(4):245–63.
32. Sartippour MR, Rao JY, Apple S, et al. A pilot clinical study of short-term isoflavone supplements in breast cancer patients. Nutr Cancer 2004;49(1):59–65.
33. Shu XO, Zheng Y, Cai H, et al. Soy food intake and breast cancer survival. JAMA 2009;302(22):2437–43.
34. Fritz H, Seely D, Flower G, et al. Soy, red clover, and isoflavones and breast cancer: a systematic review. PLoS One 2013;8(11):e81968.
35. Unfer V, Casini ML, Costabile L, et al. Endometrial effects of long-term treatment with phytoestrogens: a randomized, double-blind, placebo-controlled study. Fertil Steril 2004;82(1):145–8 [quiz: 265].
36. Alexandersen P, Toussaint A, Christiansen C, et al. Ipriflavone in the treatment of postmenopausal osteoporosis: a randomized controlled trial. JAMA 2001; 285(11):1482–8.
37. Available at: http://www.swansonvitamins.com/swanson-premium-ipriflavone-complex-wo-stivone-120-tabs. Accessed June 15, 2015.
38. Kruse SO, Löhning A, Pauli GF, et al. Fukiic and piscidic acid esters from the rhizome of Cimicifuga racemosa and the in vitro estrogenic activity of fukinolic acid. Planta Med 1999;65(8):763–4.
39. Wuttke W, Jarry H, Becker T, et al. Phytoestrogens: endocrine disrupters or replacement for hormone replacement therapy? Maturitas 2003;44(Suppl 1): S9–20 [review].
40. Newton KM, Reed SD, LaCroix AZ, et al. Treatment of vasomotor symptoms of menopause with black cohosh, multibotanicals, soy, hormone therapy, or placebo: a randomized trial. Ann Intern Med 2006;145(12):869–79.
41. Pockaj B, Gallagher JG, Loprinzi CL, et al. Phase III double-blind, randomized, placebo-controlled crossover trial of black cohosh in the management of hot flashes: NCCTG Trial N01CC1. J Clin Oncol 2006;24(18):2836–41.
42. Raus K, Brucker C, Gorkow C, et al. First-time proof of endometrial safety of the special black cohosh extract (Actaea or Cimicifuga racemosa extract) CR BNO 1055. Menopause 2006;13(4):678–91.
43. Mahady GB, Low Dog T, Barrett ML, et al. United States Pharmacopeia review of the black cohosh case reports of hepatotoxicity. Menopause 2008;15(4 Pt 1): 628–38.
44. Jenny M, Wondrak A, Zvetkova E, et al. Crinum latifolium leave extracts suppress immune activation cascades in peripheral blood mononuclear cells and proliferation of prostate tumor cells. Scientia Pharmaceutica 2011;79:323–35.
45. Wu WH, Liu LY, Chung CJ, et al. Estrogenic effect of yam ingestion in healthy postmenopausal women. J Am Coll Nutr 2005;24(4):235–43.
46. Komesaroff PA, Black CV, Cable V, et al. Effects of wild yam extract on menopausal symptoms, lipids and sex hormones in healthy menopausal women. Climacteric 2001;4(2):144–50.
47. Beinfeld H, Korngold E. Between heaven and earth: a guide to Chinese medicine. New York: Ballantine Books; 1991.
48. Circosta C, Pasquale RD, Palumbo DR, et al. Estrogenic activity of standardized extract of Angelica sinensis. Phytother Res 2006;20(8):665–9.
49. Hirata JD, Swiersz LM, Zell B, et al. Does dong quai have estrogenic effects in postmenopausal women? A double-blind, placebo-controlled trial. Fertil Steril 1997;68(6):981–6.
50. Chenoy R, Hussain S, Tayob Y, et al. Effect of oral gamolenic acid from evening primrose oil on menopausal flushing. BMJ 1994;308(6927):501–3.

51. Lewis JE, Nickell LA, Thompson LU, et al. A randomized controlled trial of the effect of dietary soy and flaxseed muffins on quality of life and hot flashes during menopause. Menopause 2006;13(4):631–42.

52. Colli MC, Bracht A, Soares AA, et al. Evaluation of the efficacy of flaxseed meal and flaxseed extract in reducing menopausal symptoms. J Med Food 2012;15(9): 840–5.

53. Pruthi S, Qin R, Terstreip SA, et al. A phase III, randomized, placebo-controlled, double-blind trial of flaxseed for the treatment of hot flashes: North Central Cancer Treatment Group N08C7. Menopause 2012;19(1):48–53.

54. Baranov AI. Medicinal uses of ginseng and related plants in the Soviet Union: recent trends in the Soviet literature. J Ethnopharmacol 1982;6(3):339–53.

55. Heyerick A, Vervarcke S, Depypere H, et al. A first prospective, randomized, double-blind, placebo-controlled study on the use of a standardized hop extract to alleviate menopausal discomforts. Maturitas 2006;54(2):164–75.

56. Erkkola R, Vervarcke S, Vansteelandt S, et al. A randomized, double-blind, placebo-controlled, cross-over pilot study on the use of a standardized hop extract to alleviate menopausal discomforts. Phytomedicine 2010;17(6):389–96.

57. Lee MS, Shin BC, Yang EJ, et al. Maca (Lepidium meyenii) for treatment of menopausal symptoms: a systematic review. Maturitas 2011;70:227–33.

58. Brooks NA, Wilcox G, Walker KZ, et al. Beneficial effects of Lepidium meyenii (maca) on psychological symptoms and measures of sexual dysfunction in postmenopausal women are not related to estrogen or androgen content. Menopause 2008;15:1157–62.

59. Meissner HO, Mscisz A, Reich-Bilinska H, et al. Hormone-balancing effect of pre-gelatinized organic maca (Lepidium peruvanum chacon): (ii) physiological and symptomatic responses of early-postmenopausal women to standardized doses of maca in double blind, randomized, placebo-controlled, multi-centre clinical study. Int J Biomed Sci 2006;2:360–74.

60. Meissner HO, Reich-Bilinska H, Mscisz A, et al. Therapeutic effects of pre-gelatinized organic maca (Lepidium peruvanum chacon) used as a nonhormonal alternative to HRT in perimenopausal women-clinical pilot study. Int J Biomed Sci 2006;2:143–59.

61. Yang HM, Liao MF, Zhu SY, et al. A randomised, double-blind, placebo-controlled trial on the effect of Pycnogenol on the climacteric syndrome in peri-menopausal women. Acta Obstet Gynecol Scand 2007;86(8):978–85.

62. Errichi S, Bottari A, Belcaro G, et al. Supplementation with Pycnogenol improves signs and symptoms of menopausal transition. Panminerva Med 2011;53(3 Suppl 1): 65–70.

63. Kohama T, Negami M. Effect of low-dose French maritime pine bark extract on climacteric syndrome in 170 perimenopausal women: a randomized, double-blind, placebo-controlled trial. J Reprod Med 2013;58(1–2):39–46.

64. Hellström AC, Muntzing J. The pollen extract Femal–a nonestrogenic alternative to hormone therapy in women with menopausal symptoms. Menopause 2012; 19(7):825–9.

65. Winther K, Rein E, Hedman C. Femal, a herbal remedy made from pollen extracts, reduces hot flushes and improves quality of life in menopausal women: a randomized, placebo-controlled, parallel study. Climacteric 2005;8(2): 162–70.

66. Wober J, Möller F, Richter T, et al. Activation of estrogen receptor-beta by a special extract of Rheum rhaponticum (ERr 731), its aglycones and structurally related compounds. J Steroid Biochem Mol Biol 2007;107(3–5):191–201.

67. Heger M, Ventskovskiy BM, Borzenko I, et al. Efficacy and safety of a special extract of Rheum rhaponticum (ERr 731) in perimenopausal women with climacteric complaints: a 12-week randomized, double-blind, placebo-controlled trial. Menopause 2006;13(5):744–59.
68. Hasper I, Ventskovskiy BM, Rettenberger R, et al. Long-term efficacy and safety of the special extract ERr 731 of Rheum rhaponticum in perimenopausal women with menopausal symptoms. Menopause 2009;16(1):117–31.
69. Kaszkin-Bettag M, Richardson A, Rettenberger R, et al. Long-term toxicity studies in dogs support the safety of the special extract ERr 731 from the roots of Rheum rhaponticum. Food Chem Toxicol 2008;46(5):1608–18.
70. Kupfersztain C, Rotem C, Fagot R, et al. The immediate effect of natural plant extract, Angelica sinensis and Matricaria chamomilla (Climex) for the treatment of hot flushes during menopause. A preliminary report. Clin Exp Obstet Gynecol 2003;30(4):203–6.
71. Haines CJ, Lam PM, Chung TK, et al. A randomized, double-blind, placebo-controlled study of the effect of a Chinese herbal medicine preparation (Dang Gui Buxue Tang) on menopausal symptoms in Hong Kong Chinese women. Climacteric 2008;11(3):244–51.
72. Verhoeven MO, van der Mooren MJ, van de Weijer PH, et al. CuraTrial Research Group. Effect of a combination of isoflavones and Actaea racemosa Linnaeus on climacteric symptoms in healthy symptomatic perimenopausal women: a 12-week randomized, placebo-controlled, double-blind study. Menopause 2005; 12(4):412–20.
73. Zhong LL, Tong Y, Tang GW, et al. A randomized, double-blind, controlled trial of a Chinese herbal formula (Er-Xian decoction) for menopausal symptoms in Hong Kong perimenopausal women. Menopause 2013;20(7):767–76.
74. Sammartino A, Tommaselli GA, Gargano V, et al. Short-term effects of a combination of isoflavones, lignans and Cimicifuga racemosa on climacteric-related symptoms in postmenopausal women: a double-blind, randomized, placebo-controlled trial. Gynecol Endocrinol 2006;22(11):646–50.
75. Xia Y, Zhao Y, Ren M, et al. A randomized double-blind placebo-controlled trial of a Chinese herbal medicine preparation (Jiawei Qing'e Fang) for hot flashes and quality of life in perimenopausal women. Menopause 2012; 19(2):234–44.
76. Liu D, Lu Y, Ma H, et al. A pilot observational study to assess the safety and efficacy of Menoprogen for the management of menopausal symptoms in Chinese women. J Altern Complement Med 2009;15(1):79–85.
77. Garcia JT, Gonzaga F, Tan D, et al. Use of a multibotanical (Nutrafem) for the relief of menopausal vasomotor symptoms: a double-blind, placebo-controlled study. Menopause 2010;17(2):303–8.
78. Rotem C, Kaplan B. Phyto-Female Complex for the relief of hot flushes, night sweats and quality of sleep: randomized, controlled, double-blind pilot study. Gynecol Endocrinol 2007;23(2):117–22.
79. Nedeljkovic M, Tian L, Ji P, et al. Effects of acupuncture and Chinese herbal medicine (Zhi Mu 14) on hot flushes and quality of life in postmenopausal women: results of a four-arm randomized controlled pilot trial. Menopause 2014;21(1): 15–24.
80. Available at: https://www.consumerlab.com/recall_detail.asp?recallid=10799. Accessed June 15, 2015.
81. Available at: http://well.blogs.nytimes.com/2015/02/03/new-york-attorney-general-targets-supplements-at-major-retailers/. Accessed June 15, 2015.

82. Available at: http://well.blogs.nytimes.com/2015/03/09/safety-of-herbal-supplements-pulls-prosecutors-together/. Accessed June 15, 2015.
83. Available at: http://www.usp.org/usp-verification-services/usp-verified-dietary-supplements/verified-supplements. Accessed June 15, 2015.
84. Available at: https://www.consumerlab.com/products.asp. Accessed June 15, 2015.
85. Available at: http://www.fda.gov/AboutFDA/Transparency/Basics/ucm194344.htm. Accessed June 15, 2015.

Menopause and Sexuality

Kimberley Thornton, MD[a], Judi Chervenak, MD[a],
Genevieve Neal-Perry, MD, PhD[b],*

KEYWORDS

- Menopause • Sexuality • Vulvovaginal atrophy • Hypoactive sexual desire disorder
- Hormone therapy

KEY POINTS

- Sexual dysfunction increases with age and is highly prevalent among menopausal women.
- Most menopausal women consider sex to be an important part of their life and strongly desire to maintain sexual activity.
- Few women disclose their concerns to health care providers; therefore, health care providers should routinely query perimenopausal and menopausal patients about their satisfaction with their sexual functioning.

INTRODUCTION

Sexuality may impact quality of life through effects on the emotional and psychological health of a woman. Consequently, clinicians who take care of women appreciate when they may be vulnerable to sexual dysfunction. The menopausal transition, a time characterized by hormonal, physiologic, and social changes, is often associated with sexual dysfunction. The physiologic mechanism by which the menopausal transition affects sexual health involves declining and fluctuating gonadal steroid hormone levels that adversely affect elasticity of the vaginal mucosa and vaginal secretions and result in vaginal atrophy and pain with sexual intercourse.[1] Additionally, social conditions or life stressors, such as divorce, lack of a partner, job loss, or declining health, may affect desire for sexual intercourse.

Improved access to medical care and nutrition has increased the average life expectancy. Therefore, the average woman making the transition into menopause can expect to live for at least 25 years.[2] With increased expectations for a longer and

The authors have nothing to disclose.
[a] Department of Obstetrics and Gynecology, Montefiore Medical Center, Albert Einstein College of Medicine, 1300 Morris Park Avenue, Mazer Building Room 322, Bronx, NY 10461, USA; [b] Department of Obstetrics and Gynecology, University of Washington, 1959 Northeast Pacific Street, Box 356460, Seattle, WA 98195-6460, USA
* Corresponding author.
E-mail address: NealPerr@uw.edu

healthier life, women are thinking more about quality-of-life issues, which include maintaining sexual function.[3] Additionally, attitudes and expectations regarding sexual function were further impacted when the Food and Drug Administration (FDA) approved phosphodiesterase type 5 inhibitors for male erectile dysfunction, which resulted in more menopausal women with male partners who have renewed sexual interest and improved function.[4,5]

ATTITUDES ABOUT SEX AND THE MENOPAUSE

Regardless of age and menopausal status, sexual interest continues for many women. Seventy-six percent of middle-aged women in the Study of Women's Health Across the Nation (SWAN) reported sex was moderately or extremely important to them.[6] Even though sex is important to reproductively senescing women, sexual activity and function decline with age. In the Women's Healthy Aging Project cohort, an extension of the Melbourne Women's Midlife Health Project, a significant decline from 74% to 56% in sexual activity (P<.001) was reported between early postmenopausal women and late postmenopausal women.[7] Short Personal Experience Questionnaire (SPEQ; a 9-item sexual-function instrument) scores also indicated that 42% of early perimenopausal women had sexual dysfunction in the Melbourne Women's Midlife Health Project at baseline. After 8 years of follow-up, the percentage of women with sexual dysfunction, as determined by SPEQ scores, more than doubled to 88%.[8] The etiology of this decline in sexual function and activity may vary and is often multifactorial. Thus, a careful evaluation is required to determine the cause and recommend the best intervention.

PHYSIOLOGY

In the regularly menstruating woman, in each month's follicular phase, follicle-stimulating hormone (FSH) stimulates follicular growth and estradiol synthesis. Increasing estradiol production from the dominant follicle mediates a negative feedback and suppressive effect on FSH and luteinizing hormone (LH). Estradiol synthesis from the dominant follicle continues until a critical level is reached and estradiol-positive feedback induces an LH surge and ovulation.[9] Estradiol synthesis during the menstrual cycle affects vaginal secretions and the vaginal mucosa.

PATHOPHYSIOLOGY

Multiple physiologic changes that occur during the menopausal transition result from reduced ovarian reserve, defined by reduced numbers of gonadotropin-responsive follicles. Menstrual cycles in late perimenopausal women are characterized by increased FSH, decreased inhibin B, and irregularly short and long cycle lengths.[10] Until the time of the last menstrual period (LMP), estradiol levels are equally variable in perimenopausal women. By the time of the LMP, women enter a persistent state of hypogonadism and hypergonadotropism (elevated FSH and LH).[11,12] After estradiol falls, estrone, primarily generated by the aromatization of androgens, becomes the main circulating estrogen. Compared with estradiol, serum androgen levels demonstrate a steady but less dramatic decline (**Fig. 1**).[8,13] The less dramatic fall in serum androgens is related to the decrease in sex hormone binding globulin associated with hypoestrogenism.[14]

SEX AND HORMONES

Hormonal changes during menopause may impact sexual functioning. A prospective, population-based study of Australian-born women, observed for 8 years as they

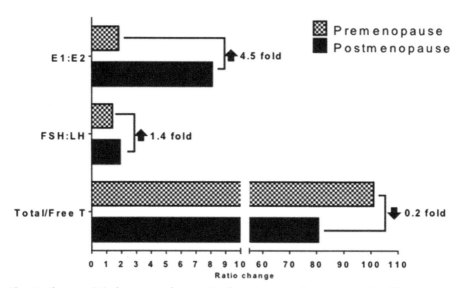

Fig. 1. Characteristic hormone changes in the menopausal as compared with premenopausal women. Compared with premenopausal women, menopausal women experience significant shifts in serum levels of gonadal steroids and gonadotropins. Reduced ovarian estradiol synthesis results in a 4.5-fold increase in the estrone to estradiol and 1.4-fold increase in the FSH to LH values in menopausal women. Menopausal women synthesize 0.2-fold less androgens than premenopausal women. However, the fold change is not nearly as great as that observed in estradiol. (*Data from* Rothman MS, Carlson NE, Xu M, et al. Re-examination of testosterone, dihydrotestosterone, estradiol and estrone levels across the menstrual cycle and in postmenopausal women measured by liquid chromatography-tandem mass spectrometry. Steroids 2011;76(1–2):177–82.)

passed through natural menopause, reported that low estrogen levels adversely affected sexual interest and responsiveness, but did not affect the frequency of sexual activity.[15] Total testosterone was not significantly affected in this cohort. Moreover, free testosterone levels did not significantly affect any sexual domains. Similarly, no significant difference in testosterone levels was observed in women undergoing natural menopause, with SPEQ scores suggesting sexual dysfunction compared with women with SPEQ scores showing no dysfunction.[8] It is worth noting that it is possible that there are differences in serum testosterone; however, it may be difficult to observe significant differences in very low levels of testosterone because of the sensitivity limitations of non–mass spectrometry-based testosterone assays.[8]

Pelvic organ prolapse (POP) is the descent of one or more of the following: anterior vaginal wall, posterior vaginal wall, uterus, or apex of the vagina. The incidence of pelvic floor weakening increases with aging and is thought to result from a combination of connective tissue degradation, pelvic denervation, and devascularization, all of which predispose to prolapse.[16] Dyspareunia, chronic pelvic pain, and modified self-image are associated with POP. Any one of these adverse symptoms can devastate sexual function.

HYPOACTIVE SEXUAL DESIRE DISORDER

Hypoactive sexual desire disorder (HSDD) occurs when there is a persistent or recurrent absence of sexual fantasies or desire for sexual activity that results in personal distress. For the diagnosis of HSDD to be made, iatrogenic or organic causes for sexual dysfunction must be ruled out and the patient must report marked distress or interpersonal difficulty.[17] Recently, the *Diagnostic and Statistical Manual of Mental Disorders, Fifth Edition* (DSM-V) grouped HSDD with female sexual arousal disorder under the category of female sexual interest/arousal disorders (FSIAD) (**Box 1**).[18]

The prevalence of HSDD has been difficult to determine and has varied among studies. Disparate estimates of prevalence may reflect differences in the age of the study group and different criteria for diagnosis and study inclusion. The Prevalence of Female Sexual Problems Associated with Distress and Determinants of Treatment Seeking survey of 31,581 US women 18 years or older found 8.9% of women aged 18 to 44 years, 12.3% of women aged 45 to 64 years, and 7.4% of women older than 65 years had low desire and distress.[19] The Global Study of Sexual Attitudes and Behavior reported a 25% to 43% prevalence of symptoms consistent with lack of sexual interest in women.[20] These numbers represent all women reporting occasional, periodic, or frequent problems with desire. If the population were restricted to women reporting frequent problems, the prevalence of low desire would vary between 5.4% and 13.6%.[21]

The risk for HSDD is greatest in women who have undergone surgical menopause. It is hypothesized that abrupt reductions in circulating 17-β-estradiol and testosterone levels significantly contribute to HSDD because testosterone replacement can increase sexual desire and arousal in this group of women.[22,23] The Women's International Study of Health and Sexuality reported surgically induced menopausal women 20 to 49 years old had significantly higher rates of HSDD compared with gonadally intact, age-matched, and regularly cycling control women (26% vs 14% respectively, $p = 0.002$).[24] In contrast, no significant difference was found in the diagnosis of HSDD between surgically or naturally postmenopausal women aged 50 to 70 years (14% and 9%, respectively, $p = 0.067$). These data suggest that health care providers should routinely assess women with surgical menopause for signs of sexual dysfunction. Androgen therapy may be considered in this population of women.

HSDD correlates with low feelings of physical and emotional satisfaction, poor self-image, and unhappiness.[25] Research suggests multiple psychological reasons why women choose to engage in sexual activity, including wanting to feel close to a partner, expression of love, and wanting to feel feminine.[26] When a diagnosis of HSDD is

---

Box 1
Hypoactive sexual desire disorder

- Clinical features occur for at least six months
- Common findings include persistently reduced or absence of
  - Sexual fantasies
  - Sexual interest
  - Responses to partner's attempts to initiate sexual activity
  - Response to external or internal sexual/erotic cues
  - Sexual excitement/pleasure during encounters
- Expressed marked personal distress or interpersonal difficulty resulting from sexual dysfunction
- No iatrogenic or organic cause for sexual dysfunction

suspected, psychosocial factors, such as conflict with a partner, history of sexual abuse, and cultural/religious factors should be considered, as they can significantly affect sexual desire.[27]

SYMPTOMATIC VULVOVAGINAL ATROPHY

Decreased levels of estrogen are associated with symptomatic vulvovaginal atrophy, a condition characterized by thin, pale, and dry vaginal and vulvar surfaces. During menopause, the decline in estrogen leads to a decrease in lactobacilli, acid-producing bacteria that play a key role in keeping the vaginal epithelial pH in the range of 3.8 to 4.5.[1] As lactobacilli decrease, the vaginal epithelium becomes more basic, leading to a change in vaginal flora. It has been noted that increased bacterial diversity is correlated with increased symptoms of vaginal dryness.[28]

Symptomatic vulvovaginal atrophy is highly prevalent in midlife and menopausal women, with as many as 45% of postmenopausal women affected.[29] Symptomatic vulvovaginal atrophy is often accompanied by diminished secretions from sebaceous glands and reduced vaginal lubrication during sexual stimulation.[1] Women with vulvovaginal atrophy experience pain with intercourse that leads to decreased interest and frank avoidance of sexual activity.[30] In the Real Women's Views on Treatment Options for Menopausal Vaginal Changes study, 63% of women with symptomatic vulvovaginal atrophy reported that their symptoms interfered with enjoyment of sexual intercourse and 47% of partnered women indicated it interfered with their relationship.[31,32] Twelve percent of women without a partner reported that they were not seeking a sexual partner because of symptoms related to vulvovaginal atrophy. Similarly, in the Vaginal Health: Insights, Views, & Attitudes study, 75% of women reported that vaginal discomfort negatively affected their sex life.[33] Despite the high prevalence of symptomatic vulvovaginal atrophy in midlife and postmenopausal women, almost half of women report that they never discuss the impact of the symptoms on their quality of life with a health care provider. Equally worrisome, only 7% reported that their health care provider ever initiated a conversation about vulvovaginal atrophy.[1,31,32] Health care providers should be vigilant about asking patients about satisfaction with their sex life and they should query patients about signs and symptoms of vulvovaginal atrophy.

CHRONIC DISEASES AND SEXUAL DYSFUNCTION

When a diagnosis of sexual dysfunction is suspected, a complete and detailed medical history should be obtained to evaluate women for chronic diseases that can adversely affect sexual health. This is especially true in menopause, because as women age they are at an increased risk for acquiring chronic diseases that impact sexual function.[22] Chronic diseases, such as hypertension, diabetes, depression, neurologic diseases, urinary incontinence, and osteoarthritis, commonly impact sexual function.[22,27,34] Some reports suggest that cardiovascular disease impacts women's sexual desire and arousal through effects on systemic blood flow. The mechanisms by which cardiovascular disease affects sexual arousal is hypothesized to be related to the fact that female genital arousal is achieved when the vascular system increases blood flow and engorges the labia via vasodilation. Vascular disease may reduce vulvovaginal vasodilation and reduce sexual arousal.[35] Reduced physical function in obese women and women with osteoarthritis also may adversely affect sexual activity. Additionally, sexual dysfunction observed in women with diabetes is attributed to reduced energy, altered body image, and suboptimal vaginal engorgement during orgasm.[22]

MEDICATIONS

Medications must be considered as a possible source of sexual dysfunction in menopausal women. Organ systems have limited homeostatic reserve with aging, resulting in decreased clearance and enhanced toxicity of many drugs.[36] For these reasons, undesired effects of medications are more prevalent in the elderly. Medications commonly associated with sexual dysfunction include serotonin reuptake inhibitors (SSRIs), neuroleptics, and cardiovascular medications.[22,34] A detailed list is shown in **Box 2**. The menopausal transition and early postmenopausal years are considered windows of vulnerability for depression; therefore, antidepressants may be a common medication among perimenopausal and early menopausal women.[37] SSRIs are associated with HSDD. When possible, the medication suspected of causing sexual side effects should be stopped or switched.

QUALITY OF LIFE IMPACT ON MENOPAUSAL WOMEN

Menopausal symptoms and sexual dysfunction can negatively impact quality of life for women. A higher sense of purpose in life is reported by midlife women who report higher levels of enjoyment with sexual activity.[38] Women more likely to engage in partnered intimate sexual activities tend to be of younger age, lower body mass index, married, and have better emotional well-being.[38] This raises the possibility that aging women affected by obesity or single status may be at high risk for experiencing an

---

Box 2
Medications associated with sexual dysfunction

Antidepressants/Mood stabilizers

  Selective serotonin reuptake inhibitors

  Tricyclic antidepressants

  Monoamine oxidase inhibitors

  Benzodiazapines

  Lithium

  Antipsychotics

Cardiovascular medications

  Beta blockers

  Digoxin

  Lipid lower medications

Other drugs

  Oral contraceptives

  Gonadotropin-releasing hormone agonists

  Antiandrogens

  Neuroleptic medications

  Steroids

  Antiepileptics

  Antihistamines

  Anticholinergics

overall decrease in quality of life. By counseling patients about the benefits of healthy diet and exercise for weight control and screening for medications and illnesses that impact sexual function, health care providers may improve overall quality of life.

Educational level and economic status impact sexual functioning and quality of life for women. Baseline data from the SWAN study suggested that women reporting financial strain were more likely to report decreased frequency of sexual desire and arousal as well as lower levels of emotional and physical satisfaction with intercourse when compared with their more financially secure counterparts.[6] Despite their decrease in desire and arousal, most of these women still reported that sex was moderately to extremely important to them. Menopausal women with some college or graduate school education have better physical and mental parameters of health that are related to quality of life compared with those with a high school education or less.[3] This demonstrates that multiple socioeconomic factors impact sexual functioning and quality of life for menopausal women. Women affected by socioeconomic stressors may benefit from increased social support.

Menopausal symptoms such as vasomotor symptoms and vaginal dryness negatively impact health-related quality of life.[39] Women with vaginal dryness, even if they do not identify the symptom as bothersome, have worse mental health composite scores as well as worse emotional well-being and social functioning.[3] These data suggest that there is a need for physician vigilance and early detection so that interventions can be used to prevent potentially debilitating effects on quality of life.

TREATMENTS
Psychological Counseling

Psychological counseling, solely or in combination with medical treatment, can be helpful to women and couples suffering from sexual dysfunction. Psychosexual therapy with the menopausal woman alone or couples sexual therapy can be considered. Couples therapy can help identify relationship issues contributing to sexual problems and allow opportunities for couples to improve communication.[40] Issues such as relationship distress, extended periods of sexual abstinence, sexual abuse history, lack of sleep, and taking care of an elderly parent can all impact sexual function.[41] Behavioral exercises may help individuals reduce anxiety associated with sexual dysfunction.[42]

Estrogen

The role of hormone therapy in consistently increasing sexual desire or activity has not been established.[25] Sexual activity analysis from the Women's Health Initiative found no statistically significant correlation between use of hormone therapy and the continuation of sexual activity, further supporting that estrogen therapy does not increase libido.[43] Current evidence does not support the use of estrogen or combined estrogen and progesterone therapy to treat sexual interest or arousal disorders in menopausal women.[44–46] Previous sexual functioning and relationship factors, such as having an attractive and available partner, a safe environment, and self-esteem, have been shown to be more important than hormonal determinants of sexual function in midlife women.[15] However, hormone therapy with estrogen may improve sexual function by increasing vaginal lubrication and reducing dyspareunia in women affected by vulvovaginal atrophy.[25] Local vaginal estrogen therapy is recommended as the treatment of choice for symptomatic vulvovaginal atrophy.[47] Low-dose vaginal estrogen formulations come in vaginal creams, tablets, and rings (**Table 1**). Systemic absorption is low for these preparations and they are not effective for the relief of vasomotor symptoms.[1] A progestin is generally not needed when low-dose vaginal estrogen

Table 1
Treatments for vulvovaginal atrophy

Delivery Route	Medication	Brand Name	Dose	Dosage Regimens Approved by the Food and Drug Administration	Typical Serum Estradiol Levels
Vaginal creams	17-β estradiol vaginal cream	Estrace vaginal cream	0.1 mg per gram of cream	2–4 g/d for 1–2 wk and then reduce to 1 g 1–3 times per week	Variable
	Conjugated estrogens vaginal cream	Premarin vaginal cream	0.625 mg per gram of cream	0.5–2 g/d for 21 d and then drug holiday for 7 d OR 0.5 g twice weekly	Variable
Vaginal rings	17-β estradiol	Estring	2 mg	7.5 μg/d for 90 d	7.8 pg/mL
	Estradiol acetate	Femring	12.4 mg[a]	50 μg/d for 90 d	40.6 pg/mL
		Femring	24.8 mg[a]	100 μg/d for 90 d	76 pg/mL
Tablet	Estradiol hemihydrate	Vagifem	10 μg	1 tablet/d for 2 wk then 1 tablet twice weekly	4.5 pg/mL

Vaginal estrogen therapy improves vulvovaginal atrophy (VVA) symptoms through multiple local vaginal effects that include increased lactobacilli colonization, decreased vaginal pH, improved vaginal blood flow and vaginal secretions, and improved vaginal thickness and elasticity through effects on vaginal epithelial cell proliferation and maturation.

[a] Treats vasomotor symptoms as well as VVA.

formulations are used, although clinical trial data supporting endometrial safety beyond 1 year are lacking.[48] Thorough evaluation of any uterine bleeding should be done in women using low-dose local estrogen therapy. For women who do not want hormonal therapy, water-based lubricants and moisturizers are available over the counter to help alleviate symptoms.

Testosterone

There are currently no FDA-approved testosterone formulations for the treatment of low sexual function in women. Despite this fact, many providers still prescribe compounded testosterone or use testosterone products off-label for this purpose. The use of testosterone to treat female sexual function is counterintuitive; free and total serum testosterone levels are not related to the scores of female sexual function assessment tests.[49] In contrast, multiple randomized controlled trials have shown promising evidence that testosterone improves sexual desire and function in some menopausal women. As discussed earlier, women who undergo surgical menopause have an approximately 50% decrease in serum testosterone and may benefit from testosterone therapy. In a randomized, double-blind, placebo-controlled trial, Shifren and colleagues[50] demonstrated that a 300-µg transdermal testosterone patch along with conjugated equine estrogens in women with oophorectomy and hysterectomy significantly increased scores for frequency and pleasure of sexual activity compared with placebo. It is important to note that several studies have now demonstrated improved sexual function with few side effects in surgically, as well as naturally, menopausal women with use of the 300-µg transdermal testosterone patch.[22,34,51] However, clinicians must seriously consider and discuss the risks and benefits of testosterone therapy in a woman who undergoes natural menopause.

Side effects of testosterone treatment tend to be mild, and commonly include application site reactions and facial hair. Statistically significant benefits of treatment are not observed until after 4 to 16 weeks of therapy, suggesting that testosterone therapy may require several months before a full assessment of benefit can be made. This is an important point to stress when counseling patients on expectations of therapy. Oral testosterone therapy increases triglycerides and low-density lipoprotein cholesterol and reduces high-density lipoprotein cholesterol. These adverse lipid effects have raised concern regarding testosterone replacement safety.[52] In 967 surgically menopausal women who were also on estrogen replacement, transdermal testosterone therapy did not affect lipid profiles over 4 years of follow-up.[53] This suggests that the route of administration affects whether or not testosterone impacts the lipid profile and suggests that transdermal testosterone is preferred over oral formulations.

Estrogen is known to increase sex hormone binding globulin levels and suppress LH secretion, decreasing testosterone availability and ovarian androgen synthesis.[54] These effects of estrogen prompted studies designed to investigate the side effects of testosterone therapy without estrogen in menopausal women. A randomized, double-blinded, placebo-controlled trial in both surgically and naturally menopausal women showed that the 300-µg testosterone patch modestly improved the mean frequency of satisfying sexual episodes to 2.1 episodes per month compared with 0.7 in the placebo group.[55] There was no significant difference in satisfying sexual episodes in those using a 150-µg testosterone patch, indicating that the 300-µg dose is needed for a clinical effect. As seen in other studies, a higher incidence of hair growth was seen in the testosterone-treated women. It was also noted that there were 3 cases of breast cancer reported in the testosterone-treated women in this study and more cases of vaginal bleeding. As these women were not on estrogen therapy, the increase in bleeding could possibly result from atrophic endometrium. Although no serious endometrial disease was found in the treatment group, the long-term safety profile of testosterone therapy without estrogen still needs additional investigation. If testosterone therapy is to be initiated for sexual dysfunction, it is generally recommended that treatment not exceed 6 months and that a patch is used.

FUTURE DIRECTIONS

Lorexys is a potential new medication for HSDD currently under investigation. Lorexys is an oral, nonhormonal medication that works by balancing the dopamine, serotonin, and norepinephrine; neurotransmitters that regulate sexual inhibition and sexual excitation.[49] It is a combination of 2 antidepressants already on the market: bupropion and trazodone. It is currently in a Phase 2a clinical study.

Flibanserin is another nonhormonal medication under investigation for treatment of HSDD. Flibanserin is a postsynaptic agonist of serotonin 5-HT receptor 1A and an antagonist of serotonin 5HT receptor 2A that has been shown to induce transient decreases in serotonin and increases in dopamine and norepinephrine in certain regions of the brain.[56] The SNOWDROP trial, a multicenter, randomized, double-blinded, placebo-controlled trial of 949 naturally menopausal women, found significant improvement in sexual desire and satisfying sexual events in postmenopausal women using flibanserin compared with placebo.[57] The most common side effects of flibanserin were dizziness, insomnia, nausea, and headache. Although flibanserin has been studied in both premenopausal and postmenopausal women, its application to the FDA is only for premenopausal women.

SUMMARY

Sexual health and function are essential components in the care of menopausal women. Most menopausal women consider sex to be an important part of their life and strongly desire to maintain a robust sexual life. However, the risk of acquiring a comorbidity that adversely affects sexual satisfaction and function as well as the risk for using medication that affects sexual function increases as women age. Although sexual dissatisfaction and dysfunction are highly prevalent in perimenopausal and postmenopausal women, few disclose their concerns to the health care provider. Thus, health care providers should be proactive and routinely query perimenopausal and menopausal patients about their satisfaction with sex and their sexual functioning. If sexual dissatisfaction or dysfunction is suspected, then a full medical and social history with focused question about factors that affect sexual function should be undertaken. Questions about living situations should be fully explored because menopause often coincides with life-stressing events, such as children leaving the home, sick parents, or loss of a partner. Discovering the etiology and identifying modifiable factors that influence sexual function will help define appropriate treatment. Finally, sexual health in menopausal women and their partners is important. Age-related declines in sexual function may significantly reduce quality of life. Increased recognition by physicians and validation of patient concerns as well as expanded discussions about sexual dysfunction with patients may offer an opportunity for effective intervention and improve the quality of life for affected women.

REFERENCES

1. Management of symptomatic vulvovaginal atrophy: 2013 position statement of The North American Menopause Society. Menopause 2013;20(9):888–902 [quiz: 903–4].

2. Murphy SL, Xu JQ, Kochanek KD. Final data for 2010. National vital statistics reports, vol. 61 no. 4. Hyattsville, MD: National Center for Health Statistics; 2013.
3. Hess R, Thurston RC, Hays RD, et al. The impact of menopause on health-related quality of life: results from the STRIDE longitudinal study. Qual Life Res 2012; 21(3):535–44.
4. Potts A, Gavey N, Grace VM, et al. The downside of viagra: women's experiences and concerns. Sociol Health Illn 2003;25(7):697–719.
5. Barnett ZL, Robleda-Gomez S, Pachana NA. Viagra: the little blue pill with big repercussions. Aging Ment Health 2012;16(1):84–8.
6. Cain VS, Johannes CB, Avis NE, et al. Sexual functioning and practices in a multi-ethnic study of midlife women: baseline results from SWAN. J Sex Res 2003; 40(3):266–76.
7. Lonnee-Hoffmann RA, Dennerstein L, Lehert P, et al. Sexual function in the late postmenopause: a decade of follow-up in a population-based cohort of Australian women. J Sex Med 2014;11(8):2029–38.
8. Dennerstein L, Randolph J, Taffe J, et al. Hormones, mood, sexuality, and the menopausal transition. Fertil Steril 2002;77(Suppl 4):S42–8.
9. Sherman BM, Korenman SG. Hormonal characteristics of the human menstrual cycle throughout reproductive life. J Clin Invest 1975;55(4):699–706.
10. Santoro N, Chervenak JL. The menopause transition. Endocrinol Metab Clin North Am 2004;33(4):627–36.
11. Santoro N, Brown JR, Adel T, et al. Characterization of reproductive hormonal dynamics in the perimenopause. J Clin Endocrinol Metab 1996;81(4):1495–501.
12. Burger HG, Hale GE, Dennerstein L, et al. Cycle and hormone changes during perimenopause: the key role of ovarian function. Menopause 2008;15(4 Pt 1):603–12.
13. Rothman MS, Carlson NE, Xu M, et al. Reexamination of testosterone, dihydrotestosterone, estradiol and estrone levels across the menstrual cycle and in postmenopausal women measured by liquid chromatography-tandem mass spectrometry. Steroids 2011;76(1–2):177–82.
14. Burger HG, Dudley EC, Cui J, et al. A prospective longitudinal study of serum testosterone, dehydroepiandrosterone sulfate, and sex hormone-binding globulin levels through the menopause transition. J Clin Endocrinol Metab 2000;85(8): 2832–8.
15. Dennerstein L, Lehert P, Burger H. The relative effects of hormones and relationship factors on sexual function of women through the natural menopausal transition. Fertil Steril 2005;84(1):174–80.
16. Mannella P, Palla G, Bellini M, et al. The female pelvic floor through midlife and aging. Maturitas 2013;76(3):230–4.
17. Brotto LA. The DSM diagnostic criteria for hypoactive sexual desire disorder in women. Arch Sex Behav 2010;39(2):221–39.
18. American Psychiatric Association. Diagnostic and statistical manual of mental disorders, 5th edition. Washington, DC: American Psychiatric Association; 2013.
19. Shifren JL, Monz BU, Russo PA, et al. Sexual problems and distress in United States women: prevalence and correlates. Obstet Gynecol 2008;112(5):970–8.
20. Laumann EO, Nicolosi A, Glasser DB, et al. Sexual problems among women and men aged 40-80 y: prevalence and correlates identified in the global study of sexual attitudes and behaviors. Int J Impot Res 2005;17(1):39–57.
21. Segraves R, Woodard T. Female hypoactive sexual desire disorder: history and current status. J Sex Med 2006;3(3):408–18.
22. Ambler DR, Bieber EJ, Diamond MP. Sexual function in elderly women: a review of current literature. Rev Obstet Gynecol 2012;5(1):16–27.

23. Davison SL, Bell R, Donath S, et al. Androgen levels in adult females: changes with age, menopause, and oophorectomy. J Clin Endocrinol Metab 2005;90(7): 3847–53.

24. Leiblum SR, Koochaki PE, Rodenberg CA, et al. Hypoactive sexual desire disorder in postmenopausal women: US results from the Women's International Study of Health and Sexuality (WISHeS). Menopause 2006;13(1):46–56.

25. Nappi RE, Wawra K, Schmitt S. Hypoactive sexual desire disorder in postmenopausal women. Gynecol Endocrinol 2006;22(6):318–23.

26. Meston CM, Buss DM. Why humans have sex. Arch Sex Behav 2007;36(4): 477–507.

27. Kingsberg SA, Rezaee RL. Hypoactive sexual desire in women. Menopause 2013;20(12):1284–300.

28. Hummelen R, Macklaim JM, Bisanz JE, et al. Vaginal microbiome and epithelial gene array in post-menopausal women with moderate to severe dryness. PLoS One 2011;6(11):e26602.

29. Santoro N, Komi J. Prevalence and impact of vaginal symptoms among postmenopausal women. J Sex Med 2009;6(8):2133–42.

30. Tan O, Bradshaw K, Carr BR. Management of vulvovaginal atrophy-related sexual dysfunction in postmenopausal women: an up-to-date review. Menopause 2012; 19(1):109–17.

31. Wysocki S, Kingsberg S, Krychman M. Management of vaginal atrophy: implications from the REVIVE survey. Clin Med Insights Reprod Health 2014;8:23–30.

32. Kingsberg SA, Wysocki S, Magnus L, et al. Vulvar and vaginal atrophy in postmenopausal women: findings from the REVIVE (REal Women's VIews of Treatment Options for Menopausal Vaginal ChangEs) survey. J Sex Med 2013;10(7): 1790–9.

33. Simon JA, Kokot-Kierepa M, Goldstein J, et al. Vaginal health in the United States: results from the vaginal health: insights, views & attitudes survey. Menopause 2013;20(10):1043–8.

34. Buster JE. Managing female sexual dysfunction. Fertil Steril 2013;100(4):905–15.

35. Nascimento ER, Maia AC, Pereira V, et al. Sexual dysfunction and cardiovascular diseases: a systematic review of prevalence. Clinics (Sao Paulo) 2013;68(11): 1462–8.

36. Camacho ME, Reyes-Ortiz CA. Sexual dysfunction in the elderly: age or disease? Int J Impot Res 2005;17(Suppl 1):S52–6.

37. Soares CN. Mood disorders in midlife women: understanding the critical window and its clinical implications. Menopause 2014;21(2):198–206.

38. Prairie BA, Scheier MF, Matthews KA, et al. A higher sense of purpose in life is associated with sexual enjoyment in midlife women. Menopause 2011;18(8):839–44.

39. Avis NE, Colvin A, Bromberger JT, et al. Change in health-related quality of life over the menopausal transition in a multiethnic cohort of middle-aged women: Study of Women's Health Across the Nation. Menopause 2009;16(5):860–9.

40. Althof SE. Sex therapy and combined (sex and medical) therapy. J Sex Med 2011;8(6):1827–8.

41. Goldstein I. Current management strategies of the postmenopausal patient with sexual health problems. J Sex Med 2007;4(Suppl 3):235–53.

42. Al-Azzawi F, Bitzer J, Brandenburg U, et al. Therapeutic options for postmenopausal female sexual dysfunction. Climacteric 2010;13(2):103–20.

43. Gass ML, Cochrane BB, Larson JC, et al. Patterns and predictors of sexual activity among women in the Hormone Therapy trials of the Women's Health Initiative. Menopause 2011;18(11):1160–71.

44. Modelska K, Cummings S. Female sexual dysfunction in postmenopausal women: systematic review of placebo-controlled trials. Am J Obstet Gynecol 2003;188(1):286–93.
45. Alexander JL, Kotz K, Dennerstein L, et al. The effects of postmenopausal hormone therapies on female sexual functioning: a review of double-blind, randomized controlled trials. Menopause 2004;11(6 Pt 2):749–65.
46. Wierman ME, Nappi RE, Avis N, et al. Endocrine aspects of women's sexual function. J Sex Med 2010;7(1 Pt 2):561–85.
47. North American Menopause Society. The 2012 hormone therapy position statement of: The North American Menopause Society. Menopause 2012;19(3): 257–71.
48. Sturdee DW, Panay N, International Menopause Society Writing Group. Recommendations for the management of postmenopausal vaginal atrophy. Climacteric 2010;13(6):509–22.
49. Davis SR, Davison SL, Donath S, et al. Circulating androgen levels and self-reported sexual function in women. JAMA 2005;294(1):91–6.
50. Shifren JL, Braunstein GD, Simon JA, et al. Transdermal testosterone treatment in women with impaired sexual function after oophorectomy. N Engl J Med 2000; 343(10):682–8.
51. Shifren JL, Davis SR, Moreau M, et al. Testosterone patch for the treatment of hypoactive sexual desire disorder in naturally menopausal women: results from the INTIMATE NM1 Study. Menopause 2006;13(5):770–9.
52. Maclaran K, Panay N. The safety of postmenopausal testosterone therapy. Womens Health (Lond Engl) 2012;8(3):263–75.
53. Nachtigall L, Casson P, Lucas J, et al. Safety and tolerability of testosterone patch therapy for up to 4 years in surgically menopausal women receiving oral or transdermal oestrogen. Gynecol Endocrinol 2011;27(1):39–48.
54. Casson PR, Elkind-Hirsch KE, Buster JE, et al. Effect of postmenopausal estrogen replacement on circulating androgens. Obstet Gynecol 1997;90(6):995–8.
55. Davis SR, Moreau M, Kroll R, et al. Testosterone for low libido in postmenopausal women not taking estrogen. N Engl J Med 2008;359(19):2005–17.
56. Borsini F, Evans K, Jason K, et al. Pharmacology of flibanserin. CNS Drug Rev 2002;8(2):117–42.
57. Simon JA, Kingsberg SA, Shumel B, et al. Efficacy and safety of flibanserin in postmenopausal women with hypoactive sexual desire disorder: results of the SNOWDROP trial. Menopause 2014;21(6):633–40.

Regulation of Body Composition and Bioenergetics by Estrogens

Rachael E. Van Pelt, PhD, Kathleen M. Gavin, PhD,
Wendy M. Kohrt, PhD*

KEYWORDS

- Menopause • Adiposity • Body composition • Estradiol • Estrogen receptor
- Energy expenditure • Energy intake • Ovariectomy

KEY POINTS

- Consistent evidence from basic and preclinical research indicates that the disruption of estradiol (E_2) signaling accelerates abdominal fat accumulation.
- Treatment of ovariectomized animals with E_2 prevents fat accumulation, thereby isolating E_2 as the regulatory ovarian factor, and transgenic studies indicate that these effects are mediated primarily through estrogen receptor alpha.
- The major system-level mechanism for excess fat accumulation in response to the loss of E_2 in animals is a decrease in energy expenditure, which occurs as a result of reductions in spontaneous physical activity and resting metabolic rate.
- Clinical evidence for the regulation of body composition by E_2 is less consistent, but the suppression of ovarian function does promote fat gain.
- If the loss of ovarian estrogens triggers a decline in physical activity and increase in abdominal adiposity in women, as it does in laboratory animals, this could increase risk for diabetes and cardiovascular disease in postmenopausal women.

INTRODUCTION

There is growing evidence that estradiol (E_2) is an important regulator of body composition and bioenergetics. The wide distribution of estrogen receptors (ERs) and their involvement in genomic and nongenomic signaling pathways[1] suggests that the

Disclosure: The authors have nothing to disclose.
The expertise of the authors on this topic was generated, in part, by research supported by the following awards: P50 HD073063, R01 DK088105, T32 AG000279, F32 AG046957, UL1 TR001082, P30 DK048520.
Division of Geriatric Medicine, Department of Medicine, University of Colorado Anschutz Medical Campus, Mailstop B179, Academic Office One, 12631 East 17th Avenue, Room 8111, Aurora, CO 80045, USA
* Corresponding author.
E-mail address: wendy.kohrt@ucdenver.edu

loss of E_2 at menopause is likely to have pronounced effects on numerous factors other than reproduction.[2] ER expression in the brain, adipose tissue, and skeletal muscle shows the potential role of E_2 in body-weight regulation and other metabolic processes. Further, the presence of mitochondrial ERs[3] suggests a role of E_2 in the regulation of cellular bioenergetics. This article discusses findings from basic, preclinical, and clinical studies that provide insight on the role of E_2 and ER signaling in the regulation of energy storage (ie, fat accrual), regional fat distribution, and energy balance (ie, energy expenditure and intake).

BASIC RESEARCH

Estrogens have many physiologic effects that were long thought to be caused by a single receptor, ERα.[4] However, the discovery of a second receptor, ERβ,[5] and the recognition that ERs are present not only in the nucleus but also in the plasma membrane,[6] have advanced the understanding of the metabolic actions of estrogens.

The systemic actions of estrogens are mediated through ER signaling. This signaling can occur through nuclear ERs and the consequent transcription of multiple genes,[7] or through membrane-bound ERs that mediate rapid, nongenomic effects of estrogens.[8] E_2 binds to ERα and ERβ with equal affinity.[9] However, ERα and ERβ have distinct and sometimes opposing actions, indicating that the ratio of ERα to ERβ may be an important determinant of tissue-specific responses to E_2.[10–12] Both ER subtypes seem to be present in most, if not all, body tissues, but in varying proportions.[13–15] Knowledge regarding the effects of ER signaling has been advanced through the use of transgenic mice that have deletions of ERα and/or ERβ throughout the body,[16,17] in specific cells or tissues,[18–20] or at the molecular level (nuclear vs membrane).[21–23]

Regulation of Adiposity by Estradiol

The importance of ER signaling in the regulation of adiposity was highlighted by the discovery of Heine and colleagues[24] that a whole-body knockout of ERα (αERKO) resulted in increased fat accrual in both females and males compared with wildtype (WT) mice. By 90 days of age, the parametrial and inguinal fat pads were 2-fold larger in female αERKO mice than in controls as a result of increased adipocyte size and number. The αERKO mice were also more insulin resistant and glucose intolerant than WT mice, consistent with the excess adiposity. Subsequent studies confirmed that the deletion of ERα increases adiposity in female mice.[21–23]

The excess fat mass in αERKO mice suggests that ERα plays a protective role against fat accumulation. However, another possibility is that removal of ERα promotes fat accumulation through increased ERβ signaling. One strategy that has been used to test this possibility is to ovariectomize αERKO (αERKO-OVX) mice to reduce circulating E_2, thereby diminishing ERβ signaling.[25] The increase in fat mass that occurred in αERKO-sham mice was attenuated in αERKO-OVX mice. Further, when αERKO-OVX mice were treated with E_2, thereby increasing ERβ signaling, fat mass increased to the level of αERKO-sham mice.[25] The deletion of ERβ in mice (ie, βERKO) does not result in excess fat mass[26] or body mass[27] compared with WT mice, providing additional evidence that the increased fat accumulation in αERKO mice is mediated, at least in part, through increased ERβ signaling. However, ERα also plays a protective role against fat accumulation. When ERα signaling was reduced in βERKO mice through ovariectomy (OVX), there was an excess gain in body mass and adiposity.[27] In addition, when both ERα and ERβ are absent (ie, double knockout; DERKO), the αERKO phenotype of increased adiposity dominates.[26]

These studies of the genetic manipulation of ERs in mice show the complex regulation of body fat accrual by E_2. In general, ERα protects against fat accumulation, whereas ERβ promotes fat gain. The actions of ERα seem to dominate among inbred mice, but this may depend on the relative density and distribution of ERs under conditions of genetic heterogeneity (eg, outbred animals, humans). Additional evidence that the net effect of E_2 is to prevent excess fat accumulation comes from studies that reduce serum E_2 through the deletion of the enzyme that converts androgens to estrogens (ie, aromatase). Regional and total body adiposity is roughly 2-fold higher in aromatase knockout (ArKO) mice than in controls by 12 weeks of age and this difference persists as mice age.[28] The regulation of adiposity by E_2 is further complicated by the discovery of G protein–coupled receptors that associate with E_2, known as G protein–coupled ER 1 (GPER1 or GPR30).[29,30] There is some evidence that deletion of this receptor increases fat gain,[31] but this has not been a consistent observation.[32]

The mechanistic signaling pathways by which E_2 regulates fat accumulation remain unclear. Studies that used tissue-specific silencing of ERs are beginning to provide some insight for the locus of regulation. The deletion of ERα in the central nervous system (CNS) (eg, ventromedial nucleus or specific neurons in the hypothalamus) seems to[18,20] play a pivotal role, but systemic deletions (eg, whole bone marrow or cells of myeloid lineage) also result in excess body-weight gain and fat accumulation.[19]

Collectively, basic research has established a solid foundation of evidence that E_2 plays an important role in the regulation of adiposity. Genetic manipulations that disrupt ERα signaling by deleting the receptor (ie, αERKO and DERKO models) or reducing the ligand (ie, ArKO model) cause excess fat gain, whereas disrupting only ERβ signaling (ie, βERKO model) does not (**Fig. 1**). Thus, the dominant action of E_2 on the regulation of body composition is to protect against fat accumulation and this is mediated primarily through ERα.

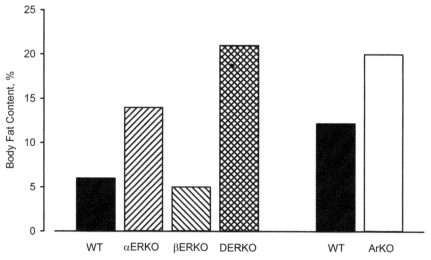

Fig. 1. Relative body fat content of WT mice and mice with whole-body knockout of ERalpha (αERKO), ERbeta (βERKO), both ERalpha and ERbeta (DERKO), and aromatase (ArKO). (*Adapted from* Lindberg MK, Weihua Z, Andersson N, et al. Estrogen receptor specificity for the effects of estrogen in ovariectomized mice. J Endocrinol 2002;174(2):167–78; and Jones ME, Thorburn AW, Britt KL, et al. Aromatase-deficient (ArKO) mice accumulate excess adipose tissue. J Steroid Biochem Mol Biol 2001;79(1–5):3–9.)

Regulation of Bioenergetics by Estradiol

The system-level mechanisms that underlie the excess adiposity triggered by disruptions in E_2 signaling include increased energy intake and/or decreased energy expenditure. There is consistent evidence that αERKO mice have little change in energy intake, but have decreased energy expenditure that is attributable to reductions in both locomotion and basal metabolic rate compared with WT mice.[21,24,33,34] In contrast, energy expenditure and intake are not altered in βERKO mice,[33,35] consistent with no change in adiposity in this model. Running-wheel activity was not different among WT-OVX, αERKO-OVX, and βERKO-OVX mice, and was increased in response to E_2 treatment in WT-OVX and βERKO-OVX but not in αERKO-OVX mice. This finding indicates that E_2 regulation of locomotor activity is mediated through ERα.[33]

Selective suppression of ERα signaling provides further insight into how E_2 mediates energy expenditure and intake. Silencing of ERα in either the CNS[20] or in the ventromedial hypothalamic nucleus[18,20] of female rodents resulted in increased energy intake, reduced basal metabolic rate, and reduced locomotor activity. These changes occurred in mice lacking ERα in the CNS despite circulating E_2 levels being increased, suggesting that ERα signaling in peripheral tissues did not compensate for the suppression of ERα signaling in the CNS. Silencing of ERα in the medial preoptic area also resulted in a decrease in locomotor activity.[36] In contrast, deleting ERα in proopiomelanocortin neurons resulted in increased energy intake and increased, rather than decreased, energy expenditure.[20]

Collectively, both whole-body and tissue-specific genetic manipulations of ER provide strong evidence that ERα-mediated signaling, in particular, plays a critical role in body-weight regulation. The finding that the specific silencing of ERα in various regions of the brain recapitulates disruptions in energy expenditure and/or increasing energy intake that occur with whole-body ERα deletion may guide the development of targeted therapies to improve weight regulation after menopause.

PRECLINICAL RESEARCH

There is a wealth of preclinical evidence that ovarian hormones play an important role in body fat accrual through the regulation of energy balance (food intake and spontaneous physical activity). Because ovaries do not fail in rodents until 11 to 18 months of age,[37,38] studies commonly use OVX to remove ovarian hormone production in young female animals as an approach to studying the effects of the loss of gonadal function. After removal of ovarian sex hormone production, animals can be treated with exogenous E_2 to isolate the action of this hormone. Using these approaches, the effects of ovarian hormones on adiposity and bioenergetics have been well documented. However, a limitation of this approach is that the removal of the ovaries at a young age may not mimic the natural loss of ovarian function at an older age.

Regulation of Adiposity by Estradiol

Compared with sham-operated mice, OVX mice gain 25% more weight and up to 5-fold more fat mass in the parametrial, retroperitoneal, and inguinal regions.[39,40] In a study that compared the effects of OVX in mice and rats,[40] the latter gain more weight than sham-operated animals, but primarily through increases in the parametrial and mesenteric (ie, intra-abdominal) fat pads, suggesting the possibility of species differences in regional fat expansion. However, this species difference has not been a consistent finding, because the expansion of subcutaneous, but not intra-abdominal, fat has been observed in OVX rats,[41] and the expansion of intra-abdominal fat has been observed in OVX mice.[42,43] Most evidence indicates that

OVX results in excess fat accumulation in laboratory animals, with a disproportionate amount stored in abdominal regions.

OVX seems to expand adipose tissue by increasing adipocyte size and preadipocyte differentiation.[39,44] Controlling food intake in OVX animals through paired feeding with sham animals attenuated, but did not prevent, the fat gain observed in OVX rats fed *ad libitum*.[40] Treatment of OVX animals with E_2 effectively prevented the gains in fat mass compared with placebo-treated animals.[37,41,45,46] The increase in total and abdominal adiposity following OVX has been found to occur under various dietary conditions, including caloric restriction, low-fat feeding, and high-fat feeding, and in all cases is markedly diminished by E_2 treatment (**Fig. 2**).[47] Other preclinical models of ovarian failure, including treatment with 4-vinylcyclohexene diepoxide[48] and gonadotropin-releasing hormone (GnRH) analogues,[49] also accelerate weight gain. Thus, there is consistent evidence in laboratory animals that the removal of ovarian hormones results in a positive energy balance and that this is prevented with E_2 treatment.

Regulation of Bioenergetics by Estradiol

The regulation of energy intake by E_2 seems to differ in mice and rats. When compared with sham-operated mice with intact ovaries, OVX mice have either no change in energy intake[39,40] or a small decrease that is reversed with E_2 treatment.[50] In contrast, rats that undergo OVX increase energy intake by $\sim 20\%$ for at least several weeks after surgery.[40,46,51] However, when Ferreira and colleagues[46] monitored food intake for 20 weeks after OVX, it returned to the level of sham-operated controls after 10 weeks. Introducing E_2 treatment 20 weeks after OVX decreased food intake to less than that of sham controls. A unique aspect of the Ferreira and colleagues[46] study was that the OVX was introduced in mature animals (ie, aged 10–12 months). It is not known whether younger animals would also show a waning of the hyperphagic effects of OVX over time.

In contrast with the discordant effects of OVX on energy intake in mice versus rats, OVX causes a marked decline in spontaneous physical activity in both mice[39,40,45,50] and rats,[40,46,52] particularly in the dark phase when activity level is typically high. The magnitude of decrease in physical activity in these studies ranged from 30% to 80% (**Fig. 3**). Importantly, Ferreira and colleagues[46] did not observe a waning of the effects

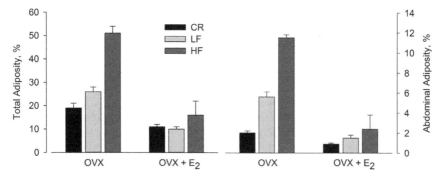

Fig. 2. Effects of OVX and treatment with E_2 on total body adiposity and abdominal adiposity in mice on caloric restriction (CR), low-fat diet (LF), or high-fat diet (HF). (*Adapted from* Stubbins RE, Holcomb VB, Hong J, et al. Estrogen modulates abdominal adiposity and protects female mice from obesity and impaired glucose tolerance. Eur J Nutr 2012;51(7):861–70.)

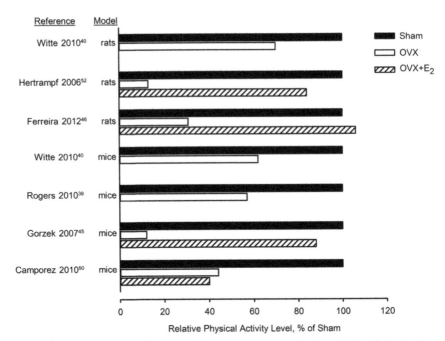

Fig. 3. Physical activity level of mice and rats in response to OVX or OVX with E_2 treatment relative to sham-operated controls. (*Adapted from* Ref.[39,40,45,46,50,52])

of OVX to reduce physical activity over 20 weeks, as they did with energy intake. Instead, there was an acute decrease in daily activity of more than 50% after OVX that persisted for 20 weeks. In most studies that treated OVX animals with E_2 within 2 to 20 weeks after surgery, there was a full rescue of physical activity by E_2.[45,46,52] One exception was a study of mice treated with E_2 at the time of OVX, in which E_2 did not prevent the OVX-related decline in physical activity.[50] Paradoxically, many of the unfavorable effects of OVX, including increased adiposity, reduced energy expenditure, and increased insulin resistance, were prevented by E_2 treatment. Energy expenditure was increased in OVX mice given E_2 (OVX+E_2) compared with OVX controls (ie, to the level of sham-operated animals), despite similar or lower activity levels, which suggests that E_2 increases basal metabolic rate. Other investigators have also found that energy expenditure is lower in OVX mice than in OVX+E_2 mice when activity is similar.[39]

The regulation of physical activity by E_2 seems to be mediated by ERα, which is consistent with results of studies that genetically manipulated ERs. Evidence for this comes from a study in which rats were treated after OVX with E_2, an ERα agonist, an ERβ agonist, or genistein, which is a phytoestrogen that is thought to bind primarily to ERβ.[53] E_2 and ERα agonist treatments increased wheel-running activity 4-fold compared with the level in OVX controls, whereas ERβ agonist and genistein treatments had no effect; the differences among treatments in physical activity mirrored differences in body weight.

In summary, OVX seems to increase energy intake in rats but not in mice. OVX causes a marked decrease in spontaneous physical activity in both mice and rats. Some studies have also reported a decrease in energy expenditure in OVX animals beyond that explained by decreased physical activity, suggesting a decrease in basal metabolic rate. Thus, preclinical studies provide convincing evidence that the loss of gonadal function via OVX in young or mature rodents disrupts energy balance in a manner that accelerates fat accumulation.

CLINICAL RESEARCH

Investigations of the potential effects of the menopause on adiposity, regional fat distribution, and bioenergetics have included cross-sectional comparisons of premenopausal and postmenopausal women, prospective cohort studies of women through the menopause, randomized trials of estrogen-based hormone therapy (HT) in postmenopausal women, and the pharmacologic suppression of ovarian function in premenopausal women. Each of these approaches has limitations. A well-recognized disadvantage of cross-sectional comparisons is that many factors other than menopausal status contribute to differences between premenopausal and postmenopausal women. Prospective cohort studies are valuable because they capture individual changes over time. However, one limitation is that, because the menopause transition is a process that can last several years, age is inextricably linked with the menopause. Thus, it is challenging (if not impossible) to distinguish effects of the menopause from those of aging. Randomized trials of menopausal HT might be considered the gold standard for evaluating the effects of the menopause, but numerous factors regarding the type of HT regimen (eg, type and dose of estrogens and progestins, oral vs transdermal delivery) may influence results. In addition, the pharmacologic suppression of ovarian function in premenopausal women with GnRH analogues is another approach for experimentally controlling ovarian hormones, but changes in hormones occur abruptly and, thus, may not mimic the effects of the natural menopause. The discussion of clinical research focuses on studies that are in the last 2 categories.

Regulation of Adiposity by Estrogens

The Postmenopausal Estrogen/Progestin Interventions (PEPI) trial was the first large randomized controlled trial of HT to show protective effects of HT against weight gain.[54] Women randomized to take conjugated equine estrogens (CEE; 0.625 mg/d) with or without a progestin gained 50% as much weight over 3 years as women randomized to placebo treatment. Body composition was not measured in this study, but HT attenuated the increase in waist girth compared with placebo treatment. Also, although differences between CEE alone and CEE plus progestin were not significantly different, the smallest increases in body weight and waist size occurred in the CEE-alone group, suggesting a regulatory role of estrogens. On average, compared with the placebo group, the increases in body weight and waist girth in the CEE group were attenuated by 67% and 61%, respectively. The Women's Health, Osteoporosis, Progestin, Estrogen (HOPE) trial also found that treatment with CEE 0.625 mg/d attenuated weight gain over 1 year by 49% compared with placebo; smaller doses of CEE were less effective.[55] The attenuation of weight gain in postmenopausal women by HT is not a consistent observation. Most notably, in a subgroup of women who participated in the CEE plus progestin and placebo arms of the Women's Health Initiative trial, there was no attenuation of weight gain by HT.[56]

Most of the large trials of HT in postmenopausal women did not assess body composition. One exception to this was the Danish Osteoporosis Prevention study, which evaluated changes in total and regional adiposity over 5 years in early postmenopausal women randomized to HT (E_2 plus progestin or E_2 alone in women with hysterectomy) or no HT.[57] A limitation of this trial was that it was not placebo controlled. In the HT group, the increases in body weight, total fat mass, and trunk fat mass after

5 years of intervention were 25% smaller than in the no-HT group. These differences increased to 35% to 40% in on-treatment analyses. Body composition was also assessed in a subset of women who participated in the CEE plus progestin and placebo arms of the Women's Health Initiative trial.[56] Although there were no differences between the groups in the change in body weight or fat mass after 3 years of intervention, the trunk/leg fat ratio decreased in the HT group, suggesting a protective effect of HT against abdominal fat distribution. Another interesting finding in this study was an attenuation of the loss of lean mass by HT. A 2006 meta-analysis of HT intervention trials found that HT reduced waist circumference by -0.8% and abdominal adiposity by -6.8%.[58] HT was also associated with reductions in insulin resistance, new-onset diabetes, and dyslipidemia. The extent to which the effects of HT to improve metabolic function are mediated indirectly by beneficial effects on body composition or fat distribution remains unclear. However, at least some of the benefit of HT to reduce insulin resistance seems to be through direct effects of estrogens.[59,60]

Several studies have evaluated the effects of 4 to 6 months of GnRH agonist (GnRH$_{AG}$) therapy on body composition (**Fig. 4**).[61–66] In general, these studies suggest that the magnitude of fat accrual increases with duration of ovarian hormone suppression. The only study that did not follow this pattern[65] was also the only study that enrolled healthy volunteers rather than women who had a clinical indication for GnRH$_{AG}$ therapy. Because the consenting process for this study disclosed weight gain as a risk of the intervention, it is possible that participants were sensitized to the possibility of gaining weight and made behavioral changes to minimize this. However, even though total adiposity did not increase after 5 months of GnRH$_{AG}$ therapy, there was a 12% increase in intra-abdominal fat area measured by computed tomography, which was prevented in women treated with GnRH$_{AG}$ plus E$_2$ add-back therapy.[65] Fat-free mass was consistently decreased in response to ovarian hormone suppression across all studies, but the magnitude of decrease was not aligned with the duration of treatment (see **Fig. 4**). This finding raises the question of whether the decreases reflected the loss of the water component of fat-free mass. However, thigh skeletal muscle area measured via computed tomography decreased in response to

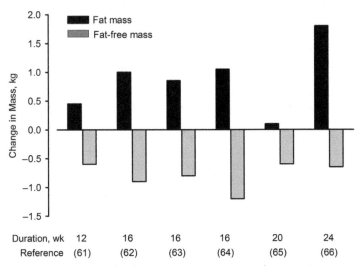

Fig. 4. Changes in fat mass and fat-free mass in premenopausal women in response to 12 to 24 weeks of GnRH$_{AG}$ therapy. (*Adapted from* Refs.[61–66])

5 months of GnRH$_{AG}$ therapy, and was prevented by GnRH$_{AG}$ plus E$_2$,[65] supporting an effect of E$_2$ on muscle mass and not just water.

Regulation of Bioenergetics by Estrogens

The regulation of energy intake and expenditure by estrogens in women has not been well studied. The scant evidence available suggests that the loss of estrogens disrupts energy balance through decreases in resting energy expenditure (REE) and physical activity, which is consistent with basic and preclinical research.

Both acute (6 days) and more chronic (5 months) ovarian hormone suppression have been found to reduce REE. In a small group of premenopausal women, REE was measured during the midluteal phase of the menstrual cycle, when E$_2$ level was increased; during the early follicular phase, when E$_2$ level was low; and after 6 days of GnRH antagonist treatment, which further reduced the E$_2$ level.[67] The changes in REE across these 3 conditions paralleled the changes in E$_2$ level. REE was highest in the midluteal phase, lower (−29 kcal/d) in the early follicular phase, and reduced further (−42 kcal/d) after GnRH antagonist treatment. There were no significant differences across the conditions in energy intake, as assessed by 3-day food records. In a larger trial, 45 premenopausal women underwent 5 months of GnRH$_{AG}$ therapy with randomization to concurrent transdermal E$_2$ or placebo treatment to isolate the effects of the loss of estrogens on bioenergetics (Melanson and colleagues; submitted for publication). REE and total energy expenditure (TEE) were measured in the early follicular phase of the menstrual cycle at baseline and again at the end of the intervention. REE decreased (−54 kcal/d) in response to ovarian hormone suppression, and this was prevented by E$_2$ treatment (+6 kcal/d). The decrease in TEE in response to GnRH$_{AG}$ (−128 kcal/d) was not prevented by E$_2$ (−96 kcal/d). Although the measurement of TEE by whole-room calorimetry in this study is state of the science, it provides only a snapshot (ie, 24 hours) of TEE and does not reflect free-living conditions. It will be important to use another approach, such as the doubly labeled water technique, which can measure free-living TEE over many days, to determine how estrogens influence bioenergetics in women.

The effects of estrogens on REE in postmenopausal women have been examined primarily through cross-sectional comparisons of premenopausal women with postmenopausal women on or not on HT, with varied results. These studies are not reviewed here because of the multiple factors other than hormone status that can influence bioenergetics. However, one intervention trial measured changes in REE in 18 younger (45–55 years) and 15 older (70–80 years) postmenopausal women after 2 months of newly initiated HT.[68] REE was lower in the older group than in the younger group, even when adjusted for fat-free mass, but was not influenced by HT in either group. Physical activity level, as assessed by questionnaire, was also unchanged in response to HT. Another short-term intervention study also found that 2 weeks of E$_2$ did not increase REE in postmenopausal women.[69] Physical activity, as assessed by questionnaire, was unchanged in both studies. Because of the consistent finding in preclinical research that spontaneous physical activity is regulated by E$_2$, it will be important to determine whether this occurs in humans using objective measures of activity. To date, we are not aware of any intervention trials of either hormone suppression in premenopausal women or HT in postmenopausal women that have done so. However, one prospective study of women going through the menopause transition measured physical activity annually by accelerometry and found that it decreased by more than 50% over the 4 years leading up to the onset of menopause.[70] Energy intake, assessed by 4-day food records, also decreased over this time interval. Thus, the limited data on the effects of estrogens on bioenergetics suggest that energy expenditure may decline as a result of the loss of ovarian function, resulting in increased risk for fat gain.

SUMMARY

There is consistent evidence from basic and preclinical research that the disruption of E_2 signaling, through either genetic manipulation (eg, ER deletion) or surgical intervention (eg, OVX), accelerates fat accumulation. The excess fat seems to accumulate disproportionately in the abdominal region and leads to insulin resistance and dyslipidemia. Treatment of OVX animals with E_2 prevents these phenotypic changes, thereby isolating E_2 as the regulatory ovarian factor, and transgenic studies indicate that the effects are mediated, in large part, through $ER\alpha$. The primary system-level mechanism for the increased fat accumulation is a decrease in energy expenditure, although energy intake also increases in some species. The lower energy expenditure is the result of a marked decline in spontaneous physical activity and a decrease in resting metabolic rate.

Clinical evidence for the regulation of body composition and bioenergetics by E_2 is less consistent. Cross-sectional comparisons of premenopausal and postmenopausal women and prospective cohort studies of women through the menopause transition have yielded evidence both for and against menopause as the mediator of changes in body composition. This finding is likely related to the prolonged nature of the menopause transition in women and the associated complexities of distinguishing effects of the loss of gonadal function from other phenomena of aging. However, even controlled interventions that evaluate changes in body composition and bioenergetics in response to HT in postmenopausal women or suppression of ovarian function in premenopausal women do not always reveal a clear role of estrogens. A myriad of factors, such as the type, dose, and duration of treatment, could contribute to the variable results. It is also possible that interindividual differences in the distribution of $ER\alpha$ and $ER\beta$ influence the changes women experience in response to the withdrawal of ovarian estrogens and in response to exogenous E_2 treatment.

The totality of evidence from basic, preclinical, and clinical research points to an important physiologic role of E_2 in the regulation of bioenergetics and body composition. Further advances in basic and preclinical research will help to elucidate the mechanistic targets of estrogens. However, it is important to recognize the limitations of translating basic and preclinical discoveries to humans. For example, dehydroepiandrosterone (DHEA) is secreted primarily by the adrenal gland in humans and it is the major progenitor for androgens and estrogens in postmenopausal women. In contrast, DHEA is secreted primarily by the gonads in rodents, which means that OVX leads to the loss of both biologically active sex hormones and prohormones. This finding suggests that the phenotypic consequences of OVX in animals may be more severe than those that occur with the loss of ovarian function in women.

There is a need to better understand the mechanisms for the metabolic actions of estrogens in women because of the potential adverse impact on health after the menopause. It is well known that the menopausal decline in estrogens accelerates the loss of bone mineral, thereby increasing risk for osteoporosis. If the loss of ovarian estrogens also triggers such changes as a decline in physical activity and an increase in abdominal adiposity in women, as it does in laboratory animals, this could contribute to increased risk for other age-related chronic diseases, such as diabetes and cardiovascular disease. Thus, it is important to continue to advance studies in women that experimentally control the sex hormone environment to better understand the metabolic and bioenergetic consequences of the menopausal loss of estrogens.

REFERENCES

1. Gruber CJ, Tschugguel W, Schneeberger C, et al. Production and actions of estrogens. N Engl J Med 2002;346(5):340–52.
2. Rettberg JR, Yao J, Brinton RD. Estrogen: a master regulator of bioenergetic systems in the brain and body. Front Neuroendocrinol 2014;35(1):8–30.
3. Yang SH, Liu R, Perez EJ, et al. Mitochondrial localization of estrogen receptor beta. Proc Natl Acad Sci U S A 2004;101(12):4130–5.
4. Jensen EV. On the mechanism of estrogen action. Perspect Biol Med 1962;6: 47–59.
5. Kuiper GG, Enmark E, Pelto-Huikko M, et al. Cloning of a novel receptor expressed in rat prostate and ovary. Proc Natl Acad Sci U S A 1996;93(12): 5925–30.
6. Pappas TC, Gametchu B, Watson CS. Membrane estrogen receptors identified by multiple antibody labeling and impeded-ligand binding. FASEB J 1995;9(5):404–10.
7. O'Malley BW, Tsai MJ. Molecular pathways of steroid receptor action. Biol Reprod 1992;46(2):163–7.
8. Sutter-Dub MT. Rapid non-genomic and genomic responses to progestogens, estrogens, and glucocorticoids in the endocrine pancreatic B cell, the adipocyte and other cell types. Steroids 2002;67(2):77–93.
9. Kuiper GG, Carlsson B, Grandien K, et al. Comparison of the ligand binding specificity and transcript tissue distribution of estrogen receptors alpha and beta. Endocrinology 1997;138(3):863–70.
10. Paech K, Webb P, Kuiper GG, et al. Differential ligand activation of estrogen receptors ERalpha and ERbeta at AP1 sites. Science 1997;277(5331):1508–10.
11. Dieudonne MN, Leneveu MC, Guidicelli Y, et al. Evidence for functional estrogen receptors α and β in human adipose cells: regional specificities and regulation by estrogens. Am J Physiol Cell Physiol 2004;286:655–61.
12. Barros RP, Gabbi C, Morani A, et al. Participation of ERalpha and ERbeta in glucose homeostasis in skeletal muscle and white adipose tissue. Am J Physiol Endocrinol Metab 2009;297(1):E124–33.
13. Sakaguchi H, Fujimoto J, Aoki I, et al. Expression of estrogen receptor alpha and beta in myometrium of premenopausal and postmenopausal women. Steroids 2003;68(1):11–9.
14. Gavin KM, Cooper EE, Hickner RC. Estrogen receptor protein content is different in abdominal than gluteal subcutaneous adipose tissue of overweight-to-obese premenopausal women. Metabolism 2013;62(8):1180–8.
15. Wend K, Wend P, Krum SA. Tissue-specific effects of loss of estrogen during menopause and aging. Front Endocrinol (Lausanne) 2012;3:19.
16. Lubahn DB, Moyer JS, Golding TS, et al. Alteration of reproductive function but not prenatal sexual development after insertional disruption of the mouse estrogen receptor gene. Proc Natl Acad Sci U S A 1993;90(23):11162–6.
17. Krege JH, Hodgin JB, Couse JF, et al. Generation and reproductive phenotypes of mice lacking estrogen receptor beta. Proc Natl Acad Sci U S A 1998;95(26): 15677–82.
18. Musatov S, Chen W, Pfaff DW, et al. Silencing of estrogen receptor alpha in the ventromedial nucleus of hypothalamus leads to metabolic syndrome. Proc Natl Acad Sci U S A 2007;104(7):2501–6.
19. Ribas V, Drew BG, Le JA, et al. Myeloid-specific estrogen receptor alpha deficiency impairs metabolic homeostasis and accelerates atherosclerotic lesion development. Proc Natl Acad Sci U S A 2011;108(39):16457–62.

20. Xu Y, Nedungadi TP, Zhu L, et al. Distinct hypothalamic neurons mediate estrogenic effects on energy homeostasis and reproduction. Cell Metab 2011;14(4): 453–65.

21. Park CJ, Zhao Z, Glidewell-Kenney C, et al. Genetic rescue of nonclassical ERalpha signaling normalizes energy balance in obese ERalpha-null mutant mice. J Clin Invest 2011;121(2):604–12.

22. Pedram A, Razandi M, Kim JK, et al. Developmental phenotype of a membrane only estrogen receptor alpha (MOER) mouse. J Biol Chem 2009;284(6):3488–95.

23. Syed FA, Fraser DG, Monroe DG, et al. Distinct effects of loss of classical estrogen receptor signaling versus complete deletion of estrogen receptor alpha on bone. Bone 2011;49(2):208–16.

24. Heine PA, Taylor JA, Iwamoto GA, et al. Increased adipose tissue in male and female estrogen receptor-alpha knockout mice. Proc Natl Acad Sci U S A 2000; 97(23):12729–34.

25. Naaz A, Zakroczymski M, Heine P, et al. Effect of ovariectomy on adipose tissue of mice in the absence of estrogen receptor alpha (ERalpha): a potential role for estrogen receptor beta (ERbeta). Horm Metab Res 2002;34(11–12):758–63.

26. Lindberg MK, Weihua Z, Andersson N, et al. Estrogen receptor specificity for the effects of estrogen in ovariectomized mice. J Endocrinol 2002;174(2):167–78.

27. Seidlova-Wuttke D, Nguyen BT, Wuttke W. Long-term effects of ovariectomy on osteoporosis and obesity in estrogen-receptor-beta-deleted mice. Comp Med 2012;62(1):8–13.

28. Jones ME, Thorburn AW, Britt KL, et al. Aromatase-deficient (ArKO) mice accumulate excess adipose tissue. J Steroid Biochem Mol Biol 2001;79(1–5):3–9.

29. Revankar CM, Cimino DF, Sklar LA, et al. A transmembrane intracellular estrogen receptor mediates rapid cell signaling. Science 2005;307(5715):1625–30.

30. Thomas P, Pang Y, Filardo EJ, et al. Identity of an estrogen membrane receptor coupled to a G protein in human breast cancer cells. Endocrinology 2005; 146(2):624–32.

31. Davis KE, Carstens EJ, Irani BG, et al. Sexually dimorphic role of G protein-coupled estrogen receptor (GPER) in modulating energy homeostasis. Horm Behav 2014;66(1):196–207.

32. Isensee J, Meoli L, Zazzu V, et al. Expression pattern of G protein-coupled receptor 30 in LacZ reporter mice. Endocrinology 2009;150(4):1722–30.

33. Ogawa S, Chan J, Gustafsson JA, et al. Estrogen increases locomotor activity in mice through estrogen receptor alpha: specificity for the type of activity. Endocrinology 2003;144(1):230–9.

34. Geary N, Asarian L, Korach KS, et al. Deficits in E2-dependent control of feeding, weight gain, and cholecystokinin satiation in ER-alpha null mice. Endocrinology 2001;142(11):4751–7.

35. Foryst-Ludwig A, Clemenz M, Hohmann S, et al. Metabolic actions of estrogen receptor beta (ERbeta) are mediated by a negative cross-talk with PPARgamma. PLoS Genet 2008;4(6):e1000108.

36. Spiteri T, Ogawa S, Musatov S, et al. The role of the estrogen receptor alpha in the medial preoptic area in sexual incentive motivation, proceptivity and receptivity, anxiety, and wheel running in female rats. Behav Brain Res 2012;230(1):11–20.

37. Felicio LS, Nelson JF, Finch CE. Longitudinal studies of estrous cyclicity in aging C57BL/6J mice: II. Cessation of cyclicity and the duration of persistent vaginal cornification. Biol Reprod 1984;31(3):446–53.

38. Durbin PW, Williams MH, Jeung N, et al. Development of spontaneous mammary tumors over the life-span of the female Charles River (Sprague-Dawley) rat: the

influence of ovariectomy, thyroidectomy, and adrenalectomy-ovariectomy. Cancer Res 1966;26(3):400–11.

39. Rogers NH, Perfield JW 2nd, Strissel KJ, et al. Reduced energy expenditure and increased inflammation are early events in the development of ovariectomy-induced obesity. Endocrinology 2009;150(5):2161–8.

40. Witte MM, Resuehr D, Chandler AR, et al. Female mice and rats exhibit species-specific metabolic and behavioral responses to ovariectomy. Gen Comp Endocrinol 2010;166(3):520–8.

41. Gloy V, Langhans W, Hillebrand JJ, et al. Ovariectomy and overeating palatable, energy-dense food increase subcutaneous adipose tissue more than intra-abdominal adipose tissue in rats. Biol Sex Differ 2011;2:6.

42. Jackson KC, Wohlers LM, Lovering RM, et al. Ectopic lipid deposition and the metabolic profile of skeletal muscle in ovariectomized mice. Am J Physiol Regul Integr Comp Physiol 2013;304(3):R206–17.

43. Yonezawa R, Wada T, Matsumoto N, et al. Central versus peripheral impact of estradiol on the impaired glucose metabolism in ovariectomized mice on a high-fat diet. Am J Physiol Endocrinol Metab 2012;303(4):E445–56.

44. Fu Y, Li R, Zhong J, et al. Adipogenic differentiation potential of adipose-derived mesenchymal stem cells from ovariectomized mice. Cell Prolif 2014;47(6):604–14.

45. Gorzek JF, Hendrickson KC, Forstner JP, et al. Estradiol and tamoxifen reverse ovariectomy-induced physical inactivity in mice. Med Sci Sports Exerc 2007;39(2):248–56.

46. Ferreira JA, Foley AM, Brown M. Sex hormones differentially influence voluntary running activity, food intake and body weight in aging female and male rats. Eur J Appl Physiol 2012;112(8):3007–18.

47. Stubbins RE, Holcomb VB, Hong J, et al. Estrogen modulates abdominal adiposity and protects female mice from obesity and impaired glucose tolerance. Eur J Nutr 2012;51(7):861–70.

48. Wright LE, Christian PJ, Rivera Z, et al. Comparison of skeletal effects of ovariectomy versus chemically induced ovarian failure in mice. J Bone Miner Res 2008;23(8):1296–303.

49. Roth CL, Neu C, Jarry H, et al. Different effects of agonistic vs. antagonistic GnRH-analogues (triptorelin vs. cetrorelix) on bone modeling and remodeling in peripubertal female rats. Exp Clin Endocrinol Diabetes 2005;113(8):451–6.

50. Camporez JP, Jornayvaz FR, Lee HY, et al. Cellular mechanism by which estradiol protects female ovariectomized mice from high-fat diet-induced hepatic and muscle insulin resistance. Endocrinology 2013;154(3):1021–8.

51. Asarian L, Geary N. Cyclic estradiol treatment normalizes body weight and restores physiological patterns of spontaneous feeding and sexual receptivity in ovariectomized rats. Horm Behav 2002;42(4):461–71.

52. Hertrampf T, Degen GH, Kaid AA, et al. Combined effects of physical activity, dietary isoflavones and 17beta-estradiol on movement drive, body weight and bone mineral density in ovariectomized female rats. Planta Med 2006;72(6):484–7.

53. Hertrampf T, Seibel J, Laudenbach U, et al. Analysis of the effects of oestrogen receptor alpha (ERalpha)- and ERbeta-selective ligands given in combination to ovariectomized rats. Br J Pharmacol 2008;153(7):1432–7.

54. Espeland MA, Stefanick ML, Kritz-Silverstein D, et al. Effect of postmenopausal hormone therapy on body weight and waist and hip girths. Postmenopausal estrogen-progestin interventions study investigators. J Clin Endocrinol Metab 1997;82(5):1549–56.

55. Utian WH, Gass ML, Pickar JH. Body mass index does not influence response to treatment, nor does body weight change with lower doses of conjugated estrogens and medroxyprogesterone acetate in early postmenopausal women. Menopause 2004;11(3):306–14.

56. Chen Z, Bassford T, Green SB, et al. Postmenopausal hormone therapy and body composition–a substudy of the estrogen plus progestin trial of the women's health initiative. Am J Clin Nutr 2005;82(3):651–6.

57. Jensen LB, Vestergaard P, Hermann AP, et al. Hormone replacement therapy dissociates fat mass and bone mass, and tends to reduce weight gain in early postmenopausal women: a randomized controlled 5-year clinical trial of the Danish Osteoporosis Prevention Study. J Bone Miner Res 2003;18(2):333–42.

58. Salpeter SR, Walsh JM, Ormiston TM, et al. Meta-analysis: effect of hormone-replacement therapy on components of the metabolic syndrome in postmenopausal women. Diabetes Obes Metab 2006;8(5):538–54.

59. Van Pelt RE, Gozansky WS, Schwartz RS, et al. Intravenous estrogens increase insulin clearance and action in postmenopausal women. Am J Physiol Endocrinol Metab 2003;285(2):E311–7.

60. Van Pelt RE, Schwartz RS, Kohrt WM. Insulin secretion and clearance after subacute estradiol administration in postmenopausal women. J Clin Endocrinol Metab 2008;93(2):484–90.

61. Nowicki M, Adamkiewicz G, Bryc W, et al. The influence of luteinizing hormone-releasing hormone analog on serum leptin and body composition in women with solitary uterine myoma. Am J Obstet Gynecol 2002;186(3):340–4.

62. Yamasaki H, Douchi T, Yamamoto S, et al. Body fat distribution and body composition during GnRH agonist therapy. Obstet Gynecol 2001;97(3):338–42.

63. Douchi T, Kuwahata R, Yamasaki H, et al. Inverse relationship between the changes in trunk lean and fat mass during gonadotropin-releasing hormone agonist therapy. Maturitas 2002;42(1):31–5.

64. Douchi T, Kuwahata T, Yoshimitsu N, et al. Changes in serum leptin levels during GnRH agonist therapy. Endocr J 2003;50(3):355–9.

65. Shea KL, Gavin KM, Melanson EL, et al. Body composition and bone mineral density after ovarian hormone suppression with or without estradiol treatment. Menopause 2015. [Epub ahead of print].

66. Revilla R, Revilla M, Villa LF, et al. Changes in body composition in women treated with gonadotropin-releasing hormone agonists. Maturitas 1998;31(1):63–8.

67. Day DS, Gozansky WS, Van Pelt RE, et al. Sex hormone suppression reduces resting energy expenditure and {beta}-adrenergic support of resting energy expenditure. J Clin Endocrinol Metab 2005;90(6):3312–7.

68. Anderson EJ, Lavoie HB, Strauss CC, et al. Body composition and energy balance: lack of effect of short-term hormone replacement in postmenopausal women. Metabolism 2001;50(3):265–9.

69. Bessesen DH, Cox-York KA, Hernandez TL, et al. Postprandial triglycerides and adipose tissue storage of dietary fatty acids: impact of menopause and estradiol. Obesity (Silver Spring) 2015;23(1):145–53.

70. Lovejoy JC, Champagne CM, de Jonge L, et al. Increased visceral fat and decreased energy expenditure during the menopausal transition. Int J Obes 2008;32(6):949–58.

Index

Note: Page numbers of article titles are in **boldface** type.

A

Acetylcholinesterase inhibitors, for cognitive impairment, 511
Addison disease, primary ovarian insufficiency vs. 549, 546
Adiposity, regulation during menopause, estradiol and, basic
    research on, 664–665
        preclinical research on, 666–667
      estrogens and, clinical research on, 669–671
      introduction to, 663–664
      key points of, 663
      summary overview of, 672
Adrenal insufficiency, primary ovarian insufficiency vs., 545–546, 549
    screening for, 554
Alternative medicine, for menopause, **619–648**. See also *Complementary*
    and alternative medicine (CAM).
    MEDLINE headings of, 620–621, 641
Alzheimer disease, with natural vs. surgical menopause, 536
Amenorrhea, primary ovarian insufficiency and, 544–545
Androgen, changes in, during menopause, 650–651
        natural vs. surgical, 534, 536
      sexuality and, 650–651
Androgen receptor (AR), in breast cancer, 591
Androgen therapies, for primary ovarian insufficiency, 553
    for sexuality, 651–652
Animal models. See also *Mice models*.
    breast cancer in, menopausal hormone therapy and, 592–593
    of body composition regulation during menopause, 666
Anovulation, 490
Antidepressants, for cognitive impairment, 511
    for hot flashes, 501
    for major depressive episode, 505–506
Anti-Mullerian hormone, in menopause endocrinology, 485, 489–490
    in primary ovarian insufficiency, 545–546
Anxiety disorders, 504–505
Apnea, sleep, as menopausal symptom, 502–503
Apoptosis, in breast cancer, animal models of, 592–593
    vitro studies of, 590–591
Atherogenesis. See *Cardiovascular disease (CVD)*.
Atherosclerosis progression, surrogate markers of, 562–563, 568, 577
Attitude studies, on sexuality and menopause, 650–652
Autoimmune disorders, primary ovarian insufficiency vs., 546–547, 549
    screening for, 554

Endocrinol Metab Clin N Am 44 (2015) 677–704
http://dx.doi.org/10.1016/S0889-8529(15)00076-6
0889-8529/15/$ – see front matter © 2015 Elsevier Inc. All rights reserved.

I

Printed and bound by CPI Group (UK) Ltd, Croydon, CR0 4YY

03/10/2024

01040487-0006